Childhood Food Allergy: Current Management, Emerging Therapies, and Prevention

Editor

RUCHI S. GUPTA

PEDIATRIC CLINICS
OF NORTH AMERICA

www.pediatric.theclinics.com

Consulting Editor
BONITA F. STANTON

December 2015 • Volume 62 • Number 6

ELSEVIER

1600 John F. Kennedy Boulevard • Suite 1800 • Philadelphia, Pennsylvania, 19103-2899

http://www.theclinics.com

THE PEDIATRIC CLINICS OF NORTH AMERICA Volume 62, Number 6
December 2015 ISSN 0031-3955, ISBN-13: 978-0-323-40262-0

Editor: Kerry Holland
Developmental Editor: Casey Jackson

The Pediatric Clinics of North America (ISSN 0031-3955) is published bimonthly by Elsevier Inc., 360 Park Avenue South, New York, NY 10010-1710. Months of issue are February, April, June, August, October, and December. Periodicals postage paid at New York, NY and additional mailing offices. Subscription prices are $200.00 per year (US individuals), $493.00 per year (US institutions), $270.00 per year (Canadian individuals), $657.00 per year (Canadian institutions), $325.00 per year (international individuals), $657.00 per year (international institutions), $100.00 per year (US students and residents), and $165.00 per year (international and Canadian residents and students). To receive students/resident rare, orders must be accompanied by name of affiliated institution, date of term, and the signature of program/residency coordinator on institution letterhead. Orders will be billed at individual rate until proof of status is received. Foreign air speed delivery is included in all *Clinics* subscription prices. All prices are subject to change without notice. **POSTMASTER:** Send address changes to *The Pediatric Clinics of North America*, Elsevier Health Sciences Division, Subscription Customer Service, 3251 Riverport Lane, Maryland Heights, MO 63043. **Customer Service: 1-800-654-2452 (US and Canada). From outside of the US and Canada: 1-314-447-8871. Fax: 1-314-447-8029. For print support, E-mail: JournalsCustomerService-usa@elsevier.com. For online support, E-mail: JournalsOnlineSupport-usa@elsevier.com.**

Reprints. For copies of 100 or more, of articles in this publication, please contact the Commercial Reprints Department, Elsevier Inc., 360 Park Avenue South, New York, NY 10010-1710. Tel.: 212-633-3874; Fax: 212-633-3820; E-mail: reprints@elsevier.com.

The Pediatric Clinics of North America is also published in Spanish by McGraw-Hill Inter-americana Editores S.A., Mexico City, Mexico; in Portuguese by Riechmann and Affonso Editores, Rua Comandante Coelho 1085, CEP 21250, Rio de Janeiro, Brazil; and in Greek by Althayia SA, Athens, Greece.

The Pediatric Clinics of North America is covered in *MEDLINE/PubMed (Index Medicus), Excerpta Medica, Current Contents, Current Contents/Clinical Medicine, Science Citation Index, ASCA, ISI/BIOMED*, and *BIOSIS*.

Printed in the United States of America.

PROGRAM OBJECTIVE

The goal of the *Pediatric Clinics of North America* is to keep practicing physicians and residents up to date with current clinical practice in pediatrics by providing timely articles reviewing the state-of-the-art in patient care.

TARGET AUDIENCE

All practicing pediatricians, physicians and healthcare professionals who provide patient care to pediatric patients.

LEARNING OBJECTIVES

Upon completion of this activity, participants will be able to:

1. Review the common signs, symptoms, and diagnostic techniques in food allergies.
2. Discuss how breast milk and early peanut exposure can affect food allergy risk later in childhood.
3. Recognize techniques in the clinical management of food allergies, as well as current options for allergy treatment at school and at home.

ACCREDITATION

The Elsevier Office of Continuing Medical Education (EOCME) is accredited by the Accreditation Council for Continuing Medical Education (ACCME) to provide continuing medical education for physicians.

The EOCME designates this enduring material for a maximum of 15 *AMA PRA Category 1 Credit*(s)™. Physicians should claim only the credit commensurate with the extent of their participation in the activity.

All other health care professionals requesting continuing education credit for this enduring material will be issued a certificate of participation.

DISCLOSURE OF CONFLICTS OF INTEREST

The EOCME assesses conflict of interest with its instructors, faculty, planners, and other individuals who are in a position to control the content of CME activities. All relevant conflicts of interest that are identified are thoroughly vetted by EOCME for fair balance, scientific objectivity, and patient care recommendations. EOCME is committed to providing its learners with CME activities that promote improvements or quality in healthcare and not a specific proprietary business or a commercial interest.

The planning committee, staff, authors and editors listed below have identified no financial relationships or relationships to products or devices they or their spouse/life partner have with commercial interest related to the content of this CME activity:

Shweta Bansil, BS; Whitney Morga Block, BS, MSN, RN, CPNP, FNP-BC; Paul J. Bryce, PhD; R. Sharon Chinthrajah, MD; Cynthia DiLaura Devore, MD, MS, FAAP; Anjali Fortna; Kerry Holland; Alice E.W. Hoyt, MD; Jennifer J. Koplin, PhD; Indu Kumari; Bruce J. Lanser, MD; Stephanie A. Leonard, MD; Mark J. Mandel, PhD; Tegan Medico, MS, MPH, RDN; Kari Nadeau, MD, PhD; Anna Nowak-Węgrzyn, MD; Kelly Orgel, MS; Barry J. Pelz, MD; Benjamin T. Prince, MD; Jaime S. Rosa, MD, PhD; Sally Schoessler, MEd, BSN, RN; Hemant P. Sharma, MD, MHS; Anne Marie Singh, MD; Bonita F. Stanton, MD; Megan Suermann; Dana Tupa, MS; Burcin Uygungil, MD, MPH; Brian P. Vickery, MD; Madeline Walkner, BS; Christopher Warren, BA; Benjamin L. Wright, MD.

The planning committee, staff, authors and editors listed below have identified financial relationships or relationships to products or devices they or their spouse/life partner have with commercial interest related to the content of this CME activity:

Katrina J. Allen, MBBS, FRACP, PhD is on the speakers' bureau for Nutricia, Nestlé, Aspen Care, Inc, and Thermo Fisher Scientific Inc.

Scott P. Commins, MD, PhD is on the speakers' bureau for Genentech, Inc. and Teva Pharmaceutical Industries Ltd., has research support from the National Institutes of Health, an employment affiliation with the The University of Virginia, and receives royalties/patents from UpToDate, Inc.

David M. Fleischer, MD has research support from DBV Technologies.

Matthew Greenhawt, MD, MBA, MSc is on the speakers' bureau for Nutricia; California Society of Allergy, Asthma, and Immunology; and Colorado Allergy and Asthma Society, is a consultant/advisor for Nutricia, has research support from the National Center for Advancing Translational Sciences, and an employment affiliation with Elsevier B.V.

Ruchi S. Gupta, MD, MPH is a consultant/advisor for Mylan N.V. and Food Allergy Research & Education, Inc., and has has research support from Mylan N.V.

Michael Pistiner, MD, MMSc, FAAP is a consultant/advisor for AllergyHome.org LLC and Allergy & Asthma Network, and receives royalties/patents from AllergyHome.org LLC and Parent Perks, Inc.

UNAPPROVED/OFF-LABEL USE DISCLOSURE

The EOCME requires CME faculty to disclose to the participants:

1. When products or procedures being discussed are off-label, unlabelled, experimental, and/or investigational (not US Food and Drug Administration [FDA] approved); and
2. Any limitations on the information presented, such as data that are preliminary or that represent ongoing research, interim analyses, and/or unsupported opinions. Faculty may discuss information about pharmaceutical agents that is outside of FDA-approved labelling. This information is intended solely for CME and is not intended to promote off-label use of these medications. If you have any questions, contact the medical affairs department of the manufacturer for the most recent prescribing information.

TO ENROLL

To enroll in the *Pediatric Clinics of North America* Continuing Medical Education program, call customer service at 1-800-654-2452 or sign up online at http://www.theclinics.com/home/cme. The CME program is available to subscribers for an additional annual fee of USD 290.

METHOD OF PARTICIPATION

In order to claim credit, participants must complete the following:

1. Complete enrolment as indicated above.
2. Read the activity.
3. Complete the CME Test and Evaluation. Participants must achieve a score of 70% on the test. All CME Tests and Evaluations must be completed online.

CME INQUIRIES/SPECIAL NEEDS

For all CME inquiries or special needs, please contact elsevierCME@elsevier.com.

Contributors

CONSULTING EDITOR

BONITA F. STANTON, MD
Vice Dean for Research and Professor of Pediatrics, School of Medicine, Wayne State University, Detroit, Michigan

EDITOR

RUCHI S. GUPTA, MD, MPH
Associate Professor of Pediatrics and Medicine, Director, Food Allergy Outcomes Research Program, Northwestern Medicine, Ann & Robert H. Lurie Children's Hospital of Chicago, Chicago, Illinois

AUTHORS

KATRINA J. ALLEN, MBBS, FRACP, PhD
Professor, Centre of Food and Allergy Research, Murdoch Children's Research Institute; Departments of Allergy and Clinical Immunology, Gastroenterology and Clinical Nutrition and Department of Paediatrics, The University of Melbourne, The Royal Children's Hospital, Melbourne, Australia; Institute of Inflammation and Repair, University of Manchester, Manchester, United Kingdom

SHWETA BANSIL, BS
Division of Allergy and Immunology, Children's National Health System, George Washington University School of Medicine and Health Sciences, Washington, DC

WHITNEY MORGAN BLOCK, BS, MSN, RN, CPNP, FNP-BC
Sean N Parker Center for Allergy Research, Stanford University School of Medicine, Stanford, California

PAUL J. BRYCE, PhD
Division of Allergy-Immunology, Feinberg School of Medicine, Northwestern University, Chicago, Illinois

REBECCA SHARON CHINTHRAJAH, MD
Clinical Assistant Professor, Department of Medicine, Division of Pulmonary and Critical Care, Sean N Parker Center for Allergy Research, Stanford University School of Medicine, Stanford, California

SCOTT P. COMMINS, MD, PhD
Associate Professor, University of North Carolina School of Medicine, Chapel Hill, North Carolina

CYNTHIA DiLAURA DEVORE, MD, MS, FAAP
Monroe 1 BOCES, Fairport, New York

DAVID M. FLEISCHER, MD
Associate Professor of Pediatrics, University of Colorado Denver School of Medicine;
Children's Hospital Colorado, Aurora, Colorado

MATTHEW GREENHAWT, MD, MBA, MSc
Assistant Professor, Division of Allergy and Clinical Immunology; Department of Internal
Medicine; Child Health Evaluation and Research Unit, Department of Pediatrics,
University of Michigan Medical School, Ann Arbor, Michigan

RUCHI S. GUPTA, MD, MPH
Ann & Robert H. Lurie Children's Hospital of Chicago, Center for Community Health,
Northwestern University Feinberg School of Medicine, Chicago, Illinois

ALICE E.W. HOYT, MD
University of Virginia, Charlottesville, Virginia

JENNIFER J. KOPLIN, PhD
Centre of Food and Allergy Research, Murdoch Children's Research Institute;
Department of Paediatrics, The University of Melbourne, The Royal Children's Hospital,
Melbourne, Australia

BRUCE J. LANSER, MD
Assistant Professor of Pediatrics, Division of Allergy and Clinical Immunology; Director of
the National Jewish Health Pediatric Food Allergy Program, National Jewish Health,
Denver; University of Colorado Denver School of Medicine, Aurora, Colorado

STEPHANIE A. LEONARD, MD
Assistant Clinical Professor, Division of Pediatric Allergy and Immunology, Rady
Children's Hospital San Diego, University of California, San Diego, San Diego,
California

MARK J. MANDEL, PhD
Assistant Professor, Department of Microbiology-Immunology, Northwestern Feinberg
School of Medicine, Northwestern University, Chicago, Illinois

TEGAN MEDICO, MS, MPH, RDN
University of Virginia, Charlottesville, Virginia

KARI NADEAU, MD, PhD
Associate Professor, Department of Pediatrics; Naddisy Family Foundation Associate
Professor, Department of Medicine, Division of Pulmonary and Critical Care, Director,
Sean N Parker Center for Allergy Research, Stanford University School of Medicine,
Stanford, California

ANNA NOWAK-WĘGRZYN, MD
Associate Professor, Division of Pediatric Allergy, Department of Pediatrics, Jaffe Food
Allergy Institute, Icahn School of Medicine at Mount Sinai, New York, New York

KELLY A. ORGEL, MS
University of North Carolina at Chapel Hill School of Medicine, Chapel Hill,
North Carolina

BARRY J. PELZ, MD
Division of Allergy-Immunology, Feinberg School of Medicine, Northwestern University,
Chicago, Illinois

MICHAEL PISTINER, MD, MMSc, FAAP
Pediatric Allergy, Harvard Vanguard Medical Associates, Boston, Massachusetts

BENJAMIN T. PRINCE, MD
Allergy and Immunology Fellow, Division of Allergy and Immunology, Department of Pediatrics, Ann & Robert H. Lurie Children's Hospital of Chicago; Division of Allergy and Immunology, Department of Medicine, Northwestern Feinberg School of Medicine, Northwestern University, Chicago, Illinois

JAIME SOU ROSA, MD, PhD
Allergy and Immunology Fellow, Department of Pediatrics, Division of Allergy, Immunology, and Rheumatology, Sean N Parker Center for Allergy Research, Stanford University School of Medicine, Stanford, California

SALLY SCHOESSLER, MEd, BSN, RN
Director of Education, Allergy and Asthma Network, Vienna, Virginia; Formerly Director of Nursing Education, National Association of School Nurses, Silver Spring, Maryland

HEMANT P. SHARMA, MD, MHS
Associate Chief, Division of Allergy and Immunology, Children's National Health System, Assistant Professor of Pediatrics, George Washington University School of Medicine and Health Sciences, Washington, DC

ANNE MARIE SINGH, MD
Assistant Professor in Pediatrics-Allergy and Immunology and Medicine-Allergy-Immunology, Division of Allergy and Immunology, Departments of Pediatrics and Medicine, Ann & Robert H. Lurie Children's Hospital of Chicago, Northwestern University Feinberg School of Medicine, Chicago, Illinois

DANA TUPA, MS
Research Assistant, Sean N Parker Center for Allergy Research, Stanford University, Stanford, California

BURCIN UYGUNGIL, MD, MPH
Attending Physician, Division of Allergy and Immunology, Children's National Health System, Assistant Professor of Pediatrics, George Washington University School of Medicine and Health Sciences, Washington, DC

BRIAN P. VICKERY, MD
Assistant Professor of Pediatrics, University of North Carolina at Chapel Hill School of Medicine, Chapel Hill, North Carolina

MADELINE WALKNER, BS
Ann & Robert H. Lurie Children's Hospital of Chicago, Chicago, Illinois

CHRISTOPHER WARREN, BA
Northwestern University Feinberg School of Medicine, Chicago, Illinois

BENJAMIN L. WRIGHT, MD
Division of Allergy, Asthma, and Clinical Immunology, Mayo Clinic, Scottsdale, Arizona; University of North Carolina at Chapel Hill School of Medicine, Chapel Hill, North Carolina; Duke University Medical Center, Durham, North Carolina

Contents

Food allergy is a growing public health problem that is estimated to affect 4% to 8% of children and 5% of adults. In this review, we discuss our current understanding of the pathophysiology of food allergy, from oral tolerance, to sensitization, and lastly the elicitation of an allergic response. As much of the existing evidence for the mechanisms of food allergy is derived from animal models, we include these studies where relevant. In addition, whenever possible, we review similar evidence involved in human disease and provide applications for consideration in clinical practice.

Food allergies are increasing in prevalence. In order for pediatric clinicians to appropriately diagnose and manage food allergies, the characteristic signs and symptoms of these potentially severe reactions must be recognized. Unlike nonimmunologic adverse food reactions (such as lactose intolerance and food poisoning), food allergies by definition are immune-mediated responses that occur reproducibly on food ingestion. The varying clinical presentations of food allergy include IgE-mediated disorders, mixed IgE- and cell-mediated disorders, and cell-mediated food allergies. This review describes the clinical manifestations of each of these categories of food allergy, with special emphasis on recognition of food-induced anaphylaxis.

The prevalence of food allergies has been on the increase over the last 2 decades. Diagnosing food allergies can be complicated, as there are multiple types that have distinct clinical and immunologic features. Food allergies are broadly classified into immunoglobulin E (IgE)-mediated, non-IgE–mediated, or mixed food allergic reactions. This review focuses on the clinical manifestations of the different categories of food allergies and the different tests available to guide the clinician toward an accurate diagnosis.

loss or poor growth. Common foods triggering FPIES include cow's milk, soy, rice, oats, fish, and egg. More detailed diagnostic criteria may help in increasing awareness of FPIES and reducing delayed diagnoses or misdiagnoses.

system must balance responses to commensal bacteria (microbiome), innocuous antigens, and pathogens. Although it is clear that specialized populations of immune cells and lymph nodes create a unique environment in the gut, there remains evidence to suggest that systemic effector sites also are critical to establishing and maintaining oral tolerance.

Food allergy is increasing in prevalence; as a result, there is intense focus on developing safe and effective therapies. Current methods of specific immunotherapy include oral, sublingual, and epicutaneous, while nonspecific methods that have been investigated include: Chinese herbal medicine, probiotics, and anti-IgE antibodies. Although some studies have demonstrated efficacy in inducing desensitization, questions regarding safety and the potential for achieving immune tolerance remain. Although some of these therapies demonstrate promise, further investigation is required before their incorporation into routine clinical practice.

PEDIATRIC CLINICS OF
NORTH AMERICA

THE CLINICS ARE AVAILABLE ONLINE!
Access your subscription at:
www.theclinics.com

Foreword

Management of Pediatric Food Allergy

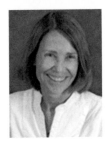

Bonita F. Stanton, MD
Consulting Editor

Every practicing pediatrician will be confronted with issues surrounding pediatric food allergies.[1–3] An estimated 6% to 8% of all children in the United States—or nearly 6 million children—are impacted by one or more food allergies. Infants and toddlers have the highest prevalence with about 10% of one-year olds demonstrating an allergic reaction to common foods, such as cow's milk, eggs, nuts, and/or fish or shellfish. The percentage of impacted children declines thereafter. Some allergies (such as to those to fish, shellfish, and peanuts) are likely to be lifelong, while others (such as those to cow's milk, soy, and eggs) tend to resolve over time.

Food allergies are an immunoglobulin E (IgE)-mediated or a non-IgE-mediated reaction. The reaction to an offending food is quite variable, ranging from mild hives to full-blown analphylaxis. IgE-mediated food allergy tends to have a rapid onset of symptoms involving the respiratory tract, skin, and sometimes the gastrointestinal tract, while non-IgE-mediated food allergy usually has a longer onset and manifests primarily in the skin and gastrointestinal tract. Underdiagnosis and overdiagnosis have been common, especially in the non-IgE-mediated gastrointestinal allergies.

Given the wide range but potential severity of the reactions, food allergies can be very debilitating to the family, impacting the child's and the family's social life. Schools and camps may be uncomfortable in managing a child with severe food allergies; children and families may sense this discomfort, further aggravating their social anxiety.

Traditionally, food allergies have been managed through avoidance of foods causing the allergic reactions and supportive treatment when exposures do occur. However, recent advances have resulted in more accurate testing, the early introduction in the diet of potentially offending foods, and the induction of tolerance to allergens.

Pediatr Clin N Am 62 (2015) xv–xvi
http://dx.doi.org/10.1016/j.pcl.2015.09.005
0031-3955/15/$ – see front matter © 2015 Published by Elsevier Inc.

The identification and treatment of pediatric food allergies and advances therein are discussed in the articles that follow. Accordingly, I anticipate that this issue of *Pediatric Clinics of North America* should be of considerable interest to the community of pediatric providers!

Bonita F. Stanton, MD
School of Medicine
Wayne State University
1261 Scott Hall
540 East Canfield, Suite 1261
Detroit, MI 48201, USA

E-mail address:
bstanton@med.wayne.edu

REFERENCES

1. Anagnostou K, Meyer R, Fox A, et al. The rapidly changing world of food allergy in children. F1000Prime Rep 2015;7:35.
2. Gupta R, Holdford D, Bilaver L, et al. The economic impact of childhood food allergy in the United States. JAMA Pediatr 2013;167(11):1026–31.
3. Dyer AA, Gupta R. Epidemiology of childhood food allergy. Pediatr Ann 2013; 42(6):91–5.

Preface

Childhood Food Allergy Update

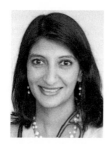

Ruchi S. Gupta, MD, MPH
Editor

Food allergy has become a major health concern worldwide. Since the last issue of *Pediatric Clinics of North America* on Food Allergy published only five years ago, much research has been conducted and has given us new insights into food allergy. This includes potential causes, experimental treatments, and better guidelines for food allergy management that include and extend beyond the clinician's office. Hopefully, these new findings help to better care for affected children and their families where they live, learn, and play. With 8% of children in the United States affected by food allergy[1] and the life-threatening nature of this condition, continual improvements to management remain imperative.

Although research on treatments has advanced, there is still no publicly available treatment or cure for food allergy. The first step in management is avoidance of the allergenic food. For many families, avoiding the allergen is complex; it takes additional time and money and adds anxiety and stress to seemingly simple everyday tasks.

The pediatrician is at the forefront of the mission to ensure proper management. Pediatricians are the first and sometimes the only physician to provide care. The National Institute of Allergy and Infectious Diseases presented *Guidelines for the Diagnosis and Management of Food Allergy* in 2010,[2] and this was followed by a publication in *Pediatrics* in 2011 on the applications of food allergy management guidelines in the pediatric population.[3] Guideline-informed care includes proper diagnosis, appropriate testing, prescribing medications, and referral to an allergist. In addition, physicians need to counsel caregivers and children alike on how to recognize a reaction, administer epinephrine, and utilize a food allergy action plan. With new data emerging rapidly, ensuring pediatricians have the tools they need to translate the evidence to the practice level and provide the best care to their patients remains essential.

In this issue, we began by exploring the pathophysiology of food allergy, signs and symptoms, diagnosis, and recommendations for pediatric management at home and at school. We then looked at important questions regarding food allergy around the globe, described quality of life for affected families, differentiated food allergy from

Pediatr Clin N Am 62 (2015) xvii–xviii
http://dx.doi.org/10.1016/j.pcl.2015.09.004
0031-3955/15/$ – see front matter © 2015 Published by Elsevier Inc.

pediatric.theclinics.com

food protein-induced enterocolitis syndrome, and explored the association of how both gut microbiome and breast feeding are associated with the development of food allergy. We then wrap up by highlighting new research on the possibility of preventing peanut allergy with early introduction, discuss mechanisms of oral tolerance, and review current work on potential treatments for food allergy.

I am so grateful and indebted to the amazing authors and coauthors for their hard work and willingness to contribute to this issue. Our goal was to develop a comprehensive update on food allergy. Thus, we hope this review will provide the pediatrician with a basic understanding as well as serve as a reference when caring for children with food allergy. I look forward to the next issue on food allergy, where the advancements in knowledge around the possible prevention and treatments may be ready for us to offer to our families.

Ruchi S. Gupta, MD, MPH
Associate Professor of Pediatrics and Medicine
Director, Food Allergy Outcomes Research Program
Northwestern Medicine
Ann & Robert H. Lurie Children's Hospital of Chicago
750 N. Lake Shore Drive, 6th Floor
Chicago, IL 60614, USA

E-mail address:
r-gupta@northwestern.edu

REFERENCES

1. Gupta RS, Springston EE, Warrier MR, et al. The prevalence, severity, and distribution of childhood food allergy in the United States. Pediatrics 2011;128:e9–17.
2. Boyce JA, Assa'ad A, Burks AW, et al. Guidelines for the diagnosis and management of food allergy in the United States: report of the NIAID-sponsored expert panel. J Allergy Clin Immunol 2010;126:S1–58.
3. Burks AW, Jones SM, Boyce JA, et al. NIAID-sponsored 2010 guidelines for managing food allergy: applications in the pediatric population. Pediatrics 2011;128:955–65.

Pathophysiology of Food Allergy

Barry J. Pelz, MD, Paul J. Bryce, PhD*

KEYWORDS

- Food allergy • Pathophysiology • Oral tolerance • Sensitization • IgE

KEY POINTS

- Our understanding of the pathogenesis of food allergy is rapidly evolving but remains incomplete.
- More insight into the pathophysiology of food allergy will be essential to improving our ability to investigate, evaluate, and ultimately treat patients affected by this complex disease.
- Our understanding of how the allergic response is elicited is evolving as we learn more about the classical pathway of anaphylaxis and continue to investigate for alternative pathways involved in human disease.

INTRODUCTION

Food allergy is a growing public health problem that is estimated to affect 4% to 8% of children and 5% of adults.[1–3] Although it is not currently understood why some individuals develop allergic sensitization whereas others have immunologic tolerance, an increasing body of evidence is helping to elucidate many of the elements involved in the development of food allergy. In this review, we discuss our current understanding of the pathophysiology of food allergy, from oral tolerance, to sensitization, and last the elicitation of an allergic response. As much of the existing evidence for the mechanisms of food allergy is derived from animal models, we include these studies where relevant. In addition, whenever possible, we review similar evidence involved in human disease and provide applications for consideration in clinical practice.

ORAL TOLERANCE

Our immune system evolved to protect us against infection, and one task essential to this defense is differentiating friend from foe. Although much of immunology focuses on self and nonself, within the immunology of allergy it seems clear that healthy

Disclosures: None.
Division of Allergy-Immunology, Feinberg School of Medicine, Northwestern University, 240 East Huron, McGaw M315, Chicago, IL 60611, USA
* Corresponding author.
E-mail address: p-bryce@northwestern.edu

Pediatr Clin N Am 62 (2015) 1363–1375
http://dx.doi.org/10.1016/j.pcl.2015.07.004
0031-3955/15/$ – see front matter © 2015 Elsevier Inc. All rights reserved.

pediatric.theclinics.com

individuals are constantly being exposed to nonself proteins yet do not elicit pathogenic responses, whereas those with allergies do. The enormity of this task is arguably most crucial at the epithelial and mucosal surfaces such as the skin, respiratory tract, and gastrointestinal tract, where the body encounters a number of proteins, both friendly and potentially pathogenic.

The gastrointestinal (GI) tract comprises an estimated 300 square meters of surface area.[4] This vast territory presents a tremendous challenge to the innate surveillance systems of the immune system. The challenge arises not only in the sheer quantity of space that the GI tract provides for potential pathogens and antigens to breach its barriers, but also in the volume of proteins that pass through it on a daily basis. The GI tract encounters an estimated 70 to 100 g of protein every day.[5] The mucosal immune system has evolved sophisticated mechanisms by which it can determine when an immune response is warranted, as well as ways to maintain control over aberrant responses, and the balance between these mechanisms is critical to health.

Oral tolerance is defined as the systemic suppression of cellular and humoral immune responses to an antigen that has already been encountered via the oral route.[6] There are a number of factors thought to contribute to the GI tract's ability to develop oral tolerance, and these include physical barriers, the digestive process, specific immune cells, and immune regulation.

The barrier function of the GI tract is aided by the presence of a protective, hydrophobic mucus-coated surface and of the secretory immunoglobulin, IgA. The mucin oligosaccharide layer helps trap antigen, whereas secretory IgA binds food proteins and prevents absorption of antigen across the intestinal epithelium.[7] One study investigating whether mucosal IgA antibodies protect against food allergy demonstrated that mice that were deficient in the polymeric immunoglobulin receptor, which secretes IgA into the intestinal lumen, were hypersensitive to IgG-mediated anaphylaxis, suggesting that mucosal IgA plays an important part in protecting against food antigen-directed immunogenicity.[8] Strait and colleagues,[9] however, suggested that systemic IgA may be more important than secretory IgA in the GI tract for protection against IgE-mediated anaphylaxis.

The digestive process also plays a role in the generation of oral tolerance.[10] Gastric acid and digestive enzymes help break down food proteins for nutrient absorption. This process also reduces some of the linear and conformational epitopes of food proteins into less immunogenic chains of dipeptides and tripeptides. Acid is also likely to play a role, because clinically, use of acid-neutralizing therapies for ulcer treatment has been demonstrated to drive IgE production against dietary allergens.[11] Further work in animal studies has shown changes in the gastric pH are important for this IgE production and lead to changes within the intestinal epithelium of the mice that are similar to those seen in human food allergy.[12,13]

Three specialized cells within the GI tract are capable of processing food proteins that survive the digestive process, and these include the microfold (M) cells, the intestinal epithelial cells, and dendritic cells. All 3 of these specialized cells of the GI tract play important roles in the presentation of antigen and in the development of oral tolerance.

M cells are specialized epithelial cells within the GI tract that are capable of transporting antigens from the lumen of the GI tract to antigen-presenting cells in the intestinal mucosa.[14] M cells are located in the dome epithelium overlying Peyer patches and other gut-associated lymphoid tissue. Their microfolds and fenestrated membranes enable them to efficiently take up antigen and deliver them unprocessed to dendritic cells. Somewhat similarly, intestinal epithelial cells are capable of translocating antigen from the lumen of the GI tract to antigen-presenting cells by transcellular mechanisms.[5] Both of these cells enable sampling of the proteins in the GI lumen and contribute to the development of oral tolerance within the intestinal milieu.

There are several different types of dendritic cells (DCs) within the GI mucosa, and it appears that these cells, involved in antigen processing and presentation, play a role in the development of tolerance.[14,15] Antigen-sampling DCs that express the integrin CD11b and the chemokine receptor CX_3CR1 are capable of extending dendritic processes into the intestinal lumen.[14] These cells are believed to collect antigen and then migrate into the mesenteric lymph nodes where they initiate activation and differentiation of effector T cells. A different class of DCs that expresses the integrin CD103 appear to be more preferentially involved in presenting antigen to naïve T cells and inducing their maturation into regulatory T cells (Tregs) for a more tolerogenic response.[14–16]

In addition to suppressing autoimmune aberrant responses, Foxp3+ Treg cells are necessary for the development of oral tolerance. Foxp3-mutant mice, DEREG mice in which Foxp3 expression can be knocked out on treatment with diphtheria toxin, and IPEX (immunodysregulation polyendocrinopathy enteropathy X-linked syndrome) patients who have a mutation in the Foxp3 gene locus all have been shown to demonstrate the importance of Foxp3+ Tregs in the development of tolerance.[17–19]

The ability for Tregs to induce a regulatory, tolerant immune response rather than an inflammatory response is facilitated in part by their elution of the inhibitory cytokines, transforming growth factor beta (TGF-ß) and interleukin-10. TGF-ß suppresses the downstream actions of T and B cells and promotes the production of secretory IgA.[20] Meanwhile, IL-10 induces T-cell anergy, sustains Treg populations, and also plays a role in promoting B-cell class switching to produce secretory IgA.[21]

Foxp3+ regulatory T cells generated in the mesenteric lymph nodes home to the mucosal surface in a manner that is dependent on retinoic-acid produced from dietary vitamin A.[22] Although the exact mechanisms by which Tregs maintain oral tolerance in the luminal surface remain somewhat elusive, they are believed to play an important role in the maintenance (and perhaps development) of tolerance. Shreffler and colleagues[23] demonstrated that milk-specific Foxp3+CD4+CD25 + Tregs were found in higher numbers in children who became tolerant to heated cow's milk protein when compared with those who remained allergic to milk (and heated milk) and to healthy controls.

SENSITIZATION

Our understanding of why some individuals develop allergic sensitization to food antigens while most individuals maintain immunologic tolerance is poor, but an increasing body of evidence suggests that the delicate balance between sensitization and tolerance may be affected at least in part by a few key determinants. These factors include the presence of adjuvants, dietary factors, doses and timing of antigen exposure, the properties of particular allergenic food components, the status of the microbiota, and the route of sensitization.

Like most humans, in the absence of an adjuvant, mice do not develop allergic sensitization to food antigens. Consequently, experimental adjuvants such as cholera toxin and staphylococcal enterotoxin B (SEB) have been required to induce hypersensitivity to food allergens.

Cholera toxin is a potent bacterial toxin that has been used as a mucosal adjuvant to break tolerance when coadministered with food antigens. Snider and colleagues[24] were among the first to demonstrate that coadministration of cholera toxin with a food antigen induces antigen-specific IgE production and subsequent anaphylaxis as demonstrated by histamine release and drop in body temperature on reexposure.

Additional studies by other investigators, including our laboratory, have demonstrated that similar protocols of coadministered cholera toxin and food antigens could be used to generate mouse models of milk-induced anaphylaxis and peanut-induced anaphylaxis.[25–27] In total, this research has demonstrated that when cholera toxin is coadministered with a variety of food antigens, it induces a robust Th2-response, with antigen-specific IgE production, and anaphylaxis on reexposure. Despite the extensive use in these models, the precise mechanisms of action remain largely unclear but are beginning to be elucidated.

Blazquez and Berin[28] demonstrated that cholera toxin alters the normally tolerogenic phenotype of CD103 + DCs, inducing their migration from the lamina propria to the mesenteric lymph nodes, where they upregulate the costimulatory surface molecules OX40L and Jagged-2 and induce Th2 cytokines, including IL-4 and IL-13, instead of undergoing their normal response of inducing Foxp3+Tregs. Blocking OX40L with neutralizing antibodies suppressed this Th2-skewed response while, in contrast, abolishment of Jagged-2 does not stop Th2-skewing,[29] suggesting that OX40L plays a dominant role in this signaling cascade.

Obviously, in humans it is unlikely that cholera toxin plays a significant role in the development of food allergy, but analogous studies using SEB, a potent endotoxin known to be involved in human allergic disease, have suggested that SEB may play a role in the development of antigen sensitization. Yang and colleagues[30] used coadministered SEB and OVA (Ovalbumin) to sensitize mice to ovalbumin and demonstrated that the combination of SEB plus OVA not only led to OVA sensitization with anaphylaxis on subsequent challenge, but also that this sensitization resulted in an upregulation of T-cell immunoglobulin and mucin domain molecule (TIM)-4 on intestinal dendritic cells. Subsequent studies demonstrated that blocking TIM-4 or its receptor TIM-1 prevented the sensitization and anaphylactic response.[31] Our own studies demonstrated that SEB drove sensitization to OVA or whole peanut extract, that there was impairment in Treg functions, and that delivery of functionally capable Tregs to these mice was capable of reversing responses.[27,32]

Our understanding of how these adjuvants lead to human food allergy remains incomplete, but the role of adjuvants seems to be an important aspect in the development of sensitization to foods. Potentially, factors that might affect the milieu in which antigen is processed within the GI tract, such as infection, intestinal injury, barrier function, mucosal integrity, and/or genetics, could have a similar influence on the immune system as adjuvants in the animal models and thereby may play an important role in breaking tolerance and skewing the immune response toward a Th2 phenotype.

Numerous studies have implicated the integrity of the skin and mucosal barrier in protecting against sensitization. The filaggrin gene is important in the development of an intact skin barrier; mutations in this gene are highly prevalent in patients with atopic dermatitis.[33] Additional research has suggested that filaggrin mutations may lead to an increased risk of peanut allergy, presumably through deficiencies in skin defenses and/or gut defenses.[34] Similarly, filaggrin mutations have been linked to eosinophilic esophagitis, a disease in which exposure to food proteins induces esophageal inflammation.[35]

In addition to an intact mucosal barrier, it appears that there are factors within the mucosal epithelium that play an active role in maintaining tolerance and regulating immune responses. One such factor is thymic stromal lymphopoietin (TSLP). TSLP is constitutively expressed by the gut epithelial cells and is also expressed by stromal cells and basophils.[36] TSLP activates OX40L on dendritic cells and generates a Th2 response that has been linked to the development of asthma and atopic dermatitis.[37,38] In the GI tract, however, TSLP appears to play a more regulatory role, as

Ziegler and Artis[39] demonstrated that TSLP limits Th1-mediated and Th17-mediated inflammation in experimental models of helminth infections and colitis. TSLP's regulatory role is complicated, however, as it is not required for sensitization or for oral tolerance.[40] Further studies are needed to elucidate the role of TSLP in human food allergy.

Multiple studies have attempted to investigate the role of dietary factors on the development of food sensitization. Studies using data from the National Health and Nutrition Examination Survey (NHANES) have independently reported that vitamin D deficiency, folate levels, and increased obesity all may be associated with food-specific IgE levels.[41–43] However, it should be noted, as has been pointed out by Keet and others,[44,45] that food-specific IgE may not by itself be an appropriate proxy for the determination of clinical food allergy. Nonetheless, the concept that dietary factors may affect the immunologic milieu and subsequently affect the balance between sensitization and tolerance seems to be supported by these epidemiologic findings. Mechanistic support for the role of diet in the development of sensitization or tolerance has been shown in animal studies. In rats, a high-fat diet led to increased intestinal permeability, increased lipopolysaccharide in the serum, increased presence of inflammatory markers in the blood, and alterations in the gut microbiota, suggesting that changes in dietary components may alter overall immune regulation.[46] However, further such studies evaluating the role of dietary factors in the development of food allergy, particularly as they relate to humans, are necessary.

Another factor that may contribute to the development of sensitization is the allergenic properties of the foods themselves. Although there is a tremendous amount and variety of food proteins in the world's diet, only a small portion of them are responsible for most food allergies.[47] These allergens are dominated by milk, soy, egg, wheat, fish, shellfish, peanut, and tree nuts. All of these foods possess a small molecular weight, an abundance of their relevant epitope(s), water solubility, glycosylation residues, and relative resistance to heat and digestion.[48] It has been proposed that each of these characteristics contributes to the food allergens' ability to survive the digestive process and to induce a Th2 response that results in IgE production and food allergy manifestations.

The timing of antigen exposure and dose of exposure also appear to be important factors in determining food antigen sensitization. Mouse models have demonstrated that high-dose exposure to an antigen early in life, even if given as a single dose, appears to induce T-cell anergy.[49] Low-dose exposure, especially in repeated doses, has been shown to lead to the development of Tregs and thereby oral tolerance.[49] In humans, numerous studies have suggested that delayed introduction of food antigens may lead to an increase in peanut allergy and wheat allergy.[50–52] In a recent landmark study, Du Toit and colleagues[53] demonstrated that early introduction of peanut to young infants who were at high risk of developing peanut allergy was protective against the development of peanut allergy. The mechanisms underlying the importance of timing and dose remain unclear, and further studies are needed in this area.

Another potentially important influence on the immune system's response to a specific food antigen is the microbiota, or the microbial flora that comprise the intestinal environment. In mice, experiments using germ-free or antibiotic-treated mice have demonstrated an increased food-allergen sensitivity, elevated serum-specific IgE, and increased levels of circulating basophils.[54,55] In humans, differences in the intestinal flora of allergic versus nonallergic children have been noted.[56] Investigators have identified certain microbes that promote the development of Tregs and certain microbes that promote the skewing toward allergic sensitization.[57–60] Although there remain a number of unknown details about the ways the microbiome affects the host's susceptibility to food allergy, it is likely that the microbiome plays a significant role in the immunologic development of the GI tract and, more specifically, in shaping the immune response toward tolerance versus sensitization.

There have been a number of recent epidemiologic observations leading to the concept that the route of exposure to an antigen may be an important determinant of whether an individual becomes sensitized or tolerant. One such observation is that the incidence of food allergy continued to increase in the face of dietary measures and anticipatory guidance suggesting delayed introduction of allergenic foods.[61,62] This finding suggests that sensitization may occur via routes other than ingestion. Another recent observation suggesting that sensitization may occur via the nonoral route arises from the discovery that most peanut-allergic children react on their first known ingestion of peanut.[63] Importantly, peanut has been shown to be present in dust in the home and to associate with increased sensitization in children with skin barrier defects.[64] These findings all suggest that the sensitization of some individuals might be occurring through nonoral exposures.

In mice, studies have found that sensitization may occur via an intragastric, sublingual, nasal, or cutaneous route.[65] However, all of these routes of exposure required adjuvant to generate allergen alpha-lactalbumin (ALA)-specific IgE; in contrast, other studies have shown that epicutaneous sensitization can occur even in the absence of adjuvant.[66,67] Interestingly, cutaneous exposure was associated with the highest level of ALA-specific IgE and the most severe anaphylactic responses in these animal models.[65]

In humans, Fox and colleagues[51] found that exposure to household peanut allergen was a risk factor for the development of peanut allergy in children, regardless of maternal ingestion during pregnancy or lactation. Their follow-up study demonstrated that peripheral blood mononuclear cells from peanut-allergic donors expressed the skin-homing integrin cutaneous lymphocyte antigen rather than the gut-homing integrin B7+, suggesting that the sensitization and subsequent lymphocyte imprinting occurred via the skin.[68] Furthermore, in an intriguing observation that preempted the recently released landmark Learning Early About Peanut Allergies (LEAP) study, Du Toit and colleagues[50] noted a 10-fold lower incidence of peanut allergy in Israeli children compared with their Jewish counterparts in London Hebrew schools. In Israel, children routinely consume a peanut-based snack, called Bamba, beginning in infancy, whereas in England (as in much of the rest of the Western world) peanut is often introduced later in childhood. Thus, the realization of Du Toit and colleagues[50] suggested that not only may sensitization occur via a nonoral route (as appeared to be the case in the British children who were not consuming peanut), but also that early exposure via the oral route may be protective against the development of sensitization. The results of the LEAP study strongly suggest that early introduction of peanut by the oral route is highly protective against the development of sensitization and allergy.[53] Additional studies will be needed to further understand the extent to which timing, dose, route of exposure, and property of the food themselves are involved in the development of sensitization or immunologic tolerance.

ELICITATION

If tolerance fails to develop or is broken, then an individual may become sensitized, which is most often characterized as the production of allergen-specific IgE antibodies after exposure to that allergen. Immunologically, sensitization involves T-cell priming after DC activation. The resultant T-cell response, when occurring in the context of the appropriate Th2-skewing milieu, leads to the production of IL-4, IL-5, and IL-13 by CD4+ T cells. These signals, in conjunction with T-cell help, prompt B cells to class switch to produce IgE. IgE then binds to its high-affinity receptor FcεRI on the surface of mast cells and basophils, thereby arming these cells for activation on reexposure to the antigen.

Once sensitization has been established, reexposure to the antigen can lead to local or systemic manifestations. Indeed, sensitization to a particular food antigen is a *necessary* step in the pathophysiology of food allergy, as classic food allergic reactions are IgE-mediated and lead to the manifestations of type 1 hypersensitivity reactions, such as urticaria, angioedema, bronchospasm, hypotension, and shock. However, it is crucial to point out that sensitization is not *sufficient* for the manifestation of food allergy. Many individuals may produce IgE antibodies (ie, be sensitized) to foods that they tolerate clinically. Therefore, the gold standard for diagnosis of food allergy is an oral food challenge, although the diagnosis can often be made when the clinical history suggests a food-induced allergic reaction and the presence of antigen-specific IgE (either by epicutaneous or serologic testing) is detected.[69]

In typical anaphylaxis, symptoms of food allergy are elicited by antigen-mediated cross-linking of antigen-specific IgE bound to the high-affinity IgE receptor, FcεRI, on mast cells.[70] Mast cells are highly granulated, tissue-resident cells that are found in the skin, GI tract, respiratory tract, and cardiovascular system. When allergen is reencountered in a sensitized individual, antigen recognition leads to adjacent FcεRI-IgE complexes moving closer together, bringing their intracellular signaling machinery closer together, and enabling the signaling events needed to promote mast cell activation and degranulation.[71] These events include a cascade of intracellular phosphorylation, which leads to calcium influx and mast cell degranulation. Activated mast cells release a plethora of preformed vasoactive compounds, such as histamine, tryptase, chymase, carboxypeptidase, platelet-activating factor (PAF), and heparin.[72] These mediators elicit the immediate symptoms of a type I hypersensitivity reaction, which clinically may include any individual or combination of the following: urticaria, angioedema, flushing, wheezing, coughing, shortness of breath, rhinorrhea, hypotension, pallor, syncope, abdominal pain, nausea, vomiting, and diarrhea.[71] Mast cells also synthesize other mediators on activation, including cysteinyl leukotrienes and prostaglandins, as well as a wide array of immunoregulatory cytokines and chemokines. These mediators are thought to play a role in the late-phase response of anaphylaxis (the potential biphasic or triphasic reactions seen clinically) that may occur several hours after antigen exposure, as these compounds lead to recruitment and activation of inflammatory mediators, which take several hours to elicit their effector response.[71]

Studies in mice have substantiated that IgE-mediated anaphylaxis is dependent on mast cells and their high-affinity IgE receptor, FcεRI.[73] Strait and colleagues[73] demonstrated that mice deficient in IL-4/IL-4 receptor alpha, mast cells, FcεRI, or IgE are protected against IgE-mediated anaphylaxis. These experiments also used drugs that block the effects of histamine and of PAF to demonstrate the role of these mediators in anaphylaxis.[73] In humans, a number of studies have supported the role of the classic pathway of anaphylaxis by detecting the presence of increased levels of several mast cell mediators, including PAF; leukotriene-B4, leukotriene-C4, and leukotriene-D4; prostaglandin D2; tryptase; chymase; and histamine in the blood of patients who have undergone anaphylaxis.[74]

Additional animal studies, however, demonstrated that systemic anaphylaxis could be induced in mice that were deficient in mast cells, FcεRI, or IgE.[75–77] These studies suggested that alternative pathways of anaphylaxis must exist and led to the discovery of a pathway of anaphylaxis in mice that is mediated by IgG antibodies acting on the low-affinity IgG receptor, FcγRIII.[73,78] Tsujimura and colleagues[79] demonstrated that basophils are important in the IgG-mediated alternative pathway of anaphylaxis, and Jonsson and colleagues[80] demonstrated that neutrophils and FcγRIV are important in this pathway as well. In total, these studies demonstrate that there is an alternative pathway of anaphylaxis in the mouse that involves IgG, FcγRIII, FcγRIV, basophils, and neutrophils.

Although the classic and alternative pathways have been described independently, work by Arias and colleagues[81] suggested that both pathways may work in concert for the generation of anaphylaxis in mice. Mice deficient in IgE or in IgG1 were only partially protected from peanut-induced anaphylaxis in their studies, whereas blockade of IgG1 in the IgE-deficient mouse completely abrogated the anaphylactic response. Along similar lines, Smit and colleagues[82] demonstrated that mice deficient in FcRγ, which is a common chain needed for both IgE and IgG receptors, were completely protected against anaphylaxis. Interestingly, although it remains unclear what, if any, role the alternative pathway of anaphylaxis plays in the pathogenesis of human disease, an intriguing study by Mancardi and colleagues[83] using humanized mice suggested that IgG may function through human receptors to elicit passive and active anaphylaxis.

Although we have learned much about the elicitation of allergic responses in individuals who have become sensitized, there remain a number of unanswered questions about the effector mechanisms and the canonical pathways involved in this complex disease. It is not yet clear whether different manifestations of human food allergy are due to different immune mechanisms, whether multiple pathways are involved in the pathophysiology, or how antigen absorption locally may lead to systemic symptoms. More insight into these complex interactions and challenging questions will be needed in developing targeted prevention strategies and treatment options for food allergy.

SUMMARY

Our understanding of the pathogenesis of food allergy is rapidly evolving but remains incomplete. Although many of the factors underlying the balance between tolerance and sensitization are incompletely understood, emerging evidence supports the role of physical barriers, digestive processes, specific immune cells, and overall immune regulation in oral tolerance. At the same time, a growing amount of data suggests that adjuvants, dietary factors, doses and timing of antigen exposure, the properties of particular allergenic food components, the status of the microbiota, and the route of sensitization all may be important factors in the development of sensitization. Last, our understanding of how the allergic response is elicited is also evolving, as we learn more about the classic pathway of anaphylaxis and continue to investigate for alternative pathways involved in human disease. As our understanding of these elements and their complex interaction evolves, many important questions remain. More insight into the pathophysiology of food allergy will be essential to improving our ability to investigate, evaluate, and ultimately treat patients affected by this complex disease.

REFERENCES

1. Branum AM, Lukacs SL. Food allergy among children in the United States. Pediatrics 2009;124:1549–55.
2. Gupta RS, Sprinston EE, Warrier MR, et al. The prevalence, severity, and distribution of childhood food allergy in the United States. Pediatrics 2011;128:e9–17.

3. Sicherer SH, Sampson HA. Food allergy: epidemiology, pathogenesis, diagnosis, and treatment. J Allergy Clin Immunol 2014;133(2):291–307.

4. Brandzaeg P. The gut as communicator between environment and host: immunological consequences. Eur J Pharmacol 2011;668(Suppl 1):S16–32.

5. Steele K, Mayer L, Berin CM. Mucosal immunology of tolerance and allergy in the gastrointestinal tract. Immunol Res 2012;54(1–3):75–82.

6. Chehade M, Mayer L. Oral tolerance and its relation to food hypersensitivities. J Allergy Clin Immunol 2005;115(1):3–12.

7. Perrier C, Corthesy B. Gut permeability and food allergies. Clin Exp Allergy 2011; 41(1):20–8.

8. Karlsson MR, Johansen FE, Kahu H, et al. Hypersensitivity and oral tolerance in the absence of a secretory immune system. Allergy 2010;65:561–70.

9. Strait RT, Mahler A, Hogan S, et al. Ingested allergens must be absorbed systemically to induce systemic anaphylaxis. J Allergy Clin Immunol 2011;127: 982–9.

10. Michael JG. The role of digestive enzymes in orally induced immune tolerance. Immunol Invest 1989;18(9–10):1049–54.

11. Untersmayr E, Bakos N, Scholl I, et al. Anti-ulcer drugs promote IgE formation toward dietary antigens in adult patients. FASEB J 2005;19(6):656–8.

12. Pali-Scholl I, Herzog R, Wallmann J, et al. Antacids and dietary supplements with an influence on the gastric pH increase the risk for food sensitization. Clin Exp Allergy 2010;40(7):1091–8.

13. Pali-Scholl I, Yildirim AO, Ackermann U, et al. Anti-acids lead to immunological and morphological changes in the intestine of BALB/c mice similar to human food allergy. Exp Toxicol Pathol 2008;60(4–5):337–45.

14. Abbas A, Lichtman AH, Pillai S. Cellular and molecular immunology. In: Abbas A, Lichtman AH, Pillai S, editors. Regional immunity: specialized immune responses in epithelial and immune privileged tissues. 7th edition. Philadelphia (PA): Elsevier; 2012. p. 295–306.

15. Johnston LK, Chien KB, Bryce PJ. The immunology of food allergy. J Immunol 2014;192:2529–34.

16. Kim JS, Sampson HA. Food allergy: a glimpse into the inner workings of gut immunology. Curr Opin Gastroenterol 2012;28:99–103.

17. Bennett CL, Christie J, Ramsfell F, et al. The immune dysregulation, polyendocrinopathy, enteropathy, X-linked syndrome (IPEX) is caused by mutations in FOXP3. Nat Genet 2001;27:20–1.

18. Wildin RS, Ramsdell F, Peake J, et al. X-linked neonatal diabetes mellitus, enteropathy and endocrinopathy syndrome is the human equivalent of mouse scurfy. Nat Genet 2001;27:18–20.

19. Kim JM, Rasmussen JP, Rudensky AY. Regulatory T cells prevent catastrophic autoimmunity throughout the lifespan of mice. Nat Immunol 2007;8:191–7.

20. Frossard CP, Hauser C, Eigenmann PA. Antigen-specific secretory IgA antibodies in the gut are decreased in a mouse model of food allergy. J Allergy Clin Immunol 2004;114:377–82.

21. Defrance T, Vanbervliet B, Briere F, et al. Interleukin 10 and transforming growth factor beta cooperate to induce anti-CD40-activated naïve human B cells to secrete immunoglobulin A. J Exp Med 1992;175:671–82.

22. Coombes JL, Siddique KR, Arancibia-Carcamo CV, et al. A functionally specialized population of mucosal CD103+ DCs induces Foxp3+ regulatory T cells via a TGF-beta and retinoic acid-dependent mechanism. J Exp Med 2007;204: 1757–64.

23. Shreffler WG, Wanich N, Moloney M, et al. Association of allergen-specific regulatory T cells with the onset of clinical tolerance to milk protein. J Allergy Clin Immunol 2009;123:43–52.

24. Snider DP, Marshall JS, Perdue MH, et al. Production of IgE antibody and allergic sensitization of intestinal and peripheral tissues after oral immunization with protein Ag and cholera toxin. J Immunol 1994;153:647–57.

25. Li XM, Schofield BH, Huang CK, et al. A murine model of IgE-mediated cow's milk hypersensitivity. J Allergy Clin Immunol 1999;103:206–14.

26. Li XM, Serebrisky D, Lee SY, et al. A murine model of peanut anaphylaxis: T- and B-cell responses to a major peanut allergen mimic human responses. J Allergy Clin Immunol 2000;106:150–8.

27. Ganeshan K, Neilsen CV, Hadsaitong A, et al. Impairing oral tolerance promotes allergy and anaphylaxis: a new murine food allergy model. J Allergy Clin Immunol 2009;123:231–8.

28. Blazquez AB, Berin MC. Gastrointestinal dendritic cells promote Th2 skewing via OX40L. J Immunol 2008;180:4441–50.

29. Krawczyk CM, Sun J, Pearce EJ. Th2 differentiation is unaffected by Jagged2 expression on dendritic cells. J Immunol 2008;180:7931–7.

30. Yang PC, Xing Z, Berin MC, et al. TIM-4 expressed by mucosal dendritic cells plays a critical role in food antigen-specific Th2 differentiation and intestinal allergy. Gastroenterology 2007;133(5):1522–33.

31. Feng BS, Chen X, He SH, et al. Disruption of T-cell immunoglobulin and mucin domain molecule [TIM]-1/TIM-4 interaction as a therapeutic strategy in dendritic cell-induced peanut allergy model. J Allergy Clin Immunol 2008;122(1):55–61. E1–7.

32. Ganeshan K, Bryce PJ. Regulatory T cells enhance mast cell production of IL-6 via surface-bound TGF-β. J Immunol 2012;188(2):594–603.

33. Irvine AD, McLean WH, Leung DY. Filaggrin mutations associated with skin and allergic disorders. N Engl J Med 2011;365(14):1315–27.

34. Brown SJ, Asai Y, Cordell HJ, et al. Loss-of-function variants in the filaggrin gene are a significant risk factor for peanut allergy. J Allergy Clin Immunol 2011;127:661–7.

35. Blanchard C, Stucke EM, Burwinkel K, et al. Coordinate interaction between IL-13 and epithelial differentiation cluster genes in eosinophilic esophagitis. J Immunol 2010;184(7):4033–41.

36. Soumelis V, Reche PA, Kanzler H, et al. Human epithelial cells trigger dendritic cell mediated allergic inflammation by producing TSLP. Nat Immunol 2002;3(7):673–80.

37. Liu YJ. Thymic stromal lymphopoietin: master switch for allergic inflammation. J Exp Med 2006;203(2):269–73.

38. Demehri S, Morimoto M, Holtzman MJ, Kopan R. Skin-derived TSLP triggers progression from epidermal-barrier defects to asthma. PLoS Biol 2009;7(5):e1000067.

39. Ziegler SF, Artis D. Sensing the outside world: TSLP regulates barrier immunity. Nat Immunol 2010;11(4):289–93.

40. Blazquez AB, Mayer L, Berin MC. Thymic stromal lymphopoietin is required for gastrointestinal allergy but not oral tolerance. Gastroenterology 2010;139(4):1301–9.

41. Sharief S, Jariwala S, Kumar J, et al. Vitamin D levels and food and environmental allergies in the United States: results from the National Health and Nutrition Examination Survey 2005–2006. J Allergy Clin Immunol 2011;127:1195–202.

42. Okupa AY, Lemanske RF Jr, Jackson DJ, et al. Early-life folate levels are associated with incident allergic sensitization. J Allergy Clin Immunol 2013;131(1):226–8.e1-2.

43. Visness CM, London SJ, Daniels JL, et al. Association of obesity with IgE levels and allergy symptoms in children and adolescents: results from the National Health and Nutrition Examination Survey 2005–2006. J Allergy Clin Immunol 2009;123:1163–9.

44. Keet CA, Wood RA, Matsui EC. Limitations of reliance on specific IgE for epidemiologic surveillance of food allergy. J Allergy Clin Immunol 2012;130:1207–9.

45. Berin MC, Sampson HA. Mucosal immunology of food allergy. Curr Biol 2013; 23(9):R389–400.

46. De La Serre CB, Ellis CL, Lee J, et al. Propensity to high-fat diet-induced obesity in rats is associated with changes in the gut microbiota and gut inflammation. Am J Physiol Gastrointest Liver Physiol 2010;299:G440–8.

47. Sicherer SH, Sampson HA. Food allergy. J Allergy Clin Immunol 2010;125: S116–25.

48. Vickery BP, Chin S. Pathogenesis of food allergy in the pediatric patient. Curr Allergy Asthma Rep 2012;12:621–9.

49. Burks AW, Laubach S, Jones SM. Oral tolerance, food allergy, and immunotherapy: implications for future treatment. J Allergy Clin Immunol 2008;121(6): 1344–50.

50. Du Toit G, Katz Y, Sasieni P, et al. Early consumption of peanuts in infancy is associated with a low prevalence of peanut allergy. J Allergy Clin Immunol 2008; 122(5):984–91.

51. Fox AT, Sasieni P, du Toit G, et al. Household peanut consumption as a risk factor for the development of peanut allergy. J Allergy Clin Immunol 2009;123(2): 417–23.

52. Poole JA, Barriga K, Leung DY, et al. Timing of initial exposure to cereal grains and the risk of wheat allergy. Pediatrics 2006;117(6):2175–82.

53. Du Toit G, Roberts G, Sayre PH, et al. Randomized trial of peanut consumption in infants at risk for peanut allergy. N Engl J Med 2015;372:803–13.

54. Hazebrouck SL, Przybylski-Nicaise S, Ah-Leung K, et al. Allergic sensitization to bovine beta-lactoglobulin: comparison between germ-free and conventional BALB/c mice. Int Arch Allergy Immunol 2009;148:65–72.

55. Hill DA, Siracusa MC, Abt MC, et al. Commensal bacteria-derived signals regulate basophil hematopoiesis and allergic inflammation. Nat Med 2012;18: 538–46.

56. Bjorksten B, Sepp E, Julge K, et al. Allergy development and the intestinal microflora during the first year of life. J Allergy Clin Immunol 2001;108(4):516–20.

57. Rakoff-Nahoum S, Paglino J, Eslami-Varzaneh F, et al. Recognition of commensal microflora by Toll-like receptors is required for intestinal homeostasis. Cell 2004; 118:229–41.

58. Round JL, Mazmanian SK. Inducible Foxp3+ regulatory T-cell development by a commensal bacterium of the intestinal microbiota. Proc Natl Acad Sci U S A 2010; 107(27):12204–9.

59. Atarashi K, Tanoue T, Shima T, et al. Induction of colonic regulatory T cells by indigenous *Clostridium* species. Science 2011;331:337–41.

60. Noval Rivas M, Burton OT, Wise P, et al. A microbiota signature associated with experimental food allergy promotes allergic sensitization and anaphylaxis. J Allergy Clin Immunol 2013;313(1):201–12.

61. Zeiger RS, Heller S. The development and prediction of atopy in high-risk children: follow up at age seven years in a prospective randomized study of combined maternal and infant food allergen avoidance. J Allergy Clin Immunol 1995;95:1179–90.

62. Lack G. Epidemiologic risks for food allergy. J Allergy Clin Immunol 2008;121: 1331–6.

63. Sicherer SH, Burks AW, Sampson HA. Clinical features of acute allergic reactions to peanut and tree nuts in children. Pediatrics 1998;102:e6.

64. Brough HA, Simpson A, Makinson K, et al. Peanut allergy: effect of environmental peanut exposure in children with filaggrin loss-of-function mutations. J Allergy Clin Immunol 2014;134(4):867–75.

65. Dunkin D, Berin MC, Mayer L. Allergic sensitization can be induced via multiple physiologic routes in an adjuvant-dependent manner. J Allergy Clin Immunol 2011;128(6):1251–8.e2.

66. Birmingham NP, Parvataneni S, Hassan HM, et al. An adjuvant-free mouse model of tree nut allergy using hazelnut as a model tree nut. Int Arch Allergy Immunol 2007;144(3):203–10.

67. Hsieh KY, Tsai CC, Wu CH, et al. Epicutaneous exposure to protein antigen and food allergy. Clin Exp Allergy 2003;33(8):1067–75.

68. Chan SM, Turcanu V, Stephens AC, et al. Cutaneous lymphocyte antigen and alpha4beta7 T-lymphocyte responses are associated with peanut allergy and tolerance in children. Allergy 2012;67:336–42.

69. Sampson HA. Utility of food-specific IgE concentrations in predicting symptomatic food allergy. J Allergy Clin Immunol 2001;107(5):891–6.

70. Gould HJ, Sutton BJ, Beavil AJ, et al. The biology of IgE and the basis of allergic disease. Annu Rev Immunol 2003;21:579–628.

71. Gould HJ, Sutton BJ. IgE in allergy and asthma today. Nat Rev Immunol 2008;8: 205–17.

72. Galli SJ, Tsai M. Mast cells in allergy and infection: versatile effector and regulatory cells in innate and adaptive immunity. Eur J Immunol 2010;40(7):1843–51.

73. Strait RT, Morris SC, Yang M, et al. Pathways of anaphylaxis in the mouse. J Allergy Clin Immunol 2002;109:658–68.

74. Hogan SP, Wang YH, Strait RT, et al. Food-induced anaphylaxis: mast cells as modulators of anaphylactic severity. Semin Immunopathol 2012;34:643–53.

75. Ha TY, Reed ND, Crowle PK. Immune response potential of mast cell-deficient W/ Wv mice. Int Arch Allergy Appl Immunol 1986;80:85–94.

76. Dombrowicz D, Flamand V, Miyajima I, et al. Absence of Fc epsilon R1 alpha chain results in upregulation of Fc gammaRIII-dependent mast cell degranulation and anaphylaxis. Evidence of competition between Fc epsilonR1 and Fc gammaRIII for limiting amounts of FcR beta and gamma chains. J Clin Invest 1997; 99:915–25.

77. Oettgen HC, Martin TR, Wynshaw-Boris A, et al. Active anaphylaxis in IgE-deficient mice. Nature 1994;370:367–70.

78. Miyajima I, Dombrowicz D, Martin TR, et al. Systemic anaphylaxis in the mouse can be mediated largely through IgG1 and Fc gammaRIII. Assessment of the cardiopulmonary changes, mast cell degranulation, and death associated with active or IgE- or IgG1-dependent passive anaphylaxis. J Clin Invest 1997;99:901–14.

79. Tsujimura Y, Obata K, Mukai K, et al. Basophils play a pivotal role in immunoglobulin-G-mediated but not immunoglobulin-E-mediated systemic anaphylaxis. Immunity 2008;28:581–9.

80. Jonsson F, Mancardi DA, Kita Y, et al. Mouse and human neutrophils induce anaphylaxis. J Clin Invest 2011;121:1484–96.

81. Arias K, Baig M, Colangelo M, et al. Concurrent blockade of platelet-activating factor and histamine prevents life-threatening peanut-induced anaphylactic reactions. J Allergy Clin Immunol 2009;124:307–14.

82. Smit JJ, Willemsen K, Hassing I, et al. Contribution of classic and alternative effector pathways in peanut-induced anaphylactic responses. PLoS One 2011; 6:e28917.
83. Mancardi DA, Albanesi M, Jonsson F, et al. The high-affinity human IgG receptor FcγRI (CD64) promotes IgG-mediated inflammation, anaphylaxis, and antitumor immunotherapy. Blood 2013;121:1563–73.

Signs and Symptoms of Food Allergy and Food-Induced Anaphylaxis

 CrossMark

Hemant P. Sharma, MD, MHS*, Shweta Bansil, BS,
Burcin Uygungil, MD, MPH

KEYWORDS

- Food allergy • Anaphylaxis • Symptoms • Presentation • History

KEY POINTS

- Unlike nonimmunologic adverse food reactions (such as lactose intolerance and food poisoning), food allergies (FAs) by definition are immune-mediated responses that occur reproducibly on food ingestion.
- There are varying clinical presentations of FA, owing to different underlying immunologic mechanisms (IgE-mediated, mixed IgE- and cell-mediated, and cell-mediated disorders).
- IgE-mediated FA may result in food-induced anaphylaxis, a potentially life-threatening severe systemic reaction, requiring prompt recognition and treatment.

INTRODUCTION

The prevalence of FAs is widespread and rising rapidly, affecting up to 8% of children in the United States.[1,2] FAs may result in significant morbidity. Among patients treated for anaphylaxis in the emergency department (ED), FA is the most common cause, accounting for one-third to half of cases.[3,4] Given this increasing prevalence and potential severity, pediatric clinicians must be able to quickly recognize the signs and symptoms of FA. The range of clinical manifestations of FAs is wide and varies based on the underlying immunopathology. Symptoms may affect the cutaneous, respiratory, gastrointestinal (GI), or cardiovascular systems. The most severe presentation of FAs is anaphylaxis, an acute systemic allergic reaction that can ultimately lead to death if untreated. This review starts by defining FAs and then discusses the range of clinical presentations of various types of FAs based on underlying immune

---

Disclosures: Consultant, Nutricia N.A.; Consultant (spokesperson for unbranded anaphylaxis educational campaign), Mylan Specialty (H.P. Sharma); None (S. Bansil & B. Uygungil).
Division of Allergy and Immunology, Children's National Health System, George Washington University School of Medicine and Health Sciences, Washington, DC, USA
* Corresponding author. Division of Allergy and Immunology, Children's National Medical Center, 111 Michigan Avenue Northwest, Washington, DC 20010.
E-mail address: hsharma@childrensnational.org

Pediatr Clin N Am 62 (2015) 1377–1392
http://dx.doi.org/10.1016/j.pcl.2015.07.008
0031-3955/15/$ – see front matter © 2015 Elsevier Inc. All rights reserved.
pediatric.theclinics.com

mechanisms. Important questions in the history of a patient with a suspected FA are also discussed.

DEFINING FOOD ALLERGIES

The term adverse food reaction is used to describe any untoward health effect that occurs after food ingestion. It can be divided into FAs, which are due to a specific immune response and occur reproducibly on food ingestion,[5] and all other reactions, which, in contrast to true FAs, are nonimmunologic in nature.[6] It is important that the pediatric clinician distinguish these nonimmunologic adverse food reactions (summarized in **Table 1**) from FA to guide appropriate treatment.

Nonimmunologic adverse food reactions can result from metabolic disorders such as lactose intolerance, galactosemia, and alcohol intolerance. Lactose intolerance manifests as a result of an inability to digest the carbohydrate lactose in milk and dairy products, owing to deficiency of the lactase enzyme. Symptoms might include abdominal pain, bloating, gas, diarrhea, and nausea. Pharmacologically active components in foods, such as caffeine and food-borne toxins, may also cause nonimmune adverse food reactions. For example, scombroid fish poisoning is a toxic adverse food

Table 1 Differential diagnosis of nonimmunologic adverse food reactions (conditions that are not food allergies)	
Host-specific metabolic disorders	Carbohydrate malabsorption • Lactase deficiency (lactose intolerance) • Sucrose-isomaltase deficiency (sucrose intolerance) Galactosemia Alcohol intolerance
Response to pharmacologically active food component	Scombroid poisoning (fish: tuna, mackerel, mahi mahi, sardines, anchovies) Histamine-like compounds (wine, sauerkraut) Caffeine Tyramine (aged cheeses, pickled fish) Theobromine (tea, chocolate) Tryptamine (tomato, plum) Serotonin (banana, tomato)
Toxic reactions (food poisoning)	Fish: ciguatera poisoning (grouper, snapper) Shellfish: saxitoxin Fungal toxins: aflatoxins, trichothecanes, ergot Other food poisoning (*Clostridium botulinum, Staphylococcus aureus*)
Gastrointestinal disorders	Structural abnormalities (hiatal hernia, pyloric stenosis, tracheoesophageal fistula, Hirschsprung disease) Gastroesophageal reflux Peptic ulcer disease
Psychological reactions	Food aversions Food phobias
Neurologic reactions	Auriculotemporal syndrome (facial redness or sweating after eating tart foods) Gustatory rhinitis (rhinorrhea after eating hot or spicy foods)

Adapted from Mansoor DK, Sharma HP. Clinical presentations of food allergy. Pediatr Clin North Am 2011;58(2):316; with permission.

reaction caused by histaminic chemicals found in spoiled dark-meat fish such as tuna, mackerel, and sardines. Exposure to these chemicals can result in cutaneous and systemic symptoms such as flushing, urticaria, angioedema, nausea, abdominal cramping, and diarrhea that closely mimic a food-allergic reaction. However, the underlying mechanism of scombroid poisoning is nonimmunologic, and thus it is not an FA.[7]

Nonimmune adverse food reactions can also be the result of GI disorders such as gastroesophageal reflux, psychological disorders such as food aversions and food phobias, or neurologic disorders such as auriculotemporal syndrome and gustatory rhinitis. Key questions in the history (discussed later) can help distinguish FA from nonimmune adverse food reactions, but referral to an allergist should be considered if uncertainty remains.

Because FAs are immune-mediated responses, an understanding of their underlying immunologic mechanisms allows food-allergic reactions to be classified into 1 of 3 groups: (1) IgE-mediated reactions, (2) non-IgE-mediated reactions, and (3) mixed IgE-mediated and non-IgE-mediated reactions.[8]

IGE-MEDIATED FOOD ALLERGIES

IgE-mediated food-allergic reactions are mediated by surface IgE on tissue mast cells and circulating basophils, which develop during initial sensitization to a food. On reexposure to the food antigen, IgE cross-linking on the surface of mast cells and basophils results in the acute release of preformed allergic mediators that cause signs and symptoms to develop rapidly. Thus, IgE-mediated FA should be considered in a patient who develops signs and symptoms minutes to 2 hours after ingesting the culprit food. Newly synthesized mediators may also be released, causing a delayed phase of symptoms several hours after the initial response.

There is one known form of IgE-mediated FA in which characteristic symptoms do not develop rapidly. Allergic reactions to mammalian meats (particularly beef, pork, and lamb) containing a carbohydrate antigen called galactose-α-1,3-galactose (alpha-gal) are typically delayed 4 to 6 hours after ingestion, likely because of the time it takes for antigen digestion and/or processing.[9] Allergic reactions to the alpha-gal antigen are the only IgE-mediated FA identified to date in which the food antigen is a carbohydrate, and not a protein. Sensitization to alpha-gal has been described following bites of *Ixodes* ticks.[10]

Patients with IgE-mediated FA can present with a variety of symptoms that involve several organ systems, including urticaria and angioedema, rhinoconjunctivitis, respiratory distress, GI disturbances, and cardiovascular compromise. Key features of each are summarized in **Table 2**.

Urticaria and Angioedema

Both urticaria and angioedema develop because of cross-linking of food-specific IgE on cutaneous mast cells. In the former, mast cells in the superficial dermis are involved, whereas in the latter, those in the deep dermis and subcutaneous tissues are implicated. Although urticaria can be the result of various processes including infection, reactions to medications, and insect bites, it is estimated that at least 20% of acute urticaria is due to FA.[11]

Urticaria or hives appear as raised erythematous wheals that are pruritic. They are usually well circumscribed or coalescing and often migrate around the body. IgE-mediated FA should be considered in patients with acute urticaria whose symptoms were preceded by a recent food exposure. If urticaria persists for greater than 6 weeks, they are classified as chronic, and FA is unlikely the cause.[12] It is important to

Table 2
IgE-mediated food allergy presentations

Symptom Complex/ Disorder	Key Points/Clinical Features	Most Common Causal Foods
Urticaria/angioedema	20% of acute urticaria (<6 wk duration) is due to FA. Chronic urticaria is unlikely related to FA Contact urticaria can occur in which hives are localized only to areas of food contact 20% of anaphylaxis, and 80% of fatal food-induced anaphylaxis, involves no hives	Cow's milk, egg, peanut, tree nuts, soy, wheat, fish, and shellfish Contact urticaria is triggered by these foods as well as raw meats and raw fruits and vegetables
Oral allergy syndrome	Pruritus, mild edema confined to oral cavity Uncommonly progresses beyond mouth (<10%) or anaphylaxis (1%–2%) Occurs in half of pollen-allergic patients	Raw fruit/vegetables (cooked forms tolerated)
Rhinoconjunctivitis and bronchospasm	Accompanies food-induced allergic reaction, but rarely isolated symptom except in occupational asthma	Major allergens (Occupational: wheat, egg, seafood)
Anaphylaxis	Rapidly progressive, multiple organ system reaction that is life threatening Respiratory symptoms: Present in up to 70% of episodes; primary cause of death in FA-induced anaphylaxis. Risk of death is higher in asthmatics GI symptoms: Present in up to 45% of episodes; upper GI symptoms are within minutes, whereas lower GI symptoms can be delayed Cardiovascular symptoms: Present in up to 45% of episodes; massive fluid shifts can cause shock within minutes	Any allergens, but more commonly peanut, tree nuts, shellfish, fish, milk, egg, and sesame
Food-dependent, exercise-induced anaphylaxis	Food triggers anaphylaxis only if ingestion followed 2–4 h by exercise	Most common: wheat, shellfish, celery

recognize that, although the route of food exposure causing acute urticaria is often ingestion, direct contact may also cause contact urticaria, in which hives are localized only to the areas of food contact. For example, a child with IgE-mediated peanut allergy may develop hives after rubbing peanut butter on his/her face without actually ingesting the food.

Angioedema is characterized by asymmetric, nonpitting edema involving nongravitationally dependent areas. It may affect the face, extremities, or upper airway. Although any food allergen may cause acute urticaria and angioedema, the most common foods to do so are cow's milk, egg, peanut, tree nuts, soy, wheat, fish, and shellfish. Contact urticaria may be triggered by these foods, as well as by raw meats, raw fruits and vegetables, and rice.

Although hives and swelling are common signs of food allergic reactions, their absence does not preclude a FA diagnosis. Skin symptoms may be absent in up to 10% to 20% of anaphylaxis.[13] About 80% of fatal food-induced anaphylaxis is not associated with skin findings,[13] which suggests that the lack of cutaneous signs may result in delayed recognition and treatment of an allergic reaction and thereby increased risk of fatality. Pediatric clinicians should be vigilant for the noncutaneous signs of IgE-mediated FA discussed later.

Oropharyngeal Symptoms: Oral Allergy Syndrome

Oropharyngeal symptoms may occur as part of a more systemic food allergic reaction or in isolation, for example, when the dose of allergen ingested is small or when the allergen is unstable or labile, as in oral allergy syndrome (OAS).

OAS, also referred to as pollen-associated FA syndrome, is a form of IgE-mediated FA in which the ingestion of raw fruits or vegetables causes oropharyngeal pruritus, tingling, and/or mild swelling of the lips, tongue, palate, and throat.[14] The reaction is most often limited to the oropharynx and subsides within minutes of ingestion. Less than 10% of patients progress to systemic involvement of symptoms, and only 1% to 2% progress to anaphylaxis. The antigen causing OAS is a heat-labile food protein of plant origin, which is structurally similar and thereby cross-reactive with pollen allergens. OAS occurs in up to half of pollen-allergic patients, and symptoms may be more prominent during the relevant pollen season. Because the antigens are heat labile, patients are usually able to tolerate cooked forms of the causative fruits and vegetables.[14]

Respiratory Tract Symptoms: Rhinoconjunctivitis and Bronchospasm

IgE-mediated FA may manifest with ocular and nasal symptoms after food exposure, such as periocular pruritis, edema, conjunctival erythema, and lacrimation, as well as sneezing, nasal itching, congestion, and rhinorrhea. Upper airway findings (hoarseness, stridor, sensation of throat tightness) and lower airway symptoms (dyspnea, tachypnea, wheezing, cough) may also be observed. Symptoms of rhinoconjunctivitis and bronchospasm are frequently observed as part of systemic IgE-mediated FA reactions (see Anaphylaxis section), but rarely as isolated findings. In a study of 480 children who underwent oral ingestion double-blind placebo-controlled food challenges, 39% of the 185 children with positive reactions experienced ocular and respiratory symptoms. Only 5% had symptoms confined to the respiratory tract alone.[15]

An exception in which isolated respiratory symptoms are observed after food exposure is occupational asthma/rhinitis among workers in the food preparation and packaging industry. These individuals may develop isolated upper and/or lower respiratory symptoms after inhalation of the culprit food allergen, such as wheat in baker's asthma.[16] The food is often tolerated on ingestion.

Gastrointestinal Symptoms

In patients with IgE-mediated FA, GI symptoms may be divided into those derived from involvement of the upper GI tract (nausea, vomiting, and/or abdominal pain typically occurring minutes to 2 hours after ingestion) versus the lower GI tract (cramping and diarrhea delayed 2–6 hours).[14,17] GI symptoms commonly occur as part of systemic FA reactions (see Anaphylaxis section). When GI symptoms occur in isolation after food allergen ingestion, this is referred to as GI anaphylaxis.

Food-Induced Anaphylaxis

The most serious clinical implication of IgE-mediated FA is anaphylaxis, a systemic allergic reaction that is rapid in onset and may cause death.[18] Anaphylaxis affects up to 2% of the population,[19,20] and FAs are responsible for up to 50% of all cases.[4,17] In children and young adults who develop anaphylaxis outside of the hospital setting, FA is the leading cause among identified triggers.[21] Several risk factors, including adolescence or young adult age, coexistent asthma, reactions due to peanut or tree nuts, and delayed administration of epinephrine, increase the risk of a fatal reaction from food-induced anaphylaxis.[4] Most cases of fatal FA reactions are preceded by prior reactions, but those were rarely severe. This finding underscores the unpredictable nature of FA in that the severity of prior reactions cannot predict future reaction severity.[22,23]

Although any food may cause anaphylaxis, in the United States (and some European countries), the most commonly implicated foods are peanut and tree nuts, followed by shellfish and fish.[24–26] Based on small series, the foods most commonly implicated in fatal food-induced anaphylaxis are peanut, tree nuts, and cow's milk.[22,27,28] A variety of other foods, including soy, egg, wheat, sesame, food additives, and spices, have also been associated with anaphylactic reactions.[29]

Rapid and massive release of allergic mediators and cytokines, including histamine, tryptase, chymase, platelet-activating factor, prostaglandin D2, cysteinyl leukotrienes, interleukin 6, and tumor necrosis factor alpha, into the systemic circulation contributes to the multiorgan compromise seen in anaphylaxis.[30] As a systemic reaction, anaphylaxis may present with a wide array of potential symptoms and signs (**Box 1**).[31,32] To assist in accurate diagnosis of anaphylaxis, formal diagnostic criteria have been developed by the National Institute of Allergy and Infectious Diseases and the Food Allergy and Anaphylaxis Network (**Box 2**).[18] In general terms, these criteria help to confirm a diagnosis of anaphylaxis after the acute development (within minutes to hours from exposure) of symptoms affecting at least 2 organ systems (or hypotension alone). These criteria have been prospectively validated in an ED population.[33] Findings suggested that the criteria are likely to be useful in the ED for the diagnosis of anaphylaxis.

Up to 90% of patients who experience anaphylaxis have urticaria/angioedema and/or rhinoconjunctivitis (see earlier discussion).[34] The other most common organ systems involved and those that contribute to the life-threatening and debilitating aspects of anaphylaxis include the respiratory, GI, and cardiovascular systems.

Children and adults with food-induced anaphylaxis differ in which of these organ systems are more characteristically affected. Compared with adults, children exhibit cardiovascular symptoms less often and respiratory symptoms more often.[26,35,36] In infants and very young children, cutaneous, GI, and respiratory symptoms are most common. Fatality is mostly due to respiratory compromise in children versus cardiovascular collapse in adults.

RESPIRATORY SYMPTOMS IN ANAPHYLAXIS

Respiratory symptoms and signs occur in up to 70% of anaphylactic episodes.[18] It is important for clinicians to recognize that respiratory symptoms, particularly laryngeal edema and bronchospasm, are the primary cause of death in children with food-induced anaphylaxis.[37] Respiratory symptoms related to FA are more likely to be severe in children with comorbid allergic conditions such as atopic dermatitis (AD) and asthma. Bronchospasm may also rarely be caused by airborne exposure to food allergens, such as inhalation of vapors from cooking of eggs, fish, and shellfish.[38]

Box 1
Common signs and symptoms of anaphylaxis

Skin or mucosal tissue

Rash

Generalized urticaria

Flushing

Pruritus

Angioedema

Piloerection

Oral pruritus or tingling

Conjunctival erythema

Respiratory

Dyspnea

Cough

Laryngeal edema

Difficulty breathing

Wheezing

Stridor

Chest tightness

Rhinorrhea

Nasal congestion

Sneezing

Nasal pruritus

Dysphonia

Hoarseness

Cardiovascular

Syncope

Feeling faint or dizzy

Confusion

Altered mental state

Chest pain

Heart palpitations

Tachycardia

Bradycardia

Urinary incontinence

Cardiac arrest

Gastrointestinal

Nausea

Vomiting

Diarrhea

Crampy abdominal pain

Difficulty swallowing

Neurologic

Anxiety

Feeling of impending doom

Seizures

Headache

Irritability

Confusion

Sudden behavioral changes (in young children: cling, cry, become irritable, cease to play)

Adapted from Simons FE. Anaphylaxis. J Allergy Clin Immunol 2010;125(2 Suppl 2):S167; and Campbell RL, Hagan JB, Manivannan V, et al. Evaluation of National Institute of Allergy and Infectious Diseases/Food Allergy and Anaphylaxis Network Criteria for the diagnosis of anaphylaxis in emergency department patients. J Allergy Clin Immunol 2012;129(3):751.

Box 2
Diagnostic criteria for anaphylaxis

Anaphylaxis is diagnosed when one of the following criteria is met:

1. Development of acute illness within minutes to hours after exposure causing skin and/or mucosal tissue involvement (eg, rash, generalized urticaria, pruritus, flushing, angioedema, laryngeal edema)
   And at least one of the following is present:
   - Evidence of respiratory compromise (eg, dyspnea, cough, difficulty breathing, wheezing, stridor)
   - Hypotension (defined later) or evidence of end-organ dysfunction (eg, syncope, hypotonia, urinary incontinence)

2. Development of 2 or more of the following within minutes to hours after exposure to a likely allergen for that patient
   - Skin or mucosal tissue involvement, including rash, generalized urticaria, pruritus, flushing, angioedema, and laryngeal edema
   - Respiratory compromise, including dyspnea, cough, difficulty breathing, wheezing, stridor, and hypoxia
   - Hypotension or symptoms causing concern for hypotension, including syncope, hypotonia, and urinary incontinence
   - Gastrointestinal symptoms, including nausea, vomiting, diarrhea, and crampy abdominal pain

3. Development of hypotension within minutes to hours after exposure to a known allergen for that patient (hypotension defined as follows)
   - Infants and children aged less than 1 year: systolic blood pressure (SBP) less than 70 mm Hg; children aged 1 to 10 years: SBP <(70 mm Hg + [2 × age in years]); children aged 11 to 17 years: SBP less than 90 mm Hg; or for all children, greater than 30% decrease from that person's baseline
   - Adults: SBP less than 90 mm Hg or greater than 30% decrease from that person's baseline

Adapted from Sampson HA, Munoz-Furlong A, Campbell RL, et al. Second symposium on the definition and management of anaphylaxis: summary report—second National Institute of Allergy and Infectious Disease/Food Allergy and Anaphylaxis Network symposium. Ann Emerg Med 2006;47(4):374.

GASTROINTESTINAL SYMPTOMS IN ANAPHYLAXIS

GI signs and symptoms occur in up to 45% of episodes of anaphylaxis and are more common in food-induced anaphylaxis than other causes.[37] GI symptoms from food-induced anaphylaxis can result in dehydration and electrolyte abnormalities, particularly in infants and very young children. The hypovolemia from GI manifestations is further exacerbated by the massive fluid shifts that occur rapidly in anaphylaxis as a result of increased vascular permeability and shift of intravascular fluid to the extravascular space.

CARDIOVASCULAR SYMPTOMS IN ANAPHYLAXIS

Cardiovascular signs and symptoms are also common in anaphylaxis, affecting up to 45% of episodes.[37] These symptoms include hypotension, dizziness, tachycardia, syncope, and urinary incontinence. Histamine-induced increases in vascular permeability cause large, rapid fluid shifts during anaphylactic episodes; up to 35% of intravascular volume can shift to the extravascular space within 10 minutes of the onset of anaphylaxis. The resulting hypotension can lead to shock and cardiac arrest.

Food-Dependent Exercise-Induced Anaphylaxis

Food-dependent exercise-induced anaphylaxis is an IgE-mediated condition in which symptoms manifest only if the patient exercises 2 to 4 hours after ingestion of a culprit food.[5] If the food is eaten without subsequent exercise or if exercise is performed without associated consumption of the food, no allergic symptoms develop. The most commonly implicated foods are wheat, shellfish, celery, fish, fruit, and milk.[39] The mechanism behind this type of anaphylaxis is presumably that exertion alters gut absorption and/or allergen digestion, resulting in allergen cross-linking of IgE and subsequent development of allergic symptoms. Risk factors for the development of this condition include female gender, late adolescent to early adult age, and coexistent atopic disease.[40]

Pitfalls in Making the Diagnosis of Food-Induced Anaphylaxis

Although formal diagnostic criteria for anaphylaxis have been developed by the National Institute of Allergy and Infectious Diseases and the Food Allergy and Anaphylaxis Network, anaphylaxis has been shown to be underdiagnosed and underreported for a variety of reasons.[41] **Box 3** lists some of the challenges in making an accurate diagnosis of anaphylaxis. One of the most common reasons that anaphylaxis is underdiagnosed is that the presentation in each individual is widely variable depending on the organ system involved, and sometimes, episodes can follow different patterns of organ involvement in the same individual.[42] Many of the signs and symptoms of anaphylaxis, including wheeze, stridor, dyspnea, confusion, and incontinence, are nonspecific, making the condition difficult to recognize clinically, particularly in the absence of a good history[37]; this is especially true when skin, nasal, and ocular symptoms are absent, which is the case in up to 10% of cases of anaphylaxis. Skin symptoms may also be masked if the patient has recently taken an H1 antihistamine.[42] Other pitfalls in making the diagnosis of anaphylaxis include reluctance among some health care professionals to label an episode as anaphylactic in the absence of hypotension or shock, despite the fact that changes in blood pressure are not required to make the diagnosis per the criteria outlined in **Box 2**. Finally, inability of young patients to communicate and recognize the presence of early symptoms also poses difficulty for clinicians in making the diagnosis of anaphylaxis.

Box 3
Pitfalls in making the diagnosis of anaphylaxis

1. Variable patterns of organ involvement between individuals and in multiple episodes of the same individual

2. Nonspecific symptoms, including dyspnea, wheeze, stridor, incontinence, and changes in mental status

3. Absence of skin, ocular, and nasal symptoms in up to 10% of cases

4. Masking of skin, ocular, and nasal symptoms if patient has recently taken an H1 antihistamine

5. Reluctance to diagnose anaphylaxis in the absence of hypotension

6. Inability of young children to communicate and recognize early signs and symptoms

---

NON-IGE-MEDIATED FOOD ALLERGIES

Unlike IgE-mediated FAs, which are acute in onset owing to their underlying immune mechanism, non-IgE-mediated FAs are driven by T cells and therefore cause delayed and more chronic clinical manifestations. These disorders include food protein–induced allergic proctocolitis (AP), food protein–induced enterocolitis syndrome (FPIES), celiac disease (CD), and food-induced pulmonary hemosiderosis (Heiner syndrome). Key clinical features of each are summarized in **Table 3**.

Food Protein–Induced Allergic Proctocolitis

AP often presents in breast-fed infants between the ages of 2 and 8 weeks and is characterized by T cell–mediated eosinophilic inflammation of the rectum and colon.[43,44] The affected infants may present with mucus and blood in their stool, as well as an increase in the frequency of bowel movements but are otherwise healthy appearing. In one prospective study of 95 breast-fed infants with AP, 88% were determined to have food-induced symptoms attributable to maternal ingestion of cow's milk, egg, corn, and soy.[45] Symptom improvement typically occurs within 48 hours of removal of the offending agent from the mother's diet. AP typically resolves after avoiding the allergen for 6 months to 2 years.[43]

Food Protein–Induced Enterocolitis Syndrome

Patients with FPIES, which is a more severe form of T cell–mediated GI FA, often present appearing ill, sometimes in shock. This disorder is underrecognized and frequently misdiagnosed in the primary care and ED settings. FPIES typically affects infants younger than 9 months of age, with a peak incidence between 1 week and 3 months.[5,14,46] This condition is rarely seen in breast-fed infants and is more common in those fed cow's milk– or soy-based formulas. Other less common culprits include grains (rice, oat, barley), vegetables (sweet potato, squash, string bean, peas), egg, and poultry (chicken, turkey).[47]

Symptoms of FPIES include profuse, repetitive vomiting and diarrhea leading to dehydration and lethargy in the short term and poor growth, anemia, and hypoproteinemia leading to failure to thrive in the long term.[48] Serious, life-threatening symptoms related to FPIES typically occur after an allergen is reintroduced into the diet after a period of restriction or on early exposure to the allergen. Clinical manifestations include profuse and repetitive vomiting approximately 1 to 3 hours after ingestion of the causative food and occasionally diarrhea after 5 to 8 hours. In addition, there is third spacing

Table 3
Non-IgE-mediated food allergy presentations

Disorder	Key Points/Clinical Features	Typical Age	Most Common Causal Foods
Food protein–induced allergic proctocolitis	Infants have mucus and blood in stool but are otherwise healthy appearing	Breast-fed infants between 2 and 8 wk	Due to maternal ingestion of foods, most commonly cow's milk, soy, egg, and corn
Food protein–induced enterocolitis syndrome	Profuse repetitive vomiting 1–8 h after ingestion Can lead to third spacing of fluid and massive inflammatory response leading to shock Chronic sequelae include poor growth, hypoproteinemia, anemia and failure to thrive	Usually infants younger than 9 mo of age; peak incidence at 1–3 mo	Rarely occurs in breast-fed infants; more common in those fed cow's milk or soy-based formulas Less commonly grains (rice, oat, barely), vegetables (sweet potato, squash, string bean, peas) and poultry (chicken, turkey)
Celiac disease	Symptoms include diarrhea, steatorrhea, abdominal discomfort Chronic consequences related to malabsorption and include growth problems and vitamin deficiencies	May occur any age after weaning	Inflammatory response to gluten in grains like wheat, rye, and barley
Food-induced pulmonary hemosiderosis (Heiner syndrome)	Rare pulmonary disease related to milk protein ingestion characterized by recurrent pneumonias, pulmonary hemosiderosis, iron deficiency anemia, and failure to thrive	Infants 4–29 mo	Cow's milk protein

of fluid and a robust systemic inflammatory response that may progress to dehydration and, in up to 20% of cases, even shock.[46] FPIES can be difficult to diagnose clinically because of the absence of skin and respiratory symptoms and a delay from food ingestion to onset. As a result, children with FPIES may undergo unnecessary tests and prolonged hospitalization for misdiagnoses of sepsis, surgical abdomen, metabolic disorder, or anaphylaxis.[49] Clinical suspicion for FPIES should be high in those children who have a history of ingestion of a new or previously avoided food within hours of characteristic symptoms. Although T cell–mediated inflammation may persist for several weeks, symptom relief is achieved with avoidance of the allergen. Children with cow's milk and soy FPIES typically become tolerant of the culprit food by the age of 3 years, but solid-food FPIES may have a more protracted course.[46]

Food Protein–Induced Enteropathy: Celiac Disease

Infants with food protein–induced enteropathy can have symptoms similar to patients with FPIES who have ingested the culprit food for long term, including chronic vomiting, diarrhea, and failure to thrive.[5] CD is an enteropathy caused by a T-cell-mediated inflammatory response to gluten in grains such as wheat, rye, and barley.[5] It is characterized histologically by mucosal inflammation, villous atrophy, and crypt hyperplasia. Symptoms include chronic diarrhea, steatorrhea, abdominal bloating, and distention as well as consequences of malabsorption such as failure to thrive, short stature, delayed puberty, iron deficiency anemia, and folate or vitamin B_{12} deficiency. When gluten-containing foods are removed from the diet, the histologic changes in the small bowel resolve, and symptoms regress within a few weeks to months.

Food-Induced Pulmonary Hemosiderosis (Heiner Syndrome)

Heiner syndrome is a rare pulmonary disease related most commonly to ingestion of cow's milk protein. It is seen in infants 4 to 29 months of age and is associated with milk-specific IgG antibodies, in contrast to IgE antibodies seen in acute FA. Complications include recurrent pneumonias, pulmonary hemosiderosis, iron deficiency anemia, and failure to thrive.[50] Radiographic evidence of pulmonary infiltrates is a common finding in those with Heiner syndrome. Milk protein elimination leads to the resolution of symptoms.

MIXED IGE-MEDIATED AND NON-IGE-MEDIATED FOOD ALLERGIES
Eosinophilic Esophagitis and Eosinophilic Gastroenteritis

Eosinophilic esophagitis (EoE) and eosinophilic gastroenteritis (EG) are considered mixed IgE and non-IgE (T cell–mediated) GI FAs. In patients with EoE, symptoms are variable depending on the age of presentation. Infants and young children may present with feeding dysfunction and failure to thrive, whereas older children and adults often manifest with vomiting, abdominal pain, dysphagia, and food impaction.[51] EoE is diagnosed by esophageal biopsy demonstrating the presence of greater than 15 eosinophils per high-powered field.[52] It is not uncommon in patients with EoE to have other allergic diseases, such as allergic rhinitis and IgE-mediated FA.[51] Food allergens, as well as possibly aeroallergens, seem to play causative roles in the immunopathology of EoE, and food-avoidance diets are often effective in inducing clinical and histologic improvement.

When eosinophils are found distal to the esophagus in the GI tract, this supports the diagnosis of EG. Symptoms of EG vary depending on the portion of the GI tract involved and may include abdominal pain, nausea, diarrhea, malabsorption, and weight loss. Unlike EoE, food-avoidance diets offer little or no benefit in EG.

Atopic Dermatitis

AD also has features of mixed IgE- and non-IgE-mediated FA immunopathology. Children with AD present with chronic pruritic rash distributed in flexor surfaces, such as the antecubital and popliteal fossa, wrists, ankles, and neck. In approximately 35% of children with AD (typically young children with severe AD), food allergens may exacerbate their rash, causing increasing erythema and pruritus, over a few hours if IgE-mediated or over days if non–IgE mediated.[53] Milk, soy, egg, wheat, and peanut are the most common culprit foods. Elimination of suspect foods often improves AD symptoms within a few weeks, and repeat exposure to them exacerbates symptoms.[53]

KEY HISTORICAL ELEMENTS IN PATIENTS WITH SUSPECTED FOOD ALLERGY

Obtaining a detailed history is crucial in providing the basis for testing and diagnosis of FA. Clinicians should consider a broad differential diagnosis and seek to identify possible trigger foods, as well as determine if the pathophysiology of the FA is IgE-mediated or otherwise. Important parts of the history are summarized in **Box 4**.

Box 4
Key history in patients with suspected food allergy

Reaction

- Symptoms including urticaria/angioedema, rhinoconjunctivitis, and respiratory, GI, and cardiovascular symptoms
- Exposure route that provoked reaction (ingestion, inhalation, contact)
- Time elapsed between ingestion of food and development of symptoms
- Course of symptoms (worsening, improving)

Suspected food

- Detailed description of foods ingested before reaction
- If patient/family unable to identify an obvious trigger, save food labels and/or review ingredients of everything ingested
- Amount of food ingested
- Form in which the food was ingested (raw, cooked)
- Whether ingested food has been tolerated previously
- Whether food was being previously avoided
- Mother's diet (for AP)

Surrounding circumstances

- Did other people who ingested the same food experience similar symptoms (rule out food poisoning such as scombroid, which can mimic FA)?
- Exercise in proximity to reaction
- Current medications
- Interventions taken to stop the reaction (medications)

Additional questions

- Whether symptoms recur consistently on reexposure to culprit food
- If food has been avoided since adverse reaction and if this has alleviated symptoms

---

SUMMARY

FAs are a common problem in the pediatric population that have serious, potentially life-threatening implications. An understanding of the underlying immune mechanisms that mediate food-allergic reactions helps delineate the characteristics of the various types of IgE-mediated, non-IgE-mediated, and mixed reactions. Although pitfalls to making the diagnosis of FAs and anaphylaxis exist, obtaining a thorough and complete history and applying available diagnostic criteria can help ensure accurate diagnosis and management. If the diagnosis of FA is unclear, patients should be referred to an allergist immunologist for further evaluation.

REFERENCES

1. Gupta RS, Springston EE, Warrier MR, et al. The prevalence, severity, and distribution of childhood food allergy in the United States. Pediatrics 2011;128(1): e9–17.
2. Rona RJ, Keil T, Summers C, et al. The prevalence of food allergy: a meta-analysis. J Allergy Clin Immunol 2007;120(3):638–46.
3. Sampson HA. Anaphylaxis and emergency treatment. Pediatrics 2003;111(6 Pt 3):1601–8.
4. Sampson HA, Mendelson L, Rosen JP. Fatal and near-fatal anaphylactic reactions to food in children and adolescents. N Engl J Med 1992;327(6):380–4.
5. Boyce JA, Assa'ad A, Burks AW, et al. Guidelines for the diagnosis and management of food allergy in the United States: report of the NIAID-sponsored expert panel. J Allergy Clin Immunol 2010;126(6 Suppl):S1–58.
6. Mansoor DK, Sharma HP. Clinical presentations of food allergy. Pediatr Clin North Am 2011;58(2):315–26, ix.
7. Hungerford JM. Scombroid poisoning: a review. Toxicon 2010;56(2):231–43.
8. Burks AW, Tang M, Sicherer S, et al. ICON: food allergy. J Allergy Clin Immunol 2012;129(4):906–20.
9. Commins SP, Platts-Mills TA. Delayed anaphylaxis to red meat in patients with IgE specific for galactose alpha-1,3-galactose (alpha-gal). Curr Allergy Asthma Rep 2013;13(1):72–7.
10. Hamsten C, Tran TA, Starkhammar M, et al. Red meat allergy in Sweden: association with tick sensitization and B-negative blood groups. J Allergy Clin Immunol 2013;132(6):1431–4.
11. Sehgal VN, Rege VL. An interrogative study of 158 urticaria patients. Ann Allergy 1973;31(6):279–83.
12. Kobza Black A, Greaves MW, Champion RH, et al. The urticarias 1990. Br J Dermatol 1991;124(1):100–8.
13. Simons FE. Anaphylaxis: recent advances in assessment and treatment. J Allergy Clin Immunol 2009;124(4):625–36 [quiz: 637–8].
14. Sampson HA, Aceves S, Bock SA, et al. Food allergy: a practice parameter update - 2014. J Allergy Clin Immunol 2014;134(5):1016–25.e43.
15. Bock SA, Atkins FM. Patterns of food hypersensitivity during sixteen years of double-blind, placebo-controlled food challenges. J Pediatr 1990;117(4):561–7.
16. Roberts G, Lack G. Relevance of inhalational exposure to food allergens. Curr Opin Allergy Clin Immunol 2003;3(3):211–5.
17. Boyce JA, Assa'ad A, Burks AW, et al. Guidelines for the diagnosis and management of food allergy in the United States: summary of the NIAID-sponsored expert panel report. J Am Diet Assoc 2011;111(1):17–27.

18. Sampson HA, Munoz-Furlong A, Campbell RL, et al. Second symposium on the definition and management of anaphylaxis: summary report–second National Institute of Allergy and Infectious Disease/Food Allergy and Anaphylaxis Network symposium. Ann Emerg Med 2006;47(4):373–80.
19. Lieberman P, Camargo CA Jr, Bohlke K, et al. Epidemiology of anaphylaxis: findings of the American College of Allergy, Asthma and Immunology Epidemiology of Anaphylaxis Working Group. Ann Allergy Asthma Immunol 2006;97(5): 596–602.
20. Lieberman P. Epidemiology of anaphylaxis. Curr Opin Allergy Clin Immunol 2008; 8(4):316–20.
21. Wang J, Sampson HA. Food anaphylaxis. Clin Exp Allergy 2007;37(5):651–60.
22. Bock SA, Munoz-Furlong A, Sampson HA. Fatalities due to anaphylactic reactions to foods. J Allergy Clin Immunol 2001;107(1):191–3.
23. Pumphrey R. Anaphylaxis: can we tell who is at risk of a fatal reaction? Curr Opin Allergy Clin Immunol 2004;4(4):285–90.
24. Sicherer SH, Munoz-Furlong A, Sampson HA. Prevalence of seafood allergy in the United States determined by a random telephone survey. J Allergy Clin Immunol 2004;114(1):159–65.
25. Sicherer SH, Sampson HA. Peanut allergy: emerging concepts and approaches for an apparent epidemic. J Allergy Clin Immunol 2007;120(3):491–503 [quiz: 504–5].
26. Hompes S, Kohli A, Nemat K, et al. Provoking allergens and treatment of anaphylaxis in children and adolescents–data from the anaphylaxis registry of German-speaking countries. Pediatr Allergy Immunol 2011;22(6):568–74.
27. Pumphrey RS, Gowland MH. Further fatal allergic reactions to food in the United Kingdom, 1999-2006. J Allergy Clin Immunol 2007;119(4):1018–9.
28. Bock SA, Munoz-Furlong A, Sampson HA. Further fatalities caused by anaphylactic reactions to food, 2001-2006. J Allergy Clin Immunol 2007;119(4):1016–8.
29. Sicherer SH, Sampson HA. Food allergy: epidemiology, pathogenesis, diagnosis, and treatment. J Allergy Clin Immunol 2014;133(2):291–307 [quiz: 308].
30. Ono E, Taniguchi M, Mita H, et al. Increased production of cysteinyl leukotrienes and prostaglandin D2 during human anaphylaxis. Clin Exp Allergy 2009;39(1): 72–80.
31. Lieberman P, Nicklas RA, Oppenheimer J, et al. The diagnosis and management of anaphylaxis practice parameter: 2010 update. J Allergy Clin Immunol 2010; 126(3):477–80.e1–42.
32. Simons FE. Anaphylaxis. J Allergy Clin Immunol 2010;125(2 Suppl 2):S161–81.
33. Campbell RL, Hagan JB, Manivannan V, et al. Evaluation of National Institute of Allergy and Infectious Diseases/Food Allergy and Anaphylaxis Network criteria for the diagnosis of anaphylaxis in emergency department patients. J Allergy Clin Immunol 2012;129(3):748–52.
34. Webb LM, Lieberman P. Anaphylaxis: a review of 601 cases. Ann Allergy Asthma Immunol 2006;97(1):39–43.
35. Brown AF, McKinnon D, Chu K. Emergency department anaphylaxis: a review of 142 patients in a single year. J Allergy Clin Immunol 2001;108(5):861–6.
36. Braganza SC, Acworth JP, McKinnon DR, et al. Paediatric emergency department anaphylaxis: different patterns from adults. Arch Dis Child 2006;91(2): 159–63.
37. Cianferoni A, Muraro A. Food-induced anaphylaxis. Immunol Allergy Clin N Am 2012;32(1):165–95.

38. Crespo JF, Pascual C, Dominguez C, et al. Allergic reactions associated with airborne fish particles in IgE-mediated fish hypersensitive patients. Allergy 1995;50(3):257–61.

39. Romano A, Di Fonso M, Giuffreda F, et al. Food-dependent exercise-induced anaphylaxis: clinical and laboratory findings in 54 subjects. Int Arch Allergy Immunol 2001;125(3):264–72.

40. Du Toit G. Food-dependent exercise-induced anaphylaxis in childhood. Pediatr Allergy Immunol 2007;18(5):455–63.

41. Lin RY, Anderson AS, Shah SN, et al. Increasing anaphylaxis hospitalizations in the first 2 decades of life: New York State, 1990-2006. Ann Allergy Asthma Immunol 2008;101(4):387–93.

42. Simons FE. Anaphylaxis, killer allergy: long-term management in the community. J Allergy Clin Immunol 2006;117(2):367–77.

43. Patenaude Y, Bernard C, Schreiber R, et al. Cow's-milk-induced allergic colitis in an exclusively breast-fed infant: diagnosed with ultrasound. Pediatr Radiol 2000; 30(6):379–82.

44. Anveden-Hertzberg L, Finkel Y, Sandstedt B, et al. Proctocolitis in exclusively breast-fed infants. Eur J Pediatr 1996;155(6):464–7.

45. Lake AM. Food-induced eosinophilic proctocolitis. J Pediatr Gastroenterol Nutr 2000;30(Suppl):S58–60.

46. Caubet JC, Ford LS, Sickles L, et al. Clinical features and resolution of food protein-induced enterocolitis syndrome: 10-year experience. J Allergy Clin Immunol 2014;134(2):382–9.

47. Ruffner MA, Ruymann K, Barni S, et al. Food protein-induced enterocolitis syndrome: insights from review of a large referral population. J Allergy Clin Immunol Pract 2013;1(4):343–9.

48. Nowak-Wegrzyn A, Muraro A. Food protein-induced enterocolitis syndrome. Curr Opin Allergy Clin Immunol 2009;9(4):371–7.

49. Sicherer SH. Food protein-induced enterocolitis syndrome: case presentations and management lessons. J Allergy Clin Immunol 2005;115(1):149–56.

50. Moissidis I, Chaidaroon D, Vichyanond P, et al. Milk-induced pulmonary disease in infants (Heiner syndrome). Pediatr Allergy Immunol 2005;16(6):545–52.

51. Greenhawt M, Aceves SS, Spergel JM, et al. The management of eosinophilic esophagitis. J Allergy Clin Immunol Pract 2013;1(4):332–40 [quiz: 341–2].

52. Furuta GT, Liacouras CA, Collins MH, et al. Eosinophilic esophagitis in children and adults: a systematic review and consensus recommendations for diagnosis and treatment. Gastroenterology 2007;133(4):1342–63.

53. Greenhawt M. The role of food allergy in atopic dermatitis. Allergy Asthma Proc 2010;31(5):392–7.

Diagnosis of Food Allergy

Rebecca Sharon Chinthrajah, MD[a],*, Dana Tupa, MS[b],
Benjamin T. Prince, MD[c,1], Whitney Morgan Block, BS, MSN, RN, CPNP, FNP-BC[d],
Jaime Sou Rosa, MD, PhD[a], Anne Marie Singh, MD[e], Kari Nadeau, MD, PhD[a]

KEYWORDS

- Food allergy • IgE-mediated • Non–IgE-mediated • Skin-prick testing
- Oral food challenge • Component testing • Elimination diets

KEY POINTS

- Food allergies consist of a group of diseases that result from immunologic, adverse reactions to foods.
- Clinical history is paramount in the diagnosis of food allergy.
- Skin tests and specific immunoglobulin E (IgE) can indicate sensitization that may not be clinically relevant.
- It is important to recognize and distinguish IgE-mediated reactions, as these can be life threatening and require significant patient education.
- Specialists, such as allergists/immunologists and gastroenterologists, play an important role in the diagnosis and management of food allergies.

INTRODUCTION

The prevalence of food allergies in children and adults has been increasing over the last few decades.[1] Food allergies are due to abnormal immunologic responses following ingestion of the offending food. Multiple food allergy entities can

The authors have no relevant conflicts of interest to disclose.

[a] Division of Allergy, Immunology, and Rheumatology, Department of Pediatrics, Sean N Parker Center for Allergy Research, Stanford University, Stanford University School of Medicine, 269 Campus Drive, CCSR 3215, MC 5366, Stanford, CA 94305-5101, USA; [b] Sean N Parker Center for Allergy Research, Stanford University, Stanford University School of Medicine, 1291 Welch Road, Grant Building S303, Stanford, CA 94305, USA; [c] Ann & Robert H. Lurie Children's Hospital of Chicago, Northwestern University, Feinberg School of Medicine, 225 East Chicago Avenue Box 60, Chicago, IL, USA; [d] Sean N Parker Center for Allergy Research, Stanford University, 2500 Grant Road, PEC, 4th Floor Tower C, Mountain View, CA 94040, USA; [e] Ann & Robert H. Lurie Children's Hospital of Chicago, Northwestern University Feinberg School of Medicine, 240 East Huron Street, M-317, McGaw Pavilion, Chicago, IL 60611, USA

[1] Present Address: 221 North Front Street, Unit 304, Columbus, OH 43215.

* Corresponding author. Division of Pulmonary and Critical Care Medicine, Department of Medicine, Sean N Parker Center for Allergy Research, Stanford University, Stanford University School of Medicine, 269 Campus Drive, CCSR 3215, MC 5366, Stanford, CA 94305.
E-mail address: schinths@stanford.edu

Pediatr Clin N Am 62 (2015) 1393–1408
http://dx.doi.org/10.1016/j.pcl.2015.07.009
0031-3955/15/$ – see front matter © 2015 Elsevier Inc. All rights reserved.

be characterized based on the immunologic response. For the purposes of this review, the diagnosis of food allergies is divided into immunoglobulin E (IgE)-mediated reactions, non–IgE-mediated reactions, and mixed allergic reactions (**Table 1**). The most important diagnostic tool is the clinical history, which is aided by diagnostic testing such as skin and blood tests to assess for food-specific IgE. When necessary, the diagnosis is confirmed with oral food challenges and elimination diets to assess for clinical symptoms related to the ingestion of an implicated food.

DIAGNOSING IMMUNOGLOBULIN E–MEDIATED FOOD ALLERGIES
Clinical History

When the clinician suspects an IgE-mediated food allergy, the medical history and physical examination can provide a good pretest probability of an IgE-mediated allergy.[2,3] It is important for the clinician to note the dietary history, foods involved at the time of the allergic event, timing of exposure to the onset of symptoms,[4] route of exposure, nature and duration of symptoms, and treatments received (**Table 2**). Supplemental factors, such as concomitant medication use or alcohol ingestion, may play a role in the reaction severity.[5] Symptoms during an IgE-mediated allergic reaction can range from mild to severe, involving one or multiple organ systems (**Table 3**). A history consistent with anaphylaxis, an immediate, severe, allergic reaction involving multiple organ systems, after the ingestion of a food is highly suggestive of an IgE-mediated food allergy. The timing and events during an allergic episode, such as the timing of exercise in food-dependent, exercise-induced anaphylaxis (FDEIAn), and the type (cooked vs raw) and amount of the suspected offending food ingested, are important parts of the history to be elicited. Comorbid conditions such as asthma, allergic rhinitis, or atopic dermatitis might indicate an increased risk of IgE-mediated food allergy.[6]

It is important to consider and rule out, if necessary, other diseases, triggers, and syndromes that may be mistaken for IgE-mediated food allergies, which may include allergic reactions caused by:

- Medications or insect stings (possibly around the same time of food ingestion)
- Metabolic disorders: gluten and lactose intolerances and sensitivities
- Toxic reactions: food poisoning caused by toxins, such as histamine in scombroid poisoning
- Chemical exposures, such as chlorine or fragrant perfumes, which may cause rhinitis, skin irritation, or exacerbation of asthma
- Viral syndromes that may cause rhinorrhea and/or urticaria

Table 1
Different types of food allergies

IgE-Mediated Reactions	Mixed Allergic Reactions	Non–IgE-Mediated Reactions
Food ingestion reactions within 2 h of ingestion	Atopic dermatitis	Food protein–induced enteropathy
"Alpha Gal" allergy	Eosinophilic esophagitis	Food protein–induced enterocolitis
Oral allergy syndrome	Eosinophilic gastritis	Food protein–induced proctitis
Food-dependent exercise-induced anaphylaxis	—	Celiac disease

Table 2
Clinical pearls of an IgE-mediated food allergy

Offending food	Cow's milk, egg, wheat, soy, peanut, tree nut, fish, shellfish (these 8 foods account for 90% of reactions)
Timing of exposure to onset of symptoms	Minutes to hours (usually within the first 2 h); however, late reactions can occur with normal foods and within 3–6 h after ingestion of red meat, such as beef, pork, and lamb in "Alpha Gal" allergy[4]
Route of exposure	Oral ingestions tend to have more severe reactions; mild skin reactions occur with cutaneous exposure
Type of food	Oral pruritus with raw forms of fruits or vegetables, but tolerance of cooked forms, would suggest oral allergy syndrome
Nature of symptoms	Cutaneous, gastrointestinal, and respiratory symptoms predominate
Duration of symptoms	Less than 1 h to several hours; however, late reactions and biphasic reactions can occur
Treatment of symptoms	Responsive to antihistamines and/or epinephrine
Dietary history	Foods eaten before and after an allergic episode without reaction are typically not the culprit of an IgE-mediated food allergy (exception is exercise-induced anaphylaxis); note avoidance patterns
Supplemental factors	Alcohol consumption, NSAID use, exercise, concurrent illness

Abbreviation: NSAID, nonsteroidal anti-inflammatory drug.

- Reactions and sensitivities to food additives such as sulfites, nitrites, and monosodium glutamate[2]
- Most cases of new-onset urticaria in children are infectious in origin and do not involve IgE-mediated mechanisms. In addition, most cases of chronic idiopathic urticaria are related to physical factors (cold, pressure, sun exposure, and so forth) rather than food ingestion[7]

Food-Dependent Exercise-Induced Anaphylaxis

FDEIAn is a disorder whereby allergic symptoms occur if exercise takes place within several hours after consumption of the causative food allergen, as identified by clinical history and allergy testing.[2,8,9] Omega-5 gliadin, a protein component of gluten,

Table 3
Examples of most common symptoms during an IgE-mediated allergic reaction

Cutaneous	Gastrointestinal	Respiratory
Erythema	Nausea	Nasal congestion
Pruritus	Abdominal pain	Rhinorrhea
Urticaria	Reflux	Sneezing
Morbilliform rash	Vomiting	Hoarseness
Angioedema	Diarrhea	Laryngeal edema
Eczematous rash (typical of late reactions)		Cough
		Chest tightness
		Dyspnea
		Wheezing
		Increased work of breathing

is a major protein involved in wheat allergy that causes exercise-induced anaphylaxis, although other foods have also been implicated, including egg, nuts, crustaceans, meats, fruits, and vegetables.[10,11] The diagnosis of FDEIAn can be made when a patient has signs and symptoms consistent with recurrent anaphylaxis upon or soon after physical exertion, and if the food allergen was consumed within 2 to 4 hours before the allergic event. There should also be an absence of symptoms during vigorous physical activities or food allergen ingestion alone.[2,8,9] The patient should demonstrate evidence of sensitization to the food allergen by skin-prick or in vitro (specific IgE [sIgE]) testing.[8,10,11] When no allergen is found, a repeat test after 6 to 12 months may increase the sensitivity of identifying the culprit food allergen.[12]

Oral Allergy Syndrome

Almost all patients with pollen-food allergy syndrome, more commonly known as oral allergy syndrome (OAS), have underlying allergic rhinoconjunctivitis caused by respiratory sensitization to airborne pollens. OAS results from IgE sensitization to aeroallergens and cross-reactive antibodies recognizing homologous epitopes in fruits (ie, Pru p 1 in peach), vegetables (ie, Api g 1 in celery), or other plant-derived, heat-labile food proteins (ie, Ara h 8 in peanut).[13–16] A local IgE-mediated response leads to an immediate sensation of oropharyngeal pruritus after food contact or ingestion, which is sometimes accompanied by angioedema of the oral mucosa and abdominal discomfort.[13,14] Cooking or factory processing of the food can denature the conformational integrity of the culprit proteins, resulting in significant reductions in IgE-binding avidity, which generally renders the food harmless when consumed.[14–16] More severe symptoms such as vomiting, diarrhea, and anaphylaxis rarely develop, and thus would be less consistent with OAS but more concerning for systemic reactions associated with heat-stable proteins.[17]

Skin-Prick Tests and Serum Tests

Diagnostic testing in suspected IgE-mediated food allergy should be guided by the clinical history. A positive skin-prick test (SPT) or positive sIgE test denotes sensitization and not necessarily clinically relevant allergy. Careful patient selection for testing is advised because of the potential for false-positive results, possibly resulting in unnecessary dietary restrictions. In general, the larger the SPT or sIgE, the more likely that the allergen is clinically relevant, although these tests correlate less with the severity of reactions.[18] Although SPTs have varying positive predictive values (PPVs), they generally have a relatively high negative predictive value. Threshold values for SPTs and sIgE have been identified for some allergens to define the 95% PPV, the point at which patients are likely to react to a food challenge **(Table 4)**.[19,20]

Table 4		
Predictive values of SPT in positive or negative oral food challenge results		
	>95% Positive Predictive Value in Children	
Food	**SPT (mm)**	**sIgE (kUA/L)**
Egg white	$\geq 7^{19}$ or $\geq 13^{20}$	≥ 7 (≥ 2 in infants <2 y old)[18]
Cow's milk	$\geq 8^{19}$ or $\geq 12.5^{20}$	≥ 15 (≥ 5 in infants <2 y old)[18]
Peanut	$\geq 8^{19}$	$\geq 14^{18}$
Fish	Undetermined	$\geq 20^{2}$

Skin and in vitro testing with commercially available, heat-labile, and easily degradable fruit and vegetable extracts often leads to false-negative results. However, the prick-prick skin test, whereby the fruit or vegetable is pricked and then the patient's skin is pricked, is a reliable method for confirming OAS, described in the previous section.[21,22]

The ratio of sIgE to total IgE has also been examined. Some have found that it does not add additional value compared with sIgE alone,[23] whereas others have found the ratio to be higher for those who failed their food challenge when compared with those who passed. This finding is particularly true for allergens that are less likely to be outgrown, such as peanuts, shellfish, tree nuts, and seeds.[24]

Component-resolved diagnosis (CRD) is now more widely available to investigate IgE against smaller, relevant peptides of the larger parent protein. This approach allows for distinction between peptides that are similar to pollens and may be heat labile.[3,25] Proteins that are degraded by digestion or heat are less likely to cause systemic reactions and are often implicated in OAS. In addition, nonspecific lipid transfer proteins have been implicated in allergic reactions associated with supplemental factors.[11,26,27] Using components may aid in understanding which patients might tolerate baked egg or milk food challenges.[28–30] Some clinical pearls using component testing are listed in **Table 5**. Of importance is that severe reactions can still occur despite negative component testing results, as all relevant peptides have not been identified.

Oral Food Challenge

The gold standard of diagnosing an IgE-mediated food allergy is the double-blind, placebo-controlled food challenge. If this is not feasible or realistic, open challenges or single-blind challenges, whereby a placebo dose is introduced into the succession of true allergen doses, may be considered. The challenge is typically done in the office of a specialist well trained in treating allergic reactions, and consists of ingesting multiple doses of a food spaced out over time to minimize the risk of severe reactions. Patients are then observed for clinical reactions, with medications to treat allergic reactions readily available in the clinic. Oral food challenges are necessary because of the poor sensitivity and specificity of SPT and sIgE; 89% of children diagnosed with food allergy based on sIgEs were able to reintroduce foods into their diet following a challenge.[31]

DIAGNOSING MIXED IMMUNOGLOBULIN E AND NON–IMMUNOGLOBULIN E FOOD REACTIONS

Some food allergy disorders can have both IgE-mediated and cellular-mediated pathology (delayed Th2 responses). Mixed disorders typically manifest in the gastrointestinal (GI) tract and the skin. The relationship between food allergies and atopic dermatitis has been reviewed comprehensively elsewhere.[32–37] This review addresses mixed food allergic GI disorders. Eosinophilic GI disorders (EGIDs) are a group of inflammatory disorders primarily classified by the presence of a high density of infiltrating eosinophils within the GI mucosal epithelium, muscularis, and serosal layers. EGIDs include eosinophilic esophagitis (EoE), eosinophilic gastroenteritis (EG), and eosinophilic colitis (EC).[38] EoE is one of the most studied of the EGIDs, while less is known about EC because of its rare occurrence. Healthy esophageal tissue is normally free of eosinophils, and the rest of the GI tract contains a low density of these cells.[39] Characteristic findings for the EGIDs are outlined in **Table 6**.[22,37–45]

Table 5
Component-resolved diagnostics: pearls

Food	Components	Clinical Pearls
Peanut	Heat-stable: Ara h 1, 2, 3 Heat-labile: Ara h 8 (Bet v 1 homologue)	Higher risk of systemic reactions Low risk of systemic reactions
Hazelnut	Heat-stable: Cor a 8, 9, 14 Heat-labile: Cor a 1 (Bet v 1 homologue)	Higher risk of systemic reactions Low risk of systemic reactions
Wheat	Omega-5 gliadin Tri a 14	Associated with wheat-dependent exercise-induced anaphylaxis
Meat	Galactose a 1,3 galactose "Alpha Gal"	Delayed anaphylaxis, 3–6 h after ingestion of red meat
Peach	Pru p 3	Associated with food-dependent exercise-induced anaphylaxis
	Pru p 1 (Bet v 1 homologue)	Low risk of systemic reactions
Apple	Mal d 3	Higher risk of systemic reactions
	Mal d 1 (Bet v 1 homologue)	Low risk of systemic reactions
Cow's milk	Caseins: Bos d 8	Casein-specific IgE <0.7 kUA/L is a very favorable prognostic factor for tolerance of baked milk
	Whey proteins: Bos d 4 α-lactalbumin Bos d 5 β-lactoglobulin	For those exclusively allergic to whey proteins, many tolerate baked milk and yogurt
	Bos d 6 serum albumin Lactoferrin	Bos d 6; can also be allergic to beef
Egg white	Heat-stable: Gal d 1 (ovomucoid)	Higher sIgE levels to ovomucoid associated with persistent egg allergy
	Heat-labile: Gal d 2: ovalbumin Gal d 3: ovotransferrin Gal d 4: lysozyme	Gal d 2: most abundant protein in egg white; heating may reduce allergenicity; lower ovalbumin sIgE/IgG4 ratio is associated with tolerance to heated egg Gal d 4: might be important in occupational asthma

Clinical History

Eosinophilic infiltration of the GI tract can be induced by drug hypersensitivities, parasitic infections, *Helicobacter pylori* infections, and cancer, and it is important to rule out these conditions.[39] In addition, gastroesophageal reflux disease (GERD) and inflammatory bowel disease can present with symptoms similar to EGIDs.[46] Individuals who have unexplained dysphagia or food impaction, a history of atopy, peripheral eosinophilia, and a family history of EGIDs should be considered for EGID. The most characteristic symptoms seen in EoE in children is failure to thrive and malnutrition,[45] whereas adults present with dysphagia, food impaction, and heartburn.[22,42] The prevalence of EoE is approximately 50 of 100,000 inhabitants in select regions of the United States and Europe, and the condition is more common in males than females, at a ratio of 3:1.[41] Several studies show that at least half of both children and adult populations with EoE and EG often suffer from other atopic conditions.[38,42,44–49] In one study, more than 40% of 381 children with EoE had first-degree family members with atopic or food allergies.[50]

Table 6
Eosinophilic gastrointestinal disorders

Disease	Location Affected	Symptoms	Endoscopic Findings	Histology/Lab Tests
Eosinophilic esophagitis	Esophagus	Adults: Dysphagia, food impaction[42] Children: Irritability, feeding difficulties, vomiting, abdominal pain, malnutrition[45]	Ringed esophagus, strictures, linear furrows, narrow esophagus, vesicles on mucosal surface	≥15 eosinophils per high-powered field (eos/hpf) in middle esophagus, peripheral eosinophilia
Eosinophilic gastritis	Stomach and duodenum, but can affect esophagus to colon	Abdominal pain, nausea, vomiting, diarrhea, weight loss, anemia, malabsorption, motility issues (affecting muscle layer), ascites (serosal layer)	Nodular gastric mucosa, erythema, erosions	≥30 eos/hpf[37] (no consensus), abnormal D-xylose, and increased fecal fat (in malabsorption)
Eosinophilic colitis	Large Intestine	Abdominal pain, bloody stools, diarrhea	Edema, patchy granularity	Eosinophilic infiltration on biopsy

Serum Testing

The pathogenesis of these diseases is not well understood, but epidemiologic and clinical features suggest allergic components.[40,44] IgE-mediated food sensitizations and elevated total and food-specific IgEs are common among patients with EoE, although they are often not correlative with the culprit food.[47] A cross-sectional study of 53 children with EoE showed that 80% had IgE sensitization to multiple food allergens and aeroallergens, and 32% had elevated total IgE levels.[51] Younger EoE patients had more sensitizations to foods, whereas older patients had more sensitizations to aeroallergens. In another study, 62% of 107 patients with EGIDs (EoE or EG) had sensitizations to an average of 10.5 food allergens.[44] However, food sensitizations detected by SPTs and atopy patch tests generally do not correlate with clinical episodes of EoE.[52] This finding indicates that food sensitizations and elevations in IgE levels detected by conventional tests may not necessarily be able to link those foods to the pathophysiology of EGID.

Endoscopic Evaluation

Along with gross endoscopic observation, histologic studies of GI biopsies are an integral part of the diagnostic process. Four to 5 biopsies should be taken from each site, including normal and grossly abnormal appearing mucosa, as either can demonstrate eosinophilic inflammation.[53] Classic endoscopic and histologic findings are presented in **Table 6**. In the case of eosinophilic esophageal findings, one must rule out GERD (a common finding includes eosinophils in the middle and distal portions of the esophagus). A trial of a proton-pump inhibitor (PPI) is given for 6 to 8 weeks. EoE is considered if eosinophils remain in the middle esophagus, which is distinguished from PPI-responsive EoE (PPI-REE) if eosinophils remit from the mid-esophagus. It is unclear whether PPI-REE is a disease distinct from EoE.[49] Repeat endoscopies are often necessary to assess the effectiveness of appropriate management of EoE, whether a patient is treated with topical steroids or elimination diets.

Elimination Diets

Food elimination diets have been highly effective at reversing the clinical severity of all types of EGIDs, and are thus a part of the diagnostic algorithm. A meta-analysis and systematic review of numerous studies published between 1995 and 2013 compared the efficacy of the various elimination diets in both pediatric and adult EoE patient populations.[49] Most studies removed specific foods from the diet for a minimum of 6 weeks, followed by clinical, endoscopic, and histologic analyses. Efficacy of the diets was defined as histologic remission, denoted by a peak eosinophil count of ≤15 eosinophils per high-powered field.[49] The summary findings of the elimination diets from this meta-analysis are presented in **Table 7**.

Overall, these studies found that cow's milk, wheat, eggs, and soy/legumes are the most common trigger foods in EoE patients.[49,54–57] Remarkably, the elemental and milk elimination diets were capable of reducing eosinophil counts to less than 1 eosinophil per high-powered field.[48,58,59] Similar rates of remission with elemental formulas were also observed in EG patients, although studies on elimination diets in this EGID are limited.[45,60]

Food Challenges

Once an elimination diet has been instituted, foods are reintroduced, typically one at a time over 6-week intervals. Symptoms are then reviewed, and endoscopy with biopsies is repeated to ascertain whether histologic remission persists. The gradual reintroduction of excluded foods into the diet was met with high failure rates.[50,61] In one study with 22 adults, only 9% of patients who had remission while on the 4-food group elimination diet were able to add all food groups back without return of EoE.[54] However, most patients only had 1 or 2 problem food groups. The postdiet remission rates were comparable in both adult and pediatric populations; however, the allergy test–directed diet seemed to be more successful in children. Although these short-term elimination diets do not resolve the condition permanently, the food challenges act as a valuable tool in identifying problem foods to avoid over the

Table 7
Elimination diets and histologic remission

Diet	Histologic Remission Rates (%)
Elemental diet (hypoallergenic, amino acid formula)	90.8 (in 411 children, 18 adults; 13 studies)
Six-food group elimination diet (milk, egg, wheat, soy, peanuts/tree nuts, fish/shellfish)	72.1 (in 75 children, 112 adults; 7 studies)
Four-food group elimination diet (dairy, wheat, egg, legumes)	53.4 (in 15 children, 13 adults; 2 studies)
Allergy-directed diet (based on positive skin prick or atopy patch testing)	45.5 (594 children, 32 adults; 14 studies) 30 (adults alone)
Gluten-free diet	58.7 (2 studies)
Milk elimination diet	68.2 (3 studies)

long term in individuals with food-related EGIDs, and provide a means for symptom management. However, elimination diets may pose social, psychological, and nutritional repercussions in the long term. Alternatives to management of EGIDs include corticosteroids (both topical and systemic), leukotriene receptor antagonists, and anti–interleukin-5 monoclonal antibodies.[62] Despite their effectiveness, these methods may lead to serious repercussions owing to their unnatural modulation of the immune system. Further investigations should focus on developing clinically relevant and standardized methods for diagnosing these complex disorders.

DIAGNOSING NON-IMMUNOGLOBULIN E–MEDIATED ADVERSE FOOD REACTIONS

Several adverse reactions to foods in children are the result of non–IgE-mediated immunologic reactions to food proteins. By definition, the pathogenesis of these diseases does not involve the production of food-specific IgE; therefore, their clinical presentation differs from IgE-mediated and mixed adverse food reactions. Similarly, testing strategies that involve the identification of food-specific IgE are not useful. Diagnosis often requires the demonstration of clinical improvement following the withdrawal of the implicated food and, occasionally, a recurrence of symptoms with a subsequent oral food challenge. There are many non–IgE-mediated diseases that can affect a variety of different tissues, including the GI tract (food protein–induced allergic proctitis [FPIAP], food protein–induced enteropathy [FPE], food protein–induced enterocolitis [FPIES], celiac disease), the skin (systemic contact dermatitis), and the lungs (Heiner syndrome).[63] Further discussion of celiac disease and extra-GI adverse reactions to foods are beyond the scope of this review, but have been discussed extensively elsewhere.[64–66]

FPIAP, FPE, and FPIES represent a spectrum of diseases can affect the entire GI tract. These disorders are thought to be the result of a T-cell–mediated immunologic response to specific food proteins, and are differentiated by the specific region of the GI tract affected.[67,68]

Food Protein–Induced Allergic Proctitis

FPIAP is the least severe non–IgE-mediated disease and is a common cause of isolated rectal bleeding in otherwise healthy infants.[69] Pathogenic inflammation is primarily limited to the rectum, although rarely it can extend further up the sigmoid colon.[70] Although FPIAP has been rarely described in older children,[69] it is more commonly found in breastfed infants and typically starts within the first few months of life.[71–73] Infants classically present with a history of stools streaked with bright red blood and mucus. Although stools may be more frequent, frank diarrhea is uncommon, and infants otherwise appear healthy. The most common causes in breastfeeding infants are milk, soy, and egg from the maternal diet, and most patients will have symptom resolution within 72 hours of strict food elimination.[73] Typically, cow's milk should be strictly eliminated first, followed by soy and then egg if symptoms do not completely resolve within 2 weeks.[71] Formula-fed infants and breastfed infants who do not respond to elimination diets should be placed on an extensively hydrolyzed or amino acid–based formula, because of the high rate of sensitization to both cow's milk and soy proteins.[74]

The diagnosis of FPIAP is based on clinical history and resolution of symptoms following food elimination; skin testing and other in vitro tests assessing for food-specific IgE are not recommended.[2,63] It may be necessary to perform a more extensive evaluation in children who continue to have symptoms despite food elimination. Colonoscopy in FPIAP generally demonstrates features of mild colitis, patchy erythema, and a loss of vascularity, and biopsies are notable for high numbers of eosinophilia in the lamina propria and muscularis mucosa.[75–77] After symptom resolution, reintroduction of home diet is generally recommended after 6 to 9 months of age, as most children have been shown to tolerate the implicated food after this time. Some studies have even demonstrated that up to 20% of breastfed infants had spontaneous resolution of symptoms without changes in the maternal diet.[78]

Food Protein–Induced Enteropathy

In contrast to FPIAP, FPE involves the small bowel and typically presents in the first 9 months of life with protracted diarrhea that can lead to failure to thrive (FTT) in more than 50% of infants.[79,80] In many infants, symptoms usually have a gradual onset within a few weeks of introduction of the implicated food. Although the most common causal food of FPE is cow's milk, other foods such as soy, egg, rice, poultry, fish, and shellfish have been described.[80–82] FPE can also occur after acute episodes of infectious gastroenteritis.[83,84]

The diagnosis of FPE is based on the presence of clinical symptoms, often with confirmation by endoscopy and biopsies. Histologic findings include mucosal changes in the proximal and distal small bowel, with villous atrophy and cellular infiltration.[79] As in other non–IgE-mediated diseases, skin testing and in vitro assessments for food-specific IgE are not recommended. Once a diagnosis is established, elimination of the implicated food generally leads to resolution of symptoms within 1 to 3 weeks, with severe cases sometimes requiring partial parenteral nutrition during the initial recovery period.[80] After 1 to 2 years, most children with FPE have been shown to tolerate reintroduction of the eliminated food without any clinical symptoms or long-term complications.

Food Protein–Induced Enterocolitis

FPIES is the most severe form of the food protein–induced GI diseases, involving the entire GI tract. It was originally described as a cause of weight loss and FTT in hospitalized infants who were regularly ingesting cow's milk and soy protein.[85,86] Complete resolution of symptoms was shown to occur after elimination of these foods; however, on reintroduction patients developed profuse, repetitive vomiting 1 to 3 hours after ingestion, often later associated with diarrhea, lethargy, and occasionally hypotension. Although there is no specific diagnostic test, some laboratory findings associated with an acute-phase FPIES reaction include leukocytosis with neutrophilia (>3500 cells/mL), thrombocytosis, metabolic acidosis, methemoglobinemia, and fecal leukocytes, eosinophils, and erythrocytes.[87,88]

Like FPE, FPIES is typically caused by direct consumption of the offending food, and reactions in strictly breastfed infants are extremely rare.[89,90] Although cow's milk and soy continue to be the most common triggers for FPIES, with up to 50% of children reacting to both, solid foods have more recently been reported and include grains (rice, oats, barley), meat (beef, chicken, turkey), eggs, vegetables, fruit, fish, shellfish, and even the probiotic *Saccharomyces boulardii*.[88,91–98] In general, the onset of cow's milk and soy FPIES occurs in infants and younger children, whereas solid food FPIES tends to occur in older children and even adults.[97–99] Children with solid food FPIES are also more likely to react to more than 1 food.[91,97] As in FPIAP and FPE, assessing for specific IgE to foods does not have any diagnostic benefit; however, up to 25% of patients with FPIES have been found to have measurable IgE to their causative food, and these patients typically have a more protracted course and the potential for developing symptoms of IgE-mediated disease.[98,100]

The diagnosis of FPIES is based on clinical symptoms, improvement after specific food elimination, and, if necessary, response to a clinician-supervised oral food challenge.[87,88] Once a diagnosis has been made, patients should be instructed on elimination of the implicated foods and provided with an emergency treatment plan for acute reactions.[101] Potentially cross-reactive foods that have not yet been introduced should also be avoided, and introduced only under physician supervision.[101–103] Although somewhat population based, resolution of classic FPIES to milk or soy generally occurs by 3 to 5 years of age, whereas solid food FPIES tends to resolve at an older age.[104] The current recommendation is to consider performing a supervised oral food challenge to the causative food every 18 to 24 months in patients without history of a recent reaction.[105]

SUMMARY

The mainstay of diagnosing food allergies is the clinical history. The differential diagnosis of food allergy consists of several immunologic and nonimmunologic diseases. The use of skin tests, blood tests, and food challenges can help narrow the differential and improve diagnostic accuracy. Obtaining the correct diagnosis often involves a multidisciplinary approach. Improved diagnostic capabilities will transform the diagnosis and management of food allergy for both patients and their care team.

REFERENCES

1. Jackson KD, Howie L, Akinbami LJ. Trends in allergic conditions among children: United States, 1997-2011. NCHS Data Brief 2013;121:1–8.
2. Sampson HA, Aceves S, Bock SA, et al. Food allergy: a practice parameter update—2014. J Allergy Clin Immunol 2014;134(5):1016–25.e43.
3. Sicherer SH, Wood RA. Advances in diagnosing peanut allergy. J Allergy Clin Immunol Pract 2013;1(1):1–13.
4. Commins SP, Satinover SM, Hosen J, et al. Delayed anaphylaxis, angioedema, or urticaria after consumption of red meat in patients with IgE antibodies specific for galactose-α-1,3-galactose. J Allergy Clin Immunol 2009;123(2):426–33. e422.
5. Biedermann T, Wölbing F. Anaphylaxis: opportunities of stratified medicine for diagnosis and risk assessment. Allergy 2013;68(12):1499–508.
6. Chafen JJ, Newberry SJ, Riedl MA, et al. Diagnosing and managing common food allergies. JAMA 2010;303(18):1848.
7. Sackesen C, Sekerel BE, Orhan F, et al. The etiology of different forms of urticaria in childhood. Pediatr Dermatol 2004;21(2):102–8.
8. Lieberman P, Nicklas RA, Oppenheimer J, et al. The diagnosis and management of anaphylaxis practice parameter: 2010 update. J Allergy Clin Immunol 2010;126(3):477–80.e1–2.
9. Du Toit G. Food-dependent exercise-induced anaphylaxis in childhood. Pediatr Allergy Immunol 2007;18(5):455–63.
10. Brockow K, Kneissl D, Valentini L, et al. Using a gluten oral food challenge protocol to improve diagnosis of wheat-dependent exercise-induced anaphylaxis. J Allergy Clin Immunol 2015;135(4):977–84.e4.
11. Zogaj D, Ibranji A, Hoxha M. Exercise-induced anaphylaxis: the role of cofactors. Mater Sociomed 2014;26(6):401–4.
12. Heaps A, Carter S, Selwood C, et al. The utility of the ISAC allergen array in the investigation of idiopathic anaphylaxis. Clin Exp Immunol 2014;177(2):483–90.
13. Ivkovic-Jurekovic I. Oral allergy syndrome in children. Int Dent J 2015;65(3):164–8.

14. Price A, Ramachandran S, Smith GP, et al. Oral allergy syndrome (pollen-food allergy syndrome). Dermatitis 2015;26(2):78–88.

15. Breiteneder H, Ebner C. Molecular and biochemical classification of plant-derived food allergens. J Allergy Clin Immunol 2000;106(1 Pt 1):27–36.

16. De Amici M, Mosca M, Vignini M, et al. Recombinant birch allergens (Bet v 1 and Bet v 2) and the oral allergy syndrome in patients allergic to birch pollen. Ann Allergy Asthma Immunol 2003;91(5):490–2.

17. Asero R, Pravettoni V. Anaphylaxis to plant-foods and pollen allergens in patients with lipid transfer protein syndrome. Curr Opin Allergy Clin Immunol 2013;13(4):379–85.

18. Sampson HA. Update on food allergy. J Allergy Clin Immunol 2004;113(5):805–19.

19. Sporik R, Hill D, Hosking C. Specificity of allergen skin testing in predicting positive open food challenges to milk, egg and peanut in children. Clin Exp Allergy 2000;30(11):1541–6.

20. Verstege A, Mehl A, Rolinck-Werninghaus C, et al. The predictive value of the skin prick test weal size for the outcome of oral food challenges. Clin Exp Allergy 2005;35(9):1220–6.

21. Tolkki L, Alanko K, Petman L, et al. Clinical characterization and IgE profiling of birch (*Betula verrucosa*)—allergic individuals suffering from allergic reactions to raw fruits and vegetables. J Allergy Clin Immunol Pract 2013;1(6):623–31.e1.

22. Potter JW, Saeian K, Staff D, et al. Eosinophilic esophagitis in adults: an emerging problem with unique esophageal features. Gastrointest Endosc 2004;59(3):355–61.

23. Mehl A, Verstege A, Staden U, et al. Utility of the ratio of food-specific IgE/total IgE in predicting symptomatic food allergy in children. Allergy 2005;60(8):1034–9.

24. Gupta RS, Lau CH, Hamilton RG, et al. Predicting outcomes of oral food challenges by using the allergen-specific IgE-total IgE ratio. J Allergy Clin Immunol Pract 2014;2(3):300–5.

25. Hansen KS, Ballmer-Weber BK, Sastre J, et al. Component-resolved in vitro diagnosis of hazelnut allergy in Europe. J Allergy Clin Immunol 2009;123(5):1134–41, 1141.e1–3.

26. Luengo O, Cardona V. Component resolved diagnosis: when should it be used? Clin Transl Allergy 2014;4:28.

27. Romano A, Scala E, Rumi G, et al. Lipid transfer proteins: the most frequent sensitizer in Italian subjects with food-dependent exercise-induced anaphylaxis. Clin Exp Allergy 2012;42(11):1643–53.

28. Caubet JC, Nowak-Węgrzyn A, Moshier E, et al. Utility of casein-specific IgE levels in predicting reactivity to baked milk. J Allergy Clin Immunol 2013;131(1):222.

29. Caubet J-C, Kondo Y, Urisu A, et al. Molecular diagnosis of egg allergy. Curr Opin Allergy Clin Immunol 2011;11(3):210–5.

30. Ando H, Movérare R, Kondo Y, et al. Utility of ovomucoid-specific IgE concentrations in predicting symptomatic egg allergy. J Allergy Clin Immunol 2008;122(3):583–8.

31. Fleischer DM, Bock SA, Spears GC, et al. Oral food challenges in children with a diagnosis of food allergy. J Pediatr 2011;158(4):578–83.e1.

32. Sicherer SH, Sampson HA. Food hypersensitivity and atopic dermatitis: pathophysiology, epidemiology, diagnosis, and management. J Allergy Clin Immunol 1999;104(3):S114–22.

33. Worth A, Sheikh A. Food allergy and atopic eczema. Curr Opin Allergy Clin Immunol 2010;10(3):226–30.
34. Kulig M, Bergmann R, Klettke U, et al. Natural course of sensitization to food and inhalant allergens during the first 6 years of life. J Allergy Clin Immunol 1999; 103(6):1173–9.
35. Du Toit G, Roberts G, Sayre PH, et al. Identifying infants at high risk of peanut allergy: the learning early about peanut allergy (LEAP) screening study. J Allergy Clin Immunol 2013;131(1):135–43.e1–12.
36. Brough HA, Simpson A, Makinson K, et al. Peanut allergy: effect of environmental peanut exposure in children with filaggrin loss-of-function mutations. J Allergy Clin Immunol 2014;134(4):867–75.e1.
37. Bergmann MM, Caubet J-C, Boguniewicz M, et al. Evaluation of food allergy in patients with atopic dermatitis. J Allergy Clin Immunol Pract 2013;1(1):22–8.
38. Talley NJ, Shorter RG, Phillips SF, et al. Eosinophilic gastroenteritis: a clinicopathological study of patients with disease of the mucosa, muscle layer, and subserosal tissues. Gut 1990;31(1):54–8.
39. Rothenberg ME. Eosinophilic gastrointestinal disorders (EGID). J Allergy Clin Immunol 2004;113(1):11–28.
40. Assa'ad A. Eosinophilic gastrointestinal disorders. Paper presented at: Allergy and Asthma Proceedings. OceanSide Publications, Inc, 2009.
41. Hruz P. Epidemiology of eosinophilic esophagitis. Dig Dis 2014;32(1–2):40–7.
42. Pasha SF, DiBaise JK, Kim HJ, et al. Patient characteristics, clinical, endoscopic, and histologic findings in adult eosinophilic esophagitis: a case series and systematic review of the medical literature. Dis Esophagus 2007;20(4): 311–9.
43. Alfadda AA, Storr MA, Shaffer EA. Eosinophilic colitis: epidemiology, clinical features, and current management. Therap Adv Gastroenterol 2011;4(5):301–9.
44. Guajardo JR, Plotnick LM, Fende JM, et al. Eosinophil-associated gastrointestinal disorders: a world-wide-web based registry. J Pediatr 2002;141(4):576–81.
45. Ko HM, Morotti RA, Yershov O, et al. Eosinophilic gastritis in children: clinicopathological correlation, disease course, and response to therapy. Am J Gastroenterol 2014;109(8):1277–85.
46. Müller S, Pühl S, Vieth M, et al. Analysis of symptoms and endoscopic findings in 117 patients with histological diagnoses of eosinophilic esophagitis. Endoscopy 2007;39(4):339–44.
47. Sugnanam KKN, Collins JT, Smith PK, et al. Dichotomy of food and inhalant allergen sensitization in eosinophilic esophagitis. Allergy 2007;62(11):1257–60.
48. Spergel JM, Andrews T, Brown-Whitehorn TF, et al. Treatment of eosinophilic esophagitis with specific food elimination diet directed by a combination of skin prick and patch tests. Ann Allergy Asthma Immunol 2005;95(4):336–43.
49. Arias Á, González-Cervera J, Tenias JM, et al. Efficacy of dietary interventions for inducing histologic remission in patients with eosinophilic esophagitis: a systematic review and meta-analysis. Gastroenterology 2014;146(7):1639–48.
50. Liacouras CA, Spergel JM, Ruchelli E, et al. Eosinophilic esophagitis: a 10-year experience in 381 children. Clin Gastroenterol Hepatol 2005;3(12):1198–206.
51. Erwin EA, James HR, Gutekunst HM, et al. Serum IgE measurement and detection of food allergy in pediatric patients with eosinophilic esophagitis. Ann Allergy Asthma Immunol 2010;104(6):496–502.
52. Castellano Mdel R, Cimbollek S, Quiralte J. Defining the role of food allergy in a population of adult patients with eosinophilic esophagitis. Inflamm Allergy Drug Targets 2010;9(4):257–62.

53. Lee M, Hodges WG, Huggins TL, et al. Eosinophilic gastroenteritis. South Med J 1996;89(2):189–94.

54. Molina-Infante J, Arias A, Barrio J, et al. Four-food group elimination diet for adult eosinophilic esophagitis: a prospective multicenter study. J Allergy Clin Immunol 2014;134(5):1093–9.e1.

55. Lucendo AJ, Arias Á, González-Cervera J, et al. Empiric 6-food elimination diet induced and maintained prolonged remission in patients with adult eosinophilic esophagitis: a prospective study on the food cause of the disease. J Allergy Clin Immunol 2013;131(3):797–804.

56. Kagalwalla AF, Shah A, Li BU, et al. Identification of specific foods responsible for inflammation in children with eosinophilic esophagitis successfully treated with empiric elimination diet. J Pediatr Gastroenterol Nutr 2011;53(2):145–9.

57. Spergel JM, Brown-Whitehorn TF, Cianferoni A, et al. Identification of causative foods in children with eosinophilic esophagitis treated with an elimination diet. J Allergy Clin Immunol 2012;130(2):461–7.e5.

58. Kagalwalla AF, Amsden K, Shah A, et al. Cow's milk elimination. J Pediatr Gastroenterol Nutr 2012;55(6):711–6.

59. Markowitz JE, Spergel JM, Ruchelli E, et al. Elemental diet is an effective treatment for eosinophilic esophagitis in children and adolescents. Am J Gastroenterol 2003;98(4):777–82.

60. Justinich C, Katz A, Gurbindo C, et al. Elemental diet improves steroid-dependent eosinophilic gastroenteritis and reverses growth failure. J Pediatr Gastroenterol Nutr 1996;23(1):81–5.

61. González-Cervera J, Angueira T, Rodriguez-Domínguez B, et al. Successful food elimination therapy in adult eosinophilic esophagitis. J Clin Gastroenterol 2012;46(10):855–8.

62. Arora AS, Yamazaki K. Eosinophilic esophagitis: asthma of the esophagus? Clin Gastroenterol Hepatol 2004;2(7):523–30.

63. Boyce JA, Assa'ad A, Burks AW, et al. Guidelines for the diagnosis and management of food allergy in the United States: summary of the NIAID-sponsored expert panel report. J Am Diet Assoc 2011;111(1):17–27.

64. Guandalini S, Assiri A. Celiac disease. JAMA Pediatr 2014;168(3):272.

65. Moissidis I, Chaidaroon D, Vichyanond P, et al. Milk-induced pulmonary disease in infants (Heiner syndrome). Pediatr Allergy Immunol 2005;16(6):545–52.

66. Fabbro SK, Zirwas MJ. Systemic contact dermatitis to foods: nickel, BOP, and more. Curr Allergy Asthma Rep 2014;14(10):463.

67. Caubet JC, Nowak-Węgrzyn A. Current understanding of the immune mechanisms of food protein-induced enterocolitis syndrome. Expert Rev Clin Immunol 2011;7(3):317–27.

68. Berin MC. Immunopathophysiology of food protein-induced enterocolitis syndrome. J Allergy Clin Immunol 2015;135(5):1108–13.

69. Ravelli A, Villanacci V, Chiappa S, et al. Dietary protein-induced proctocolitis in childhood. Am J Gastroenterol 2008;103(10):2605–12.

70. Jenkins HR, Pincott JR, Soothill JF, et al. Food allergy: the major cause of infantile colitis. Arch Dis Child 1984;59(4):326–9.

71. Lake AM, Whitington PF, Hamilton SR. Dietary protein-induced colitis in breast-fed infants. J Pediatr 1982;101(6):906–10.

72. Anveden-Hertzberg L, Finkel Y, Sandstedt B, et al. Proctocolitis in exclusively breast-fed infants. Eur J Pediatr 1996;155(6):464–7.

73. Lake AM. Food-induced eosinophilic proctocolitis. J Pediatr Gastroenterol Nutr 2000;30(Suppl):S58–60.

74. Lucarelli S, Nardo G, Lastrucci G, et al. Allergic proctocolitis refractory to maternal hypoallergenic diet in exclusively breast-fed infants: a clinical observation. BMC Gastroenterol 2011;11(1):82.
75. Arvola T. Rectal bleeding in infancy: clinical, allergological, and microbiological examination. Pediatrics 2006;117(4):e760–8.
76. Winter HS, Antonioli DA, Fukagawa N, et al. Allergy-related proctocolitis in infants: diagnostic usefulness of rectal biopsy. Mod Pathol 1990;3(1):5–10.
77. Goldman H, Proujansky R. Allergic proctitis and gastroenteritis in children. Am J Surg Pathol 1986;10(2):75–86.
78. Xanthakos SA, Schwimmer JB, Melin-Aldana H, et al. Prevalence and outcome of allergic colitis in healthy infants with rectal bleeding: a prospective cohort study. J Pediatr Gastroenterol Nutr 2005;41(1):16–22.
79. Iyngkaran N, Yadav M, Boey CG, et al. Severity and extent of upper small bowel mucosal damage in cow's milk protein-sensitive enteropathy. J Pediatr Gastroenterol Nutr 1988;7(5):667–74.
80. Kuitunen P, Visakorpi JK, Savilahti E, et al. Malabsorption syndrome with cow's milk intolerance. Clinical findings and course in 54 cases. Arch Dis Child 1975;50(5):351–6.
81. Iyngkaran N, Robinson MJ, Prathap K, et al. Cows' milk protein-sensitive enteropathy. Combined clinical and histological criteria for diagnosis. Arch Dis Child 1978;53(1):20–6.
82. Walker-Smith JA. Cow milk-sensitive enteropathy: predisposing factors and treatment. J Pediatr 1992;121(5):S111–5.
83. Iyngkaran N, Robinson MJ, Sumithran E, et al. Cows' milk protein-sensitive enteropathy. An important factor in prolonging diarrhoea of acute infective enteritis in early infancy. Arch Dis Child 1978;53(2):150–3.
84. Kleinman RE. Milk protein enteropathy after acute infectious gastroenteritis: experimental and clinical observations. J Pediatr 1991;118(4):S111–5.
85. Gryboski JD. Gastrointestinal milk allergy in infants. Pediatrics 1967;40(3):354–62.
86. Powell GK. Enterocolitis in low-birth-weight infants associated with milk and soy protein intolerance. J Pediatr 1976;88(5):840–4.
87. Powell G. Food protein-induced enterocolitis of infancy: differential diagnosis and management. Compr Ther 1986;12(2):28–37.
88. Sicherer SH, Eigenmann PA, Sampson HA. Clinical features of food protein-induced enterocolitis syndrome. J Pediatr 1998;133(2):214–9.
89. Monti G, Castagno E, Liguori SA, et al. Food protein-induced enterocolitis syndrome by cow's milk proteins passed through breast milk. J Allergy Clin Immunol 2011;127(3):679–80.
90. Tan J, Campbell D, Mehr S. Food protein-induced enterocolitis syndrome in an exclusively breast-fed infant—an uncommon entity. J Allergy Clin Immunol 2012;129(3):873.
91. Nowak-Wegrzyn A, Sampson HA, Wood RA, et al. Food protein-induced enterocolitis syndrome caused by solid food proteins. Pediatrics 2003;111(4):829–35.
92. Levy Y, Danon YL. Food protein-induced enterocolitis syndrome—not only due to cow's milk and soy. Pediatr Allergy Immunol 2003;14(4):325–9.
93. Zapatero Remón L, Alonso Lebrero E, Martín Fernández E, et al. Food protein-induced enterocolitis syndrome caused by fish. Allergol Immunopathol (Madr) 2005;33(6):312–6.
94. Hwang J-B, Kang KJ, Kang YN, et al. Probiotic gastrointestinal allergic reaction caused by *Saccharomyces boulardii*. Ann Allergy Asthma Immunol 2009;103(1):87–8.

95. Bruni F, Peroni DG, Piacentini GL, et al. Fruit proteins: another cause of food protein-induced enterocolitis syndrome. Allergy 2008;63(12):1645–6.

96. Mehr S, Kakakios A, Frith K, et al. Food protein-induced enterocolitis syndrome: 16-year experience. Pediatrics 2009;123(3):e459–64.

97. Ruffner MA, Ruymann K, Barni S, et al. Food protein-induced enterocolitis syndrome: insights from review of a large referral population. J Allergy Clin Immunol Pract 2013;1(4):343–9.

98. Caubet JC, Ford LS, Sickles L, et al. Clinical features and resolution of food protein-induced enterocolitis syndrome: 10-year experience. J Allergy Clin Immunol 2014;134(2):382–9. e384.

99. Fernandes BN, Boyle RJ, Gore C, et al. Food protein-induced enterocolitis syndrome can occur in adults. J Allergy Clin Immunol 2012;130(5):1199–200.

100. Onesimo R, Dello Iacono I, Giorgio V, et al. Can food protein induced enterocolitis syndrome shift to immediate gastrointestinal hypersensitivity? A report of two cases. Eur Ann Allergy Clin Immunol 2011;43(2):61–3.

101. Sopo SM, Iacono ID, Greco M, et al. Clinical management of food protein-induced enterocolitis syndrome. Curr Opin Allergy Clin Immunol 2014;14(3): 240–5.

102. Järvinen KM, Nowak-Węgrzyn A. Food protein-induced enterocolitis syndrome (FPIES): current management strategies and review of the literature. J Allergy Clin Immunol Pract 2013;1(4):317–22. e314.

103. Venter C, Groetch M. Nutritional management of food protein-induced enterocolitis syndrome. Curr Opin Allergy Clin Immunol 2014;14(3):255–62.

104. Katz Y, Goldberg MR. Natural history of food protein-induced enterocolitis syndrome. Curr Opin Allergy Clin Immunol 2014;14(3):229–39.

105. Sicherer SH. Food protein-induced enterocolitis syndrome: case presentations and management lessons. J Allergy Clin Immunol 2005;115(1):149–56.

Clinical Management of Food Allergy

Benjamin L. Wright, MD[a,b], Madeline Walkner, BS[c], Brian P. Vickery, MD[a], Ruchi S. Gupta, MD, MPH[d],*

KEYWORDS

- Food allergy • Treatment • Management

KEY POINTS

- There are no proactive treatments currently available for food allergy.
- Severe life-threatening reactions typically only occur following oral ingestion.
- Identifying the potential food trigger is critical, and diagnostic testing along with clinical history is needed for diagnosis, with a food challenge being confirmative.
- Providers should teach recognition and treatment of allergic reactions and provide an emergency action plan.
- Children with food allergies should be seen annually to assess for interval ingestions, provide education, and monitor for tolerance.

INTRODUCTION

Food allergy affects approximately 8% of children in the United States.[1] Of those children with food allergies, 38.7% have experienced a severe reaction.[1] At present there are no proactive treatments available for food allergy; consequently, the mainstay of therapy is education and avoidance.[2] Often pediatricians are the first physicians encountered by patients with food allergies; therefore, it is critical that pediatricians are trained in the principles of proper diagnosis, management, and referral. This article reviews the 5 main steps of food allergy management in a primary care clinic: (1) clinical history and physical examination, (2) appropriate use of diagnostic testing, (3) medication, (4) counseling/education for patients and families, and (5) referral to an allergist.

Disclosure Statement: Dr R.S. Gupta has received grants from Mylan LP and Food Allergy Research and Education.

[a] University of North Carolina at Chapel Hill School of Medicine, Campus Box 7231, Chapel Hill, NC 27599, USA; [b] Duke University Medical Center, DUMC Box 2644, Durham, NC 27710, USA; [c] Ann & Robert H. Lurie Children's Hospital of Chicago, 225 E. Chicago Ave, Chicago, IL 60611, USA; [d] Northwestern University Feinberg School of Medicine, Center for Community Health, 750 N. Lake Shore Dr. Chicago, IL 60611, USA
* Corresponding author.
E-mail address: rgupta@northwestern.edu

Pediatr Clin N Am 62 (2015) 1409–1424
http://dx.doi.org/10.1016/j.pcl.2015.07.012
0031-3955/15/$ – see front matter © 2015 Elsevier Inc. All rights reserved.

CLINICAL HISTORY

A pertinent clinical history is the single most important tool a physician should use in the diagnosis of pediatric food allergy. Many patients may report symptoms related to food ingestion, but key historical elements can distinguish food allergies from other food-related disorders. All allergic disorders have their roots in inappropriate immune responses, from immunoglobulin E (IgE)-mediated immediate hypersensitivity (eg, anaphylaxis) to non–IgE-mediated conditions.

Differential Diagnosis

The differential diagnosis of food allergy is broad, and encompasses immune-mediated and non–immune-mediated processes. **Table 1** details the differential diagnosis of adverse reactions to foods.[3]

Allergy Versus Intolerance

Food allergies are often mistakenly defined as any adverse reaction owing to ingestion of specific foods or types of food. A true food allergy is an immunologic reaction leading to effector cell (ie, mast cell, basophil, T cell) activation, which results in a

Table 1
Differential diagnosis of adverse food reactions

Mechanism	Disorder	Example
Immune mediated	Celiac disease	Wheat ingestion results in abdominal pain, diarrhea, vomiting, and weight loss
	Eosinophilic gastrointestinal disorders	Ingestion of dairy products causes eosinophilic esophagitis manifesting as failure to thrive, vomiting, dysphagia, or food impaction
	Food protein-induced enterocolitis syndromes	Severe vomiting and hypotension hours after rice ingestion
	IgE-mediated food allergy	Severe anaphylaxis caused by peanut ingestion
	Milk protein allergy	Milk ingestion leads to bloody stools, diarrhea, and failure to thrive during the first few months of life
	Pollen-food allergy syndrome	Sensitization to birch pollens results in oropharyngeal symptom following consumption of raw apple or carrots
Non–immune mediated	Auriculotemporal (Frey) syndrome	Gustatory flushing caused by foods
	Chemical effects	Gustatory rhinitis caused by hot/spicy foods
	Food intolerance/aversion	Nonspecific symptoms resulting in unwillingness to ingest a particular food
	Metabolic disorders	Lactose intolerance characterized by abdominal pain, distension, and diarrhea following milk ingestion
	Pharmacologic reactions	Adverse effects related to caffeine, tryptamine, or alcohol consumption.
	Toxic reactions	Scromboid fish toxin, food poisoning

stereotypic clinical presentation (see later discussion). Many patients and some clinicians may attribute disorders such as celiac disease or irritable bowel syndrome to food allergies. Although some of these disorders certainly have immunologic underpinnings, they can largely be distinguished from hypersensitivity reactions based on key findings in the clinical history such as timing, reproducibility, and symptom complex. For example, a teenage patient who newly develops abdominal pain and diarrhea alone 6 hours after drinking a glass of milk is more likely to have lactose intolerance than an IgE-mediated milk allergy. Adverse reactions such as these should be labeled as intolerances and managed appropriately. Described here are salient clinical features that will assist in distinguishing IgE-mediated food allergies from other adverse reactions to foods.

Suspected Triggers

Although children can be allergic to any food, the 8 most common pediatric food allergens are peanut, cow's milk, shellfish, tree nuts, egg, fin fish, wheat, and soy.[1] Often families may be unsure of the exact food that precipitates a reaction. Common food allergens are usually explicitly stated on food labels. However, in cases where a trigger is not obvious, clinicians must assess the potential for cross-contamination, which commonly occurs in bakeries, buffets, ethnic restaurants, and ice cream parlors, among other locations.

The pathogenesis of IgE-mediated food allergies requires antigen exposure for sensitization to occur. Of note, most childhood food allergies are detected when the child is first introduced to the food.[4] Recent evidence suggests that cutaneous exposure in the context of barrier disruption (ie, atopic dermatitis), presumably early in life, may lead to food sensitization.[5,6] This aspect has important implications for food allergy prevention, as recent literature suggests that early oral exposures may be important for inducing tolerance.[7] In a landmark study, Du Toit and colleagues[8] demonstrated that children 4 to 11 months of age randomized to early oral exposure to peanut versus avoidance had an 86% reduction in the incidence of peanut allergy by 5 years of age. Previous guidelines to avoid potentially allergenic foods during the first few years of life are no longer recommended,[9] and may actually lead to food sensitization.

Type of Reaction

IgE-mediated reactions are distinguished by rapid onset (usually within 2 hours of ingestion) and typically resolve within 24 hours. Characteristic symptoms may include any of the following alone or in combination: hives, swelling/angioedema, vomiting, respiratory compromise, and anaphylaxis.[10] Less common symptoms may include eczematous rash (late onset), rhinorrhea, diarrhea, or abdominal pain. Clinicians should note which medications (antihistamines, epinephrine) were administered and the type of medical care that was given. Additional factors such as alcohol ingestion, exercise, concurrent fever, and use of nonsteroidal anti-inflammatory drugs may serve to augment food-induced reactions[11] and should be noted in the patient's clinical history.

Although most patients will have rapid symptoms that resolve relatively quickly, a significant minority will have biphasic reactions, defined as a recurrence of symptoms within 72 hours of an initial reaction.[12,13] An even smaller number of patients may develop refractory or persistent anaphylaxis requiring volume resuscitation and inotropic support.

Current Diet

In addition to classifying food-induced reactions, it is also important to determine which foods a child is currently avoiding. For example, if a patient suspects a distant episode of hives was due to a peanut allergy, the clinician should ask about ingestion of peanut-containing foods since the time of reaction. In cases where the food was previously tolerated and is currently incorporated into the diet, no further testing is warranted. It is noteworthy that some children with food allergies to milk or egg proteins are able to tolerate these foods in extensively heated forms[14,15] because the IgE molecules in these individuals are likely specific for conformational epitopes, which are denatured during the heating process. As a result, some children may be able to tolerate egg in a muffin but not in an omelet. These children should continue to ingest the allergen in its baked form, as it may signal and hasten the development of oral tolerance.[16] By contrast, IgE to peanuts, tree nuts, and shellfish (among others) are specific for linear epitopes, which are not denatured with heating, and these allergies tend to persist.[17]

Physical Examination

Physical examination of the patient should focus on the signs of an allergic reaction in addition to other atopic disorders commonly associated with food allergies.[10] For example, many patients have comorbid atopic dermatitis.[18] Others may have a history of asthma, which coupled with food allergy increases the risk of mortality from childhood asthma[19] and anaphylaxis.[20–22] Photographs of acute reactions, if available, may also be helpful. The physical examination may prove useful in distinguishing other conditions with specific findings. It is also important to assess growth parameters in children with food allergy, as this is an established risk factor for growth impairment.[23–25] Children at special risk include those allergic to milk and/or multiple foods. Consultation with an experienced nutritionist may be considered for all children with food allergy, especially those with poor growth. Speech and feeding therapists may also be called upon to evaluate food-allergic children who may demonstrate dysfunctional feeding behavior.

Immunoglobulin E Mediated Versus Non–Immunoglobulin E Mediated

Although IgE-mediated food allergies are the most common, additional immune-mediated food sensitivities known as eosinophilic gastrointestinal disorders have become increasingly prevalent.[26] Eosinophilic esophagitis (EoE), a disorder characterized by eosinophilic infiltration of the esophageal lining, has emerged as a closely related disease state.[27] In contrast to the rapid symptoms of IgE-mediated food reactions, EoE is defined by a more insidious course resulting in failure to thrive, vomiting, reflux, and food aversion. Constant inflammation of the esophagus may eventually lead to dysphagia, stricture formation, and food impaction in adolescents and adults. Eosinophilic gastrointestinal disorders, however, are not confined to the esophagus and may also involve other segments of the gastrointestinal tract.

DIAGNOSTIC TESTING

Several tools are currently used to assist in the diagnosis of food allergy. **Table 2** lists available tools and the settings in which they may be utilized.

Pediatric Clinic

Specific Immunoglobulin E (ImmunoCAP)

Allergen-specific IgE (sIgE) testing measures the presence of allergic antibody to a particular antigen. This blood test can be performed at any age and is not limited by concurrent antihistamine use. As in many other clinical situations, the detection of an antibody by a highly sensitive but nonspecific immunoassay does not necessarily

Table 2
Food allergy diagnostic testing

Test	Primary Care Clinic	Allergy Clinic
sIgE	X	X
Full protein	X	X
Component[a]	X	X
Skin-prick test	—	X
Oral food challenge	—	X

[a] The utility of component testing in diagnosing food allergy is still under investigation.

equate to disease. The presence of sIgE simply denotes allergic sensitization to a particular food protein. Many individuals, especially children with atopic dermatitis, may be sensitized but not clinically allergic. Although sIgE is not routinely recommended for the diagnosis of food allergies,[10] a pediatrician may consider targeted sIgE testing to likely triggers. It is important that this testing be based on a supportive clinical history after ingestion (eg, a high pretest probability of clinical food allergy) and not be ordered indiscriminately. Bird and colleagues[28] recently demonstrated that bulk testing to multiple food antigens with food allergy panels leads to unnecessary cost and dietary restriction. Therefore, if a child tolerates a particular food in his or her diet regularly without clear evidence of allergic disease, sIgE testing should not be ordered. sIgE testing should also not generally be used to screen patients for food allergies before the first ingestion.[10] The application of serologic IgE testing in the diagnosis and management of food allergy patients by primary care physicians has been recently reviewed elsewhere.[29,30]

Traditionally sIgE has been assessed for an entire food molecule composed of multiple component proteins. Recently, component-resolved diagnostics (CRD) have become available, potentially increasing the sensitivity and specificity of IgE measurements,[31] although this is still being studied. Although CRD for milk, egg, peanut, tree nuts, fish, and shellfish are commercially available, their use is not routinely recommended in food allergy diagnostic guidelines, and many such tests are not covered by insurance carriers. Most of the data supporting CRD come from English and European studies of component IgE testing in peanut-allergic patients, a topic that has been recently reviewed elsewhere.[32]

Allergy Clinic

Skin-prick testing

In addition to sIgE, skin-prick testing (SPT) may be useful in confirming clinical food allergy. SPT is an in vivo assessment of mast cell activation whereby a small amount of allergen is placed in the epidermis. Sensitized patients usually develop a wheal and flare reaction at the site of antigen placement within minutes. Skin reactions are then compared with positive and negative controls, as recent antihistamine use or dermatographism may result in false-negative or false-positive results, respectively. This approach is a safe, rapid, and relatively inexpensive way to assess for food sensitization. In general, SPT has an excellent negative predictive value (NPV; ~95%) but a poor positive predictive value (PPV; ~50%).[33]

For those patients who successfully avoid culprit foods and for whom the persistence of food allergy remains uncertain, serial sIgE and SPT may be used to determine whether an oral food challenge is warranted to definitively establish ongoing allergy or tolerance.[3] **Table 3** gives general recommendations for the frequency of laboratory

Table 3
General recommendations for the frequency of testing patients with food allergy

Allergen	Test	≤5 y Old	>5 y Old
Milk, egg, wheat, soy, peanut	sIgE, SPT	Every 12–18 mo	Every 2–3 y
Tree nuts, fish, shellfish	sIgE, SPT	Every 2–4 y	Every 2–4 y

Data from Burks AW, Tang M, Sicherer S, et al. ICON: food allergy. J Allergy Clin Immunol 2012;129:906–20.

monitoring and SPT in children with food allergies. Interpretation of SPT and sIgE must be performed in the appropriate clinical context. Regardless of test values, patients with a recent history of anaphylaxis within the past year should not undergo oral food challenge. Conversely, children who have incorporated a food into their diet without symptoms do not require further testing.

Oral food challenge

The double-blinded placebo-controlled food challenge is the gold standard for the diagnosis of food allergy or confirming its persistence.[10] Because of its labor-intensive and time-intensive nature, open food challenges with commercially available food products are usually used in clinical practice. Before performing an oral food challenge (OFC), the patient should understand the risks associated with the procedure and also display an interest in eating the food afterward if he or she passes the challenge. Well-accepted protocols for OFCs have been published[34] but, in general, gradually increasing amounts of a food allergen are administered over successive intervals under close clinical observation. Once a designated quantity is safely consumed, a patient is allowed to incorporate the food into the diet.

Interpretation of test results

Challenge thresholds for interpretation of sIgE and SPT have been established.[3,35] **Table 4** provides the decision points used by many allergists in deciding whether to perform an OFC. These recommendations provide 95% PPV and 50% NPV for reactions to OFCs. A challenge is usually not recommended when sIgE and SPT are greater than 95% PPV. Conversely, a challenge may be considered when the sIgE and SPT are less than 50% NPV. Positive and negative predictive thresholds do not

Table 4
Predictive value of SPT and sIgE in positive or negative OFC results

Food	>95% Positive		~50% Negative	
	SPT	sIgE	SPT	sIgE
Egg white	≥7	≥7 ≥2 if age <2 y	≤3	≤2
Cow's milk	≥8	≥15 ≥5 if age <1 y	—	≤2
Peanut	≥8	≥14	≤3	≤2 (history of prior reaction) ≤5 (no history of prior reaction)
Fish	—	≥20	—	—

Data from Sampson HA. Update on food allergy. J Allergy Clin Immunol 2004; 113:805–19; [quiz: 20]; and Sampson HA, Aceves S, Bock SA, et al. Food allergy: a practice parameter update—2014. J Allergy Clin Immunol 2014;134(5):1016–25.e43.

exist for many food allergens, and those listed cannot be extrapolated to antigens such as wheat and soy. These foods typically have much higher sIgE reaction thresholds. It should be noted that most predictive cutoffs were developed using the ImmunoCAP system in children with a high pretest probability of food allergy presenting to a tertiary care allergy subspecialty clinic[36]; therefore, values generated using other testing platforms cannot be reliably compared with these thresholds.[37] In addition, population-based estimates have shown that these cutoffs may be much higher if testing is performed indiscriminately or in the general population,[38] whereby the tests may detect sensitization more readily than clinical allergy.

MEDICATIONS
Prescription of Epinephrine

As a provider it is important to identify those patients most likely to develop fatal or near-fatal anaphylaxis and to prescribe injectable epinephrine.[10] **Box 1** presents clinical scenarios known to represent increased risk, although it is well established that allergic reactions to food are inherently unpredictable, making risk stratification difficult. Therefore, epinephrine prescription may be considered in any patient with IgE-mediated food allergy, as the severity of subsequent reactions cannot be predicted. Additional factors to consider, in addition to those listed in **Box 1**, include the age of the patient (adolescents and young adults at higher risk for fatality) and the distance from the patient's home to an appropriate medical facility.[33] Dosing of available autoinjector devices is detailed in **Table 5**.

First-line treatment of anaphylaxis is always epinephrine.[2] Second-line medications such as albuterol or antihistamines may also be prescribed for treatment of mild symptoms or adjunctive therapy, but unlike epinephrine they have no direct effect on the mast cells or basophils themselves. Prompt treatment with epinephrine is encouraged, as this may slow or halt progression of severe anaphylaxis. Furthermore, most fatalities from food-induced anaphylaxis are associated with delayed administration of epinephrine[22]; however, despite this knowledge there is a persistent and well-established underutilization of epinephrine in the treatment of anaphylaxis. When an epinephrine autoinjector is prescribed, families should be taught how and when to administer it. Written anaphylaxis action plans are encouraged, listing medications and their doses, and detailing emergency follow-up procedures including activation of emergency medical services.

Box 1
Guidelines for prescription of an epinephrine autoinjector

Prescribe epinephrine if a child has any one of the following:

- History of anaphylaxis

- Prior history of systemic allergic reaction

- History of food allergy and asthma

- Known food allergy to peanut, tree nuts, fish, and crustacean shellfish (ie, allergens known to be associated with more fatal and near-fatal allergic reactions)

[a] Consider epinephrine prescription in any child with a history of IgE-mediated food allergy.

Data from Boyce JA, Assa'ad A, Burks AW, et al. Guidelines for the diagnosis and management of food allergy in the United States: summary of the NIAID-sponsored expert panel report. J Allergy Clin Immunol 2010;126:1105–18.

Table 5	
Dosing of available epinephrine autoinjectors	
Brand	**Dose**
Adrenaclick (generic)	0.15 mg (for children 15–30 kg), 0.3 mg (for children ≥30 kg)
Auvi-Q	0.15 mg (for children 15–30 kg), 0.3 mg (for children ≥30 kg)
EpiPen	0.15 mg (for children 15–30 kg), 0.3 mg (for children ≥30 kg)
Ensure that the child has 2 autoinjectors accessible at all times	

Other Medications: Antihistamines, Albuterol, and Steroids

Antihistamines such as diphenhydramine and cetirizine are commonly given for mild food-induced reactions. Although these medications may be useful in relieving symptoms, such as itch, they do not halt the progression of an allergic reaction, and are best considered an adjunctive therapy. Albuterol should be used as adjunctive therapy for respiratory symptoms, especially in patients with a history of bronchospasm or asthma. Asthmatic individuals experiencing lower respiratory symptoms such as cough or wheeze during an allergic reaction to food should always receive epinephrine. Corticosteroids have a delayed onset of effect, making them unhelpful in immediate management. Although commonly used in this context, there is little evidence supporting their effectiveness.

COUNSELING AND EDUCATION

Despite their best efforts, most patients with food allergies will be exposed to culprit foods.[39,40] Therefore it is incumbent on health care providers to prepare families to recognize and treat anaphylaxis.[3] Food-induced reactions may be subtle, and it is useful to teach patients that anaphylaxis may present anywhere on a spectrum of symptoms ranging from a few hives and throat clearing to respiratory failure and cardiac arrest. Because anaphylaxis may progress rapidly, early detection and action is a critical step in successful management. Patients and families should be encouraged to inject epinephrine at the first sign of anaphylaxis, even if relatively mild. More educational and counseling food allergy resources for providers and caregivers can be found at http://www.ruchigupta.com/i-will-thrive-video/.

Epinephrine Use

Patients, or their caregivers, should immediately inject epinephrine for any obvious signs of a potentially severe systemic reaction, including: cardiovascular collapse (lethargy, pallor, behavioral changes); respiratory distress (wheezing, coughing, increased work of breathing); or laryngeal edema (drooling, difficulty swallowing, throat tightness). It is important to convey to affected individuals and caregivers that anaphylaxis may not present with such potentially life-threatening symptoms at the onset. Operationally, a generalized allergic reaction involving symptoms affecting more than 1 organ system can be identified as anaphylaxis. For example, a child experiencing urticaria and vomiting after a likely or confirmed allergen exposure can be considered as having anaphylaxis, and such a child should receive epinephrine even if symptoms are not considered to be immediately life-threatening. More specific indications can be individualized based on the patient's medical history.

Use of an epinephrine autoinjector first requires removal of the safety lock. Once removed, the epinephrine should be injected into the lateral thigh. Clothing need not be removed, as the needle of the autoinjector should pass through without difficulty.

The autoinjector should be held in place for at least 10 seconds to ensure complete dose delivery. One removed from the thigh, a protective sheath will cover the needle. If symptoms do not resolve within 5 to 15 minutes, patients experiencing anaphylaxis should be given a second dose. The patient should be placed in the recumbent position with the lower extremities elevated.[41] Patients and families should be instructed to call the emergency services once epinephrine has been administered. Trainer devices from several manufacturers are available for demonstration and testing of proficiency.

Emergency Action Plan

Once a provider is comfortable with a patient's and caregiver's competency using the device, its indications for use should be discussed. Formulating an emergency action plan may facilitate this. Personalized action plan forms are available in English and Spanish through the American Academy of Allergy, Asthma and Immunology (www.aaaai.org) and Food Allergy Research and Education (www.foodallergy.org) Web sites. These forms list patients' food triggers and provide guidelines for treatment.

Avoidance

Strict avoidance of allergens is the only sure way to prevent food-induced reactions. Relatively small amounts of food can trigger acute reactions in highly sensitized individuals.[42] However, reactions may vary considerably depending on the patient and the allergen,[43] resulting in misdiagnosis or a false sense of security if small amounts of food can be ingested without symptoms. One must be aware that the severity of a food-induced reaction does not predict the severity of future reactions; therefore, a child with a peanut allergy who only develops hives after an initial ingestion might develop life-threatening anaphylaxis following subsequent exposure.

Although patients may be exposed to food antigens through a variety of routes (cutaneous, respiratory, oral), typically only oral ingestion causes severe reactions. Investigators have examined the potential for food-induced reactions through casual contact.[44,45] In 2003, Simonte and colleagues[44] performed a randomized, double-blind, placebo-controlled trial of 30 children with significant peanut allergy. Subjects underwent cutaneous and inhalation challenge with peanut, and none experienced a systemic or respiratory reaction. Mild cutaneous symptoms were noted in a minority of patients. A notable exception is that in children with asthma and food allergy, bronchial challenge with aerosolized food allergens can provoke respiratory symptoms, particularly in those with allergy to fish or crustacea.[46] For symptoms to occur, protein antigens must be vigorously aerosolized during food preparation (eg, cooking seafood in a rolling boil) and come in direct contact with the respiratory mucosa. An important distinction is that the smell of foods produced by volatile organic compounds does not cause clinical reactions.

Food Labeling

To properly adhere to recommended elimination diets, patients and families should be instructed to pay careful attention to ingredient lists and food labels.[3] The Food Allergen Labeling and Consumer Protection Act (FALCPA)[47] of 2004 was passed in an effort to make food labels more accurate and understandable for consumers with food allergies. This legislation requires manufactures to label in plain English foods containing any of the 8 major food allergens (peanut, milk, crustacean shellfish, tree nuts, egg, fin fish, wheat, and soy). Major implications of this law are listed in **Box 2**.

In addition to those foods listed containing allergens, patients should also be counseled to avoid products that are processed in a facility where other food allergens are

---

Box 2
Major implications of the Food Allergen Labeling and Consumer Protection Act (FALCPA) of 2004

1. Food allergens in products must be declared in plain English by one of the following:
   a. Placing the word "Contains" followed by the name of food source from which the allergen is derived. (ie, "Contains milk, egg, peanut")
   b. Including the common or usual name in parentheses next to food source in the ingredient list (ie, "albumin [eggs]")

2. Manufacturers are subject to penalties in the Federal Food, Drug and Cosmetic Act if food allergens do not appear on labels

3. FALCPA does not establish standards for the use of "May Contain" statements

4. FALCPA only applies to packaged foods sold in the United States (Except meat, poultry, certain egg products, and alcoholic beverages)

5. Companies may receive exemptions from labeling requirements if the allergen satisfies one of the following requirements:
   a. Highly refined oils are exempt (ie, peanut oil)
   b. Scientific evidence establishes that the food ingredient does not contain the allergenic protein
   c. The Food and Drug Administration determines that the food allergen does not elicit an allergic response in sensitized individuals

---

processed, causing cross-contamination. It should be noted that use of the phrases "may contain," "may contain traces of," and "manufactured in a facility that also processes" are voluntary; therefore, families must be aware of the potential for cross-contamination. A recent study in Canada[48] found that 17% of accidental exposures resulted from unintentional cross-contamination during manufacturing or packaging, with no precautionary statement being provided. Unfortunately, widespread and inconsistent use of these phrases has also resulted in a devaluation of this warning; consequently, up to 40% of individuals ignore "may contain" statements and consume foods with potential food allergens.[49] Helpful patient information to assist with food allergen avoidance is available through the Food Allergy Research and Education Network (www.foodallergy.org) and the Consortium of Food Allergy Research (www.cofargroup.org).

Different Environments

Although most food-induced reactions occur in the home,[50] many families find that eating out at a restaurant or a friend's home can be difficult. At home, ingredient lists can be screened and meals carefully prepared to prevent cross-contamination, but eating away from home may pose unique challenges. Studies suggest that 40% to 100% of fatalities from food-induced reactions are due to food prepared or catered outside the home.[33] Although risks can be mitigated with advance planning, it is important to identify high-risk situations. Ice cream parlors, ethnic restaurants, bakeries (peanut, egg, milk, and tree nuts), and buffets (all foods) are common places where cross-contamination or occult exposure may occur.[51] Such environments seem to pose a special risk to adolescents and young adults,[20,21] who may be relatively inexperienced in self-management and have been shown to willfully engage in risk-taking behavior pertaining to food allergen exposure.[52]

REFERRAL TO AN ALLERGIST

If a food allergy is suspected or diagnosed, the patient should be referred to an allergist. As mentioned previously, allergists can provide additional diagnostic testing (ie, SPT, OFC) and are equipped to manage anaphylaxis in the clinic. In addition to assisting with diagnosis, allergists can monitor and assess for the development of tolerance and can help manage the comorbid conditions commonly encountered in food-allergic children, such as atopic dermatitis and asthma.

Monitoring for Tolerance

An OFC, performed in the allergist's office, is the gold-standard test to determine whether tolerance has occurred. Serial measurements indicating a decline in the patient's allergen-specific IgE level often provide useful predictive power that a patient is outgrowing a food allergy, and that a challenge is indicated. IgE-based online calculators developed by the Consortium of Food Allergy Research are available for public use to generate individualized probabilities for outgrowing milk and egg allergies.[53] Often the patient's interval history can provide important clues; for example, a child may accidentally be exposed to a trigger food without developing symptoms. If a significant quantity of the food has been tolerated several times without ill effect, the food allergy has likely resolved. Acquisition of tolerance is more likely to occur in younger children, who are allergic to foods such as wheat, soy, milk, or egg.[54,55] By contrast, allergies to nuts including peanut, fish, and shellfish are much less commonly outgrown.[17]

Tolerance of Extensively Heated Allergens

As mentioned previously, some children with milk or egg allergy may be able to tolerate these allergens in their baked forms.[14,15] Researchers hypothesize that this is due to sensitization to conformational epitopes that are unable to cross-link surface IgE molecules when extensively heated.[56] Some data suggest that tolerance to baked milk or egg may be an early intermediate step in the development of immunologic tolerance to the food antigen, and that consumption of baked allergens may actually hasten the resolution of clinical allergy.[16] OFCs with products containing baked milk or egg are routinely performed in the allergist's office.

Routine Follow-Up

A specialist in allergy and immunology should see patients with food allergies at least annually. Periodic visits allow for the following:

- Assessment of interval progress including a history of accidental ingestions
- Renewal of epinephrine prescription
- Renewal and revision of emergency action plans
- Additional education regarding avoidance and recognition/treatment of anaphylaxis, and transition to self-management for teenagers
- Assessment of nutritional status
- Monitoring of coexisting conditions, such as asthma or atopic dermatitis
- Monitoring for development of tolerance to food antigens

Allergen-specific immunotherapy as a proactive treatment strategy for food allergy is currently being developed in phase II/III clinical trials.[57] Its use is not recommended outside of research settings at present,[10] but allergists may be able to routinely provide this life-changing clinical treatment in coming years (Appendices 1 and 2).

SUMMARY

Successful diagnosis and management of food allergies is complex, and demands collaboration from both pediatricians and board-certified allergists, in addition to skilled nurses, nutritionists, and occasionally other team members such as psychologists and feeding therapists. It is hoped that these 5 steps for primary care providers will provide a more straightforward approach: (1) clinical history and physical examination, (2) diagnostic testing, (3) medication, (4) counseling/education for patients and families, and (5) referral to an allergist. Although some clinical trials of interventional food allergy treatments have generated promising preliminary data,[58] the standard of care continues to focus on prescribing the proper elimination diet, education, and training in the recognition and management of accidental allergic reactions.

REFERENCES

1. Gupta RS, Springston EE, Warrier MR, et al. The prevalence, severity, and distribution of childhood food allergy in the United States. Pediatrics 2011;128:e9–17.
2. Panel NI-SE, Boyce JA, Assa'ad A, et al. Guidelines for the diagnosis and management of food allergy in the United States: report of the NIAID-sponsored expert panel. J Allergy Clin Immunol 2010;126:S1–58.
3. Sampson HA, Aceves S, Bock SA, et al. Food allergy: a practice parameter update—2014. J Allergy Clin Immunol 2014;134:1016–25.e43.
4. Sicherer SH, Burks AW, Sampson HA. Clinical features of acute allergic reactions to peanut and tree nuts in children. Pediatrics 1998;102:e6.
5. Tordesillas L, Goswami R, Benede S, et al. Skin exposure promotes a Th2-dependent sensitization to peanut allergens. J Clin Invest 2014;124:4965–75.
6. Brough HA, Liu AH, Sicherer S, et al. Atopic dermatitis increases the effect of exposure to peanut antigen in dust on peanut sensitization and likely peanut allergy. J Allergy Clin Immunol 2015;135:164–70.
7. Palmer DJ, Metcalfe J, Makrides M, et al. Early regular egg exposure in infants with eczema: a randomized controlled trial. J Allergy Clin Immunol 2013;132:387–92.e1.
8. Du Toit G, Roberts G, Sayre PH, et al. Randomized trial of peanut consumption in infants at risk for peanut allergy. N Engl J Med 2015;372:803–13.
9. Greer FR, Sicherer SH, Burks AW. Effects of early nutritional interventions on the development of atopic disease in infants and children: the role of maternal dietary restriction, breastfeeding, timing of introduction of complementary foods, and hydrolyzed formulas. Pediatrics 2008;121:183–91.
10. Boyce JA, Assa'ad A, Burks AW, et al. Guidelines for the diagnosis and management of food allergy in the united states: summary of the NIAID-sponsored expert panel report. J Allergy Clin Immunol 2010;126:1105–18.
11. Niggemann B, Beyer K. Factors augmenting allergic reactions. Allergy 2014;69:1582–7.
12. Lee JM, Greenes DS. Biphasic anaphylactic reactions in pediatrics. Pediatrics 2000;106:762–6.
13. Lee S, Bellolio MF, Hess EP, et al. Time of onset and predictors of biphasic anaphylactic reactions: a systematic review and meta-analysis. J Allergy Clin Immunol Pract 2015;3:408–16.e1-2.
14. Nowak-Wegrzyn A, Bloom KA, Sicherer SH, et al. Tolerance to extensively heated milk in children with cow's milk allergy. J Allergy Clin Immunol 2008;122:342–7, 7.e1–2.

15. Peters RL, Dharmage SC, Gurrin LC, et al. The natural history and clinical predictors of egg allergy in the first 2 years of life: a prospective, population-based cohort study. J Allergy Clin Immunol 2014;133:485–91.
16. Leonard SA, Sampson HA, Sicherer SH, et al. Dietary baked egg accelerates resolution of egg allergy in children. J Allergy Clin Immunol 2012;130:473–80.e1.
17. Sicherer SH. Epidemiology of food allergy. J Allergy Clin Immunol 2011;127: 594–602.
18. Eigenmann PA, Sicherer SH, Borkowski TA, et al. Prevalence of IgE-mediated food allergy among children with atopic dermatitis. Pediatrics 1998;101:E8.
19. Vogel NM, Katz HT, Lopez R, et al. Food allergy is associated with potentially fatal childhood asthma. J Asthma 2008;45:862–8.
20. Bock SA, Munoz-Furlong A, Sampson HA. Fatalities due to anaphylactic reactions to foods. J Allergy Clin Immunol 2001;107:191–3.
21. Bock SA, Munoz-Furlong A, Sampson HA. Further fatalities caused by anaphylactic reactions to food, 2001-2006. J Allergy Clin Immunol 2007; 119:1016–8.
22. Sampson HA, Mendelson L, Rosen JP. Fatal and near-fatal anaphylactic reactions to food in children and adolescents. N Engl J Med 1992;327:380–4.
23. Christie L, Hine RJ, Parker JG, et al. Food allergies in children affect nutrient intake and growth. J Am Diet Assoc 2002;102:1648–51.
24. Robbins KA, Guerrerio AL, Hauck SA, et al. Growth and nutrition in children with food allergy requiring amino acid-based nutritional formulas. J Allergy Clin Immunol 2014;134:1463–6.e5.
25. Hobbs CB, Skinner AC, Burks AW, et al. Food allergies affect growth in children. J Allergy Clin Immunol Pract 2015;3:133–4.e1.
26. Dellon ES. Epidemiology of eosinophilic esophagitis. Gastroenterol Clin North Am 2014;43:201–18.
27. Kelly KJ, Lazenby AJ, Rowe PC, et al. Eosinophilic esophagitis attributed to gastroesophageal reflux: improvement with an amino acid-based formula. Gastroenterology 1995;109:1503–12.
28. Bird JA, Crain M, Varshney P. Food allergen panel testing often results in misdiagnosis of food allergy. J Pediatr 2015;166:97–100.
29. Fleischer DM, Burks AW. Pitfalls in food allergy diagnosis: serum IgE testing. J Pediatr 2015;166:8–10.
30. Sicherer SH, Wood RA. Allergy testing in childhood: using allergen-specific IgE tests. Pediatrics 2012;129:193–7.
31. Lieberman JA, Glaumann S, Batelson S, et al. The utility of peanut components in the diagnosis of IgE-mediated peanut allergy among distinct populations. J Allergy Clin Immunol Pract 2013;1:75–82.
32. Sicherer SH, Wood RA. Advances in diagnosing peanut allergy. J Allergy Clin Immunol Pract 2013;1:1–13 [quiz: 4].
33. Burks AW, Tang M, Sicherer S, et al. ICON: food allergy. J Allergy Clin Immunol 2012;129:906–20.
34. Bock SA, Sampson HA, Atkins FM, et al. Double-blind, placebo-controlled food challenge (DBPCFC) as an office procedure: a manual. J Allergy Clin Immunol 1988;82:986–97.
35. Sampson HA. Update on food allergy. J Allergy Clin Immunol 2004;113:805–19 [quiz: 20].
36. Sampson HA, Ho DG. Relationship between food-specific IgE concentrations and the risk of positive food challenges in children and adolescents. J Allergy Clin Immunol 1997;100:444–51.

37. Wang J, Godbold JH, Sampson HA. Correlation of serum allergy (IgE) tests performed by different assay systems. J Allergy Clin Immunol 2008;121: 1219–24.

38. Peters RL, Allen KJ, Dharmage SC, et al. Skin prick test responses and allergen-specific IgE levels as predictors of peanut, egg, and sesame allergy in infants. J Allergy Clin Immunol 2013;132:874–80.

39. Fleischer DM, Perry TT, Atkins D, et al. Allergic reactions to foods in preschool-aged children in a prospective observational food allergy study. Pediatrics 2012;130:e25–32.

40. Boyano-Martinez T, Garcia-Ara C, Pedrosa M, et al. Accidental allergic reactions in children allergic to cow's milk proteins. J Allergy Clin Immunol 2009;123:883–8.

41. Pumphrey RS. Fatal posture in anaphylactic shock. J Allergy Clin Immunol 2003; 112:451–2.

42. Blom WM, Vlieg-Boerstra BJ, Kruizinga AG, et al. Threshold dose distributions for 5 major allergenic foods in children. J Allergy Clin Immunol 2013;131:172–9.

43. Eller E, Hansen TK, Bindslev-Jensen C. Clinical thresholds to egg, hazelnut, milk and peanut: results from a single-center study using standardized challenges. Ann Allergy Asthma Immunol 2012;108:332–6.

44. Simonte SJ, Ma S, Mofidi S, et al. Relevance of casual contact with peanut butter in children with peanut allergy. J Allergy Clin Immunol 2003;112:180–2.

45. Wainstein BK, Kashef S, Ziegler M, et al. Frequency and significance of immediate contact reactions to peanut in peanut-sensitive children. Clin Exp Allergy 2007;37:839–45.

46. Roberts G, Golder N, Lack G. Bronchial challenges with aerosolized food in asthmatic, food-allergic children. Allergy 2002;57:713–7.

47. Food Allergen Labeling and Consumer Protection Act (FALCPA). 2004. Available at: http://www.fda.gov/downloads/Food/GuidanceRegulation/UCM179394.pdf. Accessed December 26, 2014.

48. Sheth SS, Waserman S, Kagan R, et al. Role of food labels in accidental exposures in food-allergic individuals in Canada. Ann Allergy Asthma Immunol 2010;104:60–5.

49. Hefle SL, Furlong TJ, Niemann L, et al. Consumer attitudes and risks associated with packaged foods having advisory labeling regarding the presence of peanuts. J Allergy Clin Immunol 2007;120:171–6.

50. Versluis A, Knulst AC, Kruizinga AG, et al. Frequency, severity and causes of unexpected allergic reactions to food: a systematic literature review. Clin Exp Allergy 2015;45(2):347–67.

51. Furlong TJ, DeSimone J, Sicherer SH. Peanut and tree nut allergic reactions in restaurants and other food establishments. J Allergy Clin Immunol 2001;108:867–70.

52. Sampson MA, Munoz-Furlong A, Sicherer SH. Risk-taking and coping strategies of adolescents and young adults with food allergy. J Allergy Clin Immunol 2006; 117:1440–5.

53. Consortium of Food Allergy Research. Available at: http://www.cofargroup.org. Accessed April 4, 2015.

54. Skripak JM, Matsui EC, Mudd K, et al. The natural history of IgE-mediated cow's milk allergy. J Allergy Clin Immunol 2007;120:1172–7.

55. Sicherer SH, Wood RA, Vickery BP, et al. The natural history of egg allergy in an observational cohort. J Allergy Clin Immunol 2014;133:492–9.

56. Vila L, Beyer K, Jarvinen KM, et al. Role of conformational and linear epitopes in the achievement of tolerance in cow's milk allergy. Clin Exp Allergy 2001;31: 1599–606.

57. Jones SM, Burks AW, Dupont C. State of the art on food allergen immunotherapy: oral, sublingual, and epicutaneous. J Allergy Clin Immunol 2014;133:318–23.

58. Lanser BJ, Wright BL, Orgel KA, et al. Current Options for the Treatment of Food Allergies. Pediatr Clin North Am 2015, in press.

APPENDIX 1: QUESTIONNAIRE FOR PATIENTS

Patient's Name: DOB:___/___/___

Provider's Name: Today's Date: ___/___/___

FOR PATIENTS:

Take this Food Allergy History Test to help your provider determine if your child has a food allergy. If your child is here for a follow up visit please complete the questions also.

Step 1: Answer every question on this page to the best of your ability. There is no right or wrong answer.

Step 2: Take the test to your healthcare provider to talk about whether your child has a new food allergy.

1. Does your child have a current diagnosis of food allergy?   Yes or No If No, proceed to #5.

2. Has your child had a food allergy reaction since their last visit?   Yes or No If No, complete #3 and #4 then stop.

    Details of the reaction: _____

3. Does your child have an up-to-date prescription for an epinephrine auto-injector?   Yes or No

4. Does your child have an up-to-date food allergy & anaphylaxis emergency care plan?   Yes or No

5. What food do you think was responsible for your child's reaction? _____

Peanut	Shellfish	Milk	Soy
Tree nut	Fin fish	Egg	Wheat
Other food: _____			

6. What happened to your child after eating the food?

Trouble breathing	Belly pain	Fainting	Tingling Mouth
Throat tightening	Nausea	Hives	Itching (Location: _____)
Repetitive cough	Vomiting	Swelling	Rash (Location: _____)
Other reaction: _____			

7. How long after eating the food did your child have the reaction?

    ____hour(s) and ___ minutes.

8. How did you respond?

Self-management	Called 911
Phone call to doctor or nurse	Emergency Department (ED) or urgent care
Primary care provider's office visit	Hospital admission

9. What medications were given to your child?

Antihistamine (Brand: Benadryl®   Claritin®   Allergra®   Zyrtec®   Other brand:_____)
Epinephrine auto-injector (Brand: EpiPen®   Auvi-Q®   Adrenaclick®   Generic)
Steroid
No medications
Other medications: _____

10. Other comments about today's visit:

APPENDIX 2: CHECKLIST FOR HEALTH CARE PROVIDERS

FOR HEALTHCARE PROVIDERS ONLY:

Plan for food allergy

Prescribe epinephrine auto-injector
Brand: EpiPen®   Auvi-Q®   Adrenaclick®   Generic
Dose: 0.15 mg (for children <25 kg)   0.3 mg (for children ≥ 25kg)

Prescribe antihistamines
Medication: Diphenhydramine   Loratadine   Cetirizine   Fexofenadine
Other: _____
Dose: _____

Prescribe other medication: _____

Order allergen-specific IgE (sIgE) testing for: _____

Provide food allergy & anaphylaxis emergency care plan

Provide educational pamphlet

Refer to allergist

Counseling for food allergy

Counsel patient and family on:
Allergen avoidance
How to recognize an allergic reaction
When to use epinephrine auto injector versus antihistamine
How to use the epinephrine auto injector (Provide brand-specific instructions)
Discuss food allergy & anaphylaxis emergency care plan
Discuss school and camp management
Medication identification jewelry
Food allergy prognosis (Provide allergen-specific prognosis)

Other notes:

Healthcare Provider's Signature_____   Date__/__/__

School Food Allergy and Anaphylaxis Management for the Pediatrician—Extending the Medical Home with Critical Collaborations

Michael Pistiner, MD, MMSc[a],*, Cynthia DiLaura Devore, MD, MS[b],
Sally Schoessler, MEd, BSN, RN[c,d]

KEYWORDS

- Food allergy • Primary care pediatrician • Anaphylaxis • Emergency response
- School health

KEY POINTS

- Community pediatricians participate in critical collaborations within schools that support families and children with food allergy and other potentially life-threatening allergies.
- Community pediatricians can provide leadership and guidance to both families and schools to safeguard children and adolescents with food allergy and other potentially life-threatening allergies, thereby extending the medical home goals into the school setting.

INTRODUCTION

Primary care pediatrician are the managers and facilitators of the patient-centered medical home and serve as the glue in a series of critical collaborations within schools that support the family and child with food allergy and other potentially life-threatening allergies. When primary care pediatricians include the school health professional team into a child's overall medical plan for managing life-threatening food allergies and anaphylaxis, they can further the goals of the medical home. They can provide leadership and guidance to extend the medical home goals into the school setting, by

[a] Harvard Vanguard Medical Associates, 133 Brookline Ave, Boston, MA 02215, USA; [b] Monroe 1 BOCES, 25 O'Connor Rd, Fairport, NY 14450, USA; [c] Allergy & Asthma Network, 8229 Boone Boulevard, Suite 260, Vienna, VA 22182, USA; [d] National Association of School Nurses, 1100 Wayne Ave, Suite 925, Silver Spring, MD 20910, USA
* Corresponding author. Harvard Vanguard Medical Associates, 133 Brookline Ave, Boston, MA 02215.
E-mail address: michaelpistiner@gmail.com

Pediatr Clin N Am 62 (2015) 1425–1439
http://dx.doi.org/10.1016/j.pcl.2015.07.016
0031-3955/15/$ – see front matter © 2015 Elsevier Inc. All rights reserved.

educating the family to partner with their schools and encouraging the school to provide reasonable and effective accommodations, as per state or federal guidelines. In fact, the most effective management of life-threatening food allergies and anaphylaxis occurs when the medical home, the family home, and the educational home work together as a team for the benefit of the child or adolescent, ultimately affording the student the least restrictive environment with the greatest chance for safety and maximal opportunity to learn and thrive.

Families of children with food allergies are reliant on many individuals when it comes to the school community. The pediatrician and the pediatric allergist play a critical role in clearly defining the food allergy management strategies necessary for the child. They work with parents and schools to ensure that these important strategies are applied to the specific student while taking school resources and policies into account and collaborating with the school team. Pediatricians can coordinate and foster mutually beneficial relationships, a spirit of trust, and positive interactions among all stakeholders, especially the family. The school nurse, school physician, and others on the school health team are key members of the multidisciplinary school teams that include nutrition services, school administration, teachers, counselors, transportation directors, special subject areas, physical education teachers, and all others who interact with students.

The purpose of this article is two fold. The first is to guide community pediatricians by strengthening their understanding of essential principles and components in effective food allergy management in the school setting and to direct readers to additional resources to support this goal.[1–3] The second is to empower pediatricians to be the stewards in collaborations that bridge the medical, family, and educational homes for the sake of children with food allergies and other potential life threatening allergies.

FOOD ALLERGY MANAGEMENT PRINCIPLES: THE PILLARS OF PREVENTION AND PREPAREDNESS

Effective food allergy management is necessary at all times and in all situations. The pillars of food allergy management are prevention and emergency preparedness. Very small amounts of food allergen can cause anaphylaxis (severe, life-threatening, allergic reaction). To prevent accidental exposure, those responsible for students must effectively read labels, prevent ingestion of hidden ingredients, prevent cross-contact, use efficient cleaning strategies, and communicate clearly. It is equally necessary to be prepared for an allergic emergency. Adults who are responsible for students must be able to recognize an allergic reaction and have epinephrine (first-line treatment of choice for anaphylaxis) available. They must also know when and how to use it and know to contact emergency services immediately. These strategies are always necessary, and the school setting is no exception. Implementing solid food allergy management is challenging and takes knowledgeable administration, school nurses, school staff, and school community.[2,4]

Prevention

It is important for pediatricians to understand the different routes of exposure and the risks of these exposures and apply this understanding to the school setting. Pediatricians should be aware of challenges and solutions as they apply to preventing accidental exposures in the school setting. **Table 1** contains a list of potential routes of exposure, challenges to preventing these exposures, and solutions to these challenges.[5] Pediatricians, as individuals and/or as American Academy of Pediatrics

Table 1
Types of routes of exposure to food allergens in the school setting

Type of Exposure	Relevant Concepts/Facts/Studies	Practical Challenges	Practical Interventions (See CDC, NSBA and/or State Guidelines)
Oral exposure	Unable to visualize allergens; they can be hidden ingredients Labels and ingredients can change without warning[7] Items with advisory labels can contain allergens[8] Trace amounts can cause severe allergic reactions Allergens can be detectable in saliva[9] Cross-contact of food allergen can occur from one surface to another, food to food, and with transfer of saliva. If a person is then exposed to these allergens, especially by mouth, it may be enough of an exposure to cause a serious allergic reaction[7,9]	Without labels, it is impossible to know avoidance practices of those responsible for preparation of foods brought in to school Classroom celebrations are common source of outside food and high risk for cross-contact In schools, most allergic reactions that occur start in classroom[10] Resources and manpower in schools to read labels vary among schools *Additional consideration for preschool/early elementary* Young children can pass saliva to each other via developmentally appropriate exploration[9] In some schools, children eat in their classrooms/learning environments Supervision during meal/snack time depends on resources and staff *Additional consideration for adolescent/teenage students* Older students under less supervision and more reliant on self-management Increased risk taking, peer pressure, bullying,[11,12] kissing with salivary exchange	If food is not from home then all labels must be accurately read by an assigned reader Classrooms should have safe nonperishable snack or celebration items available if needed Cafeterias should prepublish menus and offer meal options without known allergens Food allergic children who are eating from the cafeteria should be assisted in selection of safe food No sharing of food, drinks, and utensils anywhere No unlabeled food in classroom or cafeteria Nonfood celebrations and rewards are optimal/safest If meal/snack is in the learning environment, then effective strategies must be in place to clean and prevent accidental exposure/cross-contact In some cases, food-free classrooms or selective allergen restriction (lower age groups) may be appropriate and practical if label reading is not possible Periodic check ins to ensure continued self-management and safety from bullying Discussion of intimate kissing and allergen exposure and evidence-based preventive measures

(continued on next page)

Table 1
(continued)

Type of Exposure	Relevant Concepts/Facts/Studies	Practical Challenges	Practical Interventions (See CDC, NSBA and/or State Guidelines)
Skin exposure	Isolated skin contact on intact skin did not cause severe or systemic reactions in 2 small studies, although skin reactions did occur[13,14] Soap and water and commercial hand wipes are effective in cleaning hands; alcohol- and nonalcohol-based hand sanitizers are not[15] Soap and water, commercial cleaners, and commercial wipes were effective in cleaning table tops[15] Young children frequently place their hands and objects in their mouth (age 1–2 y, 80×/h; age 2–5 y, 40×/h)[16] Adults touch their eyes, nose, and mouth regularly (15×/h)[17]	Hand washing in young grades can take 20–30 min Resources and manpower available to clean allergens and prevent cross-contact varies school by school and classroom by classroom Some nonedible items contain some food allergens; finger paint, play dough, shaving cream, paste, bean bags, furniture, pet food, bird feed, as well as others[18] Skin exposure can result in mucosal exposure in adults and children *Additional consideration for preschool/early elementary* Skin exposure that can quickly turn into mucosal exposure or oral ingestion[16] Less effective cleaning skills (hands or eating surfaces)	Hand washing with soap/water or wipes before and after eating is optimal[15] Appropriate cleaning of eating areas decreases risk Curricular activities can be food free, or comparable, but alternate activities can be provided for children with life-threatening food allergies. Attention to avoid allergens with crafts/lessons/pets is optimal Establish a cleaning protocol to avoid cross-contact In some cases, food-free classrooms or selective allergen restriction in lower age groups may be appropriate and practical Adult supervision of hand cleaning is optimal Adults have responsibility for cleaning surfaces, toys
Inhalation exposure	Aerosolized proteins in cooking are the most common cause of allergic reactions by inhalation.[13] Odors are caused by volatile organic compounds, not protein, and odors alone do not cause allergic reactions[13,18] Inhaling proteins can cause allergic reactions. There have been deaths associated with the inhalation of actively cooked foods[13,18,19]	Experiments involving burning/heating of allergens create risk Some field trips are in areas where foods are actively cooked or aerosolized Some activities involve using food powders or grinding/crushing fresh foods	Use caution with cooking foods, flours, powders, and other small particles of food that can go up in the air[13,18,19] Avoid food in curricular science experiments or classroom activities. All field trips to have prior assessment from school nurse to determine need for special accommodations

Abbreviations: CDC, Centers for Disease Control and Prevention; NSBA, National School Boards Association.

Adapted with permission from Pistiner, AllergyHome.org (found at http://www.allergyhome.org/schools/) and previously published as Pistiner M, Devore C. The role of pediatricians in school food allergy management. Pediatr Ann 2013;42(8):334–40.

(AAP) Chapters, can provide guidance, such as school-related food allergy articles like as this current one and state and federal guidance documents,[1-3,5,6] to those administrators in schools responsible for students with life-threatening food allergies on ways to try to prevent inadvertent exposure to food allergens.[3,6] Pediatricians provide guidance for what parents expect from schools based on state and/or federal guidelines. Dietary guidance and medical orders for school diet restrictions can be challenging for both prescribers and school food services directors and staff. Under 7 CFR 15b.3, students with a disability that restricts their diet, which, according to the Americans with Disabilities Act (ADA) Amendments Act of 2008 (http://www.eeoc.gov/laws/statutes/adaaa.cfm) includes food allergy, are entitled to substitutions in lunches and after school snacks on a case-by-case basis. This occurs only when supported by a written statement of the need for substitutions from a licensed physician or, in some states, other state-allowed health care providers (US Department of Agriculture's recent memo, SP32-2015, issued March 30, 2015: http://www.fns.usda.gov/nslp/policy). The written statement must include recommended alternate foods, unless otherwise exempted by the Food and Nutrition Service (www.fns.usda.gov/sites/default/files/special_dietary_needs.pdf).

Preparedness and Emergency Response

Despite everyone's best efforts to prevent exposures to allergens through avoidance, exposures can and do occur. Therefore, it is equally necessary for schools to be prepared for allergic emergencies. The pediatrician or allergist should provide schools with an emergency care plan that includes a list of specific food and other triggers to avoid and emergency medical orders for epinephrine in the event of anaphylaxis. Alternately, physicians may write these orders as a prescription for school nurses who create the emergency care plan (ECP).[3]

Anaphylaxis Emergency Care Plans

ECPs are a collaborative effort of the medical, family, and school homes. They are created by the pediatrician, allergist, and/or school nurse and serve as simplified criteria to assist parents, school personnel, and anyone caring for a child with life-threatening allergies to identify signs and symptoms of anaphylaxis and treat appropriately with epinephrine.[21] It should be understandable to an unlicensed assistive personnel or other laypersons that epinephrine is the treatment of choice for anaphylaxis and administering other medications, like antihistamines, should never delay treatment with epinephrine.[20] It is also helpful to address the potential need for a second dose of epinephrine and the need to be evaluated in the emergency room.[2,5]

In all cases of life-threatening food allergy, unlicensed persons who function as a supervisor of a child or adolescent with a life-threatening food allergy at any time during the school day need to be willing and trained to carry out the ECP. This is a document created by the prescriber and/or the school nurse based on the provider's written medical orders, providing in simple language directions to unlicensed staff on what to do in an emergency. The format is typically "If you see this…then do this…." Emergency contact information and a photo of the student usually accompany the action plan.[5] The Centers for Disease Control and Prevention (CDC) recommends that the ECP includes information about signs and symptoms of an allergic reaction, how to respond, and what medications should be given.[1] There are multiple templates available from the American Academy of Allergy, Asthma and Immunology, AAP, as well as other respected sources.[1]

Leadership

Ultimately, pediatricians and allergists can educate, support, and empower parents to ensure that sound school policies and protocols exist and that there is clear leadership when it comes to the management of life-threatening allergies. They can guide administrators to understand that all school staff responsible for a student with a food allergy must be educated and prepared to recognize and play their specific role in an allergic emergency during a regular school day, as well as during other school situations, such as extended sheltering in place, emergency evacuations, lockdowns, and on day or extended field trips.[2,3,5] **Table 2** contain strategies to prepare for allergic emergencies in those with known and unknown allergic conditions.[5]

Epinephrine

It is critical that families and schools understand that in the event of a life-threatening allergic reaction, epinephrine is the treatment of choice.[6,20] Pediatricians may remind families that relying on antihistamines alone may delay use of epinephrine and leave a child at risk for life-threatening anaphylaxis.[6,21] Antihistamines are not first-line treatment of anaphylaxis and do not stop or prevent it. They are slow to act (30–60 minutes),

Table 2 **School strategies in place for management of allergic emergencies**	
Strategies in Place for Known History of Food Allergy	**Strategies in Place for Unknown Food Allergy (Approximately 25% of Epinephrine Administrations)[8]**

• Identification of students with life-threatening allergies via medical documentation
• Food allergy emergency care plan based on medical orders
  ○ Updated at least annually, reviewed periodically, always accessible
  ○ Shared on a need-to-know basis with all staff in a supervisory role, with education in its use given by an appropriate health professional.
• [C2] child-specific dual pack auto-injectors
  ○ Kept with supervising adult or in a known and secure but accessible location
• Delegate medication administration[a]
  ○ School nurse trains nonlicensed staff to administer auto-injector and arrange immediate transportation to ED when school nurse is not immediately available
	• Full-time school nurse
	  ○ Standing epinephrine orders[a]
	  ○ Stock epinephrine[a]
	• Supervisory staff trained to rapidly identify allergic reactions and immediate contact of school nurse and/or 911(especially if nurse not immediately available) and/or give non–patient-specific epinephrine auto-injector if allowed by state

Strategies in Place for All Students and Staff (with Known and Unknown History of Life-Threatening Allergies)	
• School physician in every district, full-time school nurse in every building • Universal staff training • Include anaphylaxis emergency in periodic school/staff-wide emergency preparedness drills • Communication access for all staff in supervisory roles available to contact 911 for ambulance transport to ED and school nurse if available	

Abbreviations: ED, emergency department; RN, registered nurse.

   [a] Regulations and guidance vary state by state. Confirm that school practices conform to state and local regulations and guidance.

   Adapted with permission from Pistiner, AllergyHome.org (found at http://www.allergyhome.org/schools/) and previously published as Pistiner M, Devore C. The role of pediatricians in school food allergy management. Pediatr Ann 2013;42(8):334–40.

and nonlicensed responders may not be able to give antihistamines in some states and schools. Delays in administration of epinephrine are associated with increased mortality[6,20–23] and increased rate of hospitalization (reference). At present, the available doses for epinephrine auto-injectors for community use are the 0.3- and 0.15-mg doses. Current recommendations are to upsize to 0.3 mg for greater than or equal to 25 kg (55 lb).[6,24] Pediatricians should consider supporting school communities by writing nonspecific/stock epinephrine standing orders in addition to student-specific prescriptions for the school that ensure the availability of two doses of 0.15 and 0.3 mg dosing (appropriate doses available for students and staff in the case of stock epinephrine), as 10% to 20% of students may require more than 1 dose.[25,26] Non specific/stock epinephrine and orders and training to administer it are important as up to 25% of epinephrine administrations are to those with no known allergy to the school.[8] Delegated staff need to be trained for the specific student's auto-injector and those designated and trained to administer to those experiencing first time anaphylaxis need to be trained for use of the specific stock auto-injectors available.

The CDC: Voluntary Guidelines for the Management of Food Allergy in Schools and Early Care and Education Programs

The CDC: Voluntary Guidelines for the Management of Food Allergy in Schools and Early Care and Education Programs[1] is a comprehensive and practical set of federal guidelines drafted to assist in the management of food allergies in school. The guidelines call for leadership in schools to develop comprehensive plans for managing food allergies in that setting. These voluntary guidelines serve as an excellent ground work for schools to implement individual school policies, practices, and protocols especially useful in states without state guidelines. The CDC guidelines have been written in a way that allows for variation in implementation, because schools have different resources and cultures, as well as strengths and challenges. The guidelines name five priority areas that should be addressed in each school's food allergy management plan. These include the following:

1. Appropriate food allergy management for the individual student
2. Preparation for allergic emergencies
3. Food allergy training/professional development for staff
4. Food allergy education for students and families
5. Healthy and safe educational environments

School Physician

Besides emphasizing the importance of excellent communication among all stakeholders and developing role-specific expectations for everyone involved, the section in this CDC guidance document regarding school medical directors warrants comment. The American Medical Association (H-60.991 Providing Medical Services through School-Based Health Programs) and the AAP[27] recommend physician oversight of all school health programs. Unfortunately, not all schools hire school physicians. Therefore, community pediatricians, who play a vital role in ensuring the health and safety of not only their patients: but also all children in their community, can actively participate on School Wellness Councils and guide school boards to understand the importance of medical oversight by a school physician. Community pediatricians can also collaborate directly in peer-to-peer deliberation with school physicians, when present, reducing time spent talking to multiple school staff. The school physician can serve as a school health leader and can contribute to the overall operations of both patient-specific and non–patient-specific (unassigned stock epinephrine) care by addressing various aspects of allergy management in school, such as

1. Participate in the school's coordinated approach to managing food allergies.
2. Ensure the daily management of food allergies for individual students.
3. Prepare for food allergy emergencies.
4. Support professional development on food allergies for staff.
5. Educate students and family members about food allergies.
6. Create and maintain a healthy and safe school environment. (excerpt from Ref.[1]).

School Nurse

Every school benefits from a school nurse, but especially in a building with a child with a life-threatening food allergy or other life-threatening conditions.[28] The NASN states that the registered school nurse, as the daily health professional in the school setting, "serves in a pivotal role to provide expertise and oversight for the provision of school health services and promotion of health education" through provision of comprehensive management, planning, and coordination of care; education of staff; collaboration with medical professionals; individualization of care; and assurance of a safe environment with prompt emergency response.[29–34] A recent study by Wang and colleagues[35] demonstrated that full-time school nurses saved money, changing the way some think about school health economics and nurse staffing.

A school nurse's education positions them to have a leadership role in managing life-threatening allergies as well as implementing or overseeing the implementation of the individualized health care plan (IHP) and ECPs. They serve as care coordinators, advocates, responders, and educators while leading and guiding the school community in food allergy and anaphylaxis management. School nurses make assessments of their students' health situation. Their role in the school and their nursing background also allow them to train and prepare others to recognize these reactions if they are unavailable and efficiently implement school-wide policies aimed at delivering emergency treatment and preventing these reactions.

The school health team, led by the school physician, provides leadership in the planning and implementation of a school district's health policies and food allergy management plan, while supporting partnerships among the student's family and health care providers and school staff.[1]

Food Allergy Policies and Protocol

School policies and protocols that directly address epinephrine are important to establish and to couple with general and comprehensive food allergy policies and management plans in the school setting. Policies and protocols delineate roles and responsibilities for key stakeholders. All schools need to make basic steps to ensure the safety of a student with life-threatening food allergy and anaphylaxis. For example, required annual generalized (non–patient specific) staff training, by a competent medical or nursing professional, is an important first step for all staff to understand the importance of prevention and preparedness. Staff need to be aware of the emotional and social impact of food allergies and the potential for food allergy–related bullying.[36–39] Staff must also recognize quickly when something is not right and take action or seek medical assistance immediately. Staff must understand that timing is critical and that giving epinephrine by auto-injector cannot be delayed, understanding there is greater risk at withholding it than giving it when not needed. Patient-specific training and updates should be offered to staff who work directly with the child and might be called upon to provide assistance in a life-threatening emergency.[2,3] Finally, policies should include a statement about liability for staff who volunteer to assist a student in a life-threatening emergency. A template of a comprehensive school anaphylaxis policy can be found at http://www.nasn.org/ToolsResources/Food AllergyandAnaphylaxis/EpinephrinePoliciesProtocolsandReporting (NASN/NASSNC/ AAP Policies and Protocols work group).

A sound protocol guides the emergency response that school physicians and nurses direct in the school setting. A sample protocol, developed by a work group that consisted of a school physician, pediatric allergist, state school nurse consultants, and school nurses has been created as a template to guide the creation of a tool that can be adapted for any school district to align with state law. Before use, these protocols must be vetted by school physician or designee according to school district health procedures. The protocol can be accessed at http://www.nasn.org/portals/0/ resources/Sample_Anaphylaxis_Epinephrine_Administration_Protocol.pdf. When school personnel, other than health care professionals, use a protocol, they must be thoroughly trained by a school health professional training that includes their specific role in the school emergency protocol, identification of anaphylaxis, and how to administer an epinephrine auto-injector. This training should be more extensive than general staff or delegate training and should include a face-to-face and hands-on component.

Understanding School Care Plans

In order for pediatricians and allergists as well as parents to make specific requests of schools, it is helpful to understand how schools develop student programs. There are three main types of student plans in the school setting: Individualized Healthcare Plan (IHPs), 504s, and individualized education plans (IEPs).

Individualized health care plans

An IHP is a standard of nursing care that outlines the nurse's plan of care for a student with any kind of special need. It clarifies clinical practice and becomes the foundation for the health portion of the other educational and emergency plans.[40] The components of the IHP include assessment data, nursing diagnosis, student goals, expected outcomes, and evaluation, including documentation of the nursing process. The IHP is based on the health care provider's orders given to the school, including documented diagnoses, medication orders, treatment orders, and other identified needed accommodations, in collaboration with the family. An IHP is written by a nurse for licensed persons. In some cases, the IHP becomes an official component of the child's 504 Plan, but by itself an IHP is not legally binding. Community pediatricians or allergists do not need to request an IHP, because it is a professional responsibility of the school nurse to prepare. However, it may be useful for the pediatrician or allergist to encourage parents to participate in the development of student goals for the IHP.

Section 504 Plan

Some students need more support and accommodations in addition to the core curriculum and the IHP. When a longer-term school plan is required because of an expected prolonged medical condition that might interfere with a child's or adolescent's ability to receive general education (regular curriculum) instruction, formalized accommodations may be considered. Section 504 of the ADA is part of the Individuals with Disabilities Education Act (IDEA) that can spell out the specific needs of a child or adolescent with a life-threatening food allergy that may interfere with instruction. The 504 requires the school to provide those accommodations based on guidance from the treating prescriber and could be useful if a building does not have a school nurse or food allergy or anaphylaxis emergency preparedness plans or a school is either having challenges with or not implementing food allergy management strategies. To create a 504 Plan, a parent makes a written request to the school district,

Table 3
A team model: critical collaborations for pediatricians in school food allergy and anaphylaxis management. How can community pediatricians partner with stakeholders in student care?

Necessary Components in Food Allergy Management	Collaborator/Partner: Family	Collaborator/Partner: School Health Team (Physician/Nurse)	Collaborator/Partner: School Nutrition Team	Collaborator/Partner: Board Certified Allergist
Patient/family-centered care	Foster and support relationship between school nurse and others in school health and the family and student	Individual student: Encourage a school culture and resources that promote a safe environment for students with allergies Provide school with detailed health history of allergies and necessary orders to medicate student when experiencing symptoms All students: Encourage a school environment that is prepared to care for everyone in the school community with life-threatening allergies	Support school collaborations to ensure optimal nutrition/diet beyond just dietary restriction	Refer patients with suspected food allergy for further evaluation and management (eg, confirmation of food allergy, monitoring for resolution) Develop a collaborative relationship and approach to comanaged patients Learn most updated approach Support allergist's care with additional anticipatory guidance Ensure routine follow-ups
Care coordination	Communicate with school nurse regularly Encourage family to update school nurse with new allergies, new ECPs and any changes in student condition	Confirm that licensed health professionals (school physician, RN) are available in the school setting to make assessments and manage both emergent and nonemergent situations Partner with school physician to promote policy and direct care Partner with school nurse who acts as care coordinator between home, school, and the medical home	Improve and maximize nutrition especially for children getting most of their meals in school Ensure that food substitutions are offered and accepted	Share responsibility for providing support for food allergy management in all settings, especially in school (eg, ECPs, auto-injector prescriptions, medication orders) Coordinate with allergist to work as team and decrease redundancy and inconsistency

Care plans	Assist in creation and implementation Plan should reflect and support food allergy management strategies implemented in all settings Check in and modify as appropriate	Provide school with ECP Collaborate with licensed school health professional to adjust care plan to unique school setting and individual student needs Partner with school stakeholders in supporting development of IHP, 504, or other plans as needed	Assist in implementation with allergist as well Get familiar with state laws and requirements as per USDA Provide statement of allergy diagnosis to food services to allow for food substitutions	For this shared responsibility, coordinate with allergist to work as team and decrease redundancy and inconsistency
Prevention	Teach and reinforce evidence-based and best practice strategies to avoid allergen exposure. Keep in mind that family has expectation that these strategies are implemented in the school setting Involve patient education in all prevention strategies	Communicate specific child capability and comorbid conditions to school Partner with school stakeholders to determine school-specific resources and preexisting policies to determine accommodations to promote a school environment where the student is safe, healthy, and ready to learn	Collaborate to ensure well-balanced healthy meals and snacks in school that avoid allergen If difficulties reaching nutritional needs in the home, question of family resources, then collaborate and use school resources and expertise of school nutrition and school dietician if available	For this shared responsibility, coordinate with allergist to work as team and decrease redundancy and inconsistency
Emergency preparedness	Strongly encourage family to provide school with 2 auto-injectors and up-to-date ECP that can be implemented in the school setting Encourage student to wear emergency ID jewelry	Partner with the school to ensure that all members of the school community are appropriately trained to respond to an emergent situation	Ensure all nutrition service staff are trained to recognize and deal with allergic reaction Encourage partnering between school nutrition and school health and being included in school-wide policies	For this shared responsibility, coordinate with allergist to work as team and decrease redundancy and inconsistency
School education/ training	Encourage family to check in with school nurse about current school community education and training that is specific to their child prevention and emergency care strategies	Consider offering services to school to support and encourage staff training Consider sharing available resources	Consider offering educational resources and guidelines to school nutrition to support and encourage staff training and encourage staff training if these trainings are not provided by school physician or nurse	If you determine schools identified without staff education then consider partnering with allergists to work toward staff training

(continued on next page)

Table 3 (continued)					
Necessary Components in Food Allergy Management	Collaborator/Partner: Family	Collaborator/Partner: School Health Team (Physician/Nurse)	Collaborator/Partner: School Nutrition Team	Collaborator/Partner: Board Certified Allergist
Undesignated epinephrine	Check in with the school as to whether stock epinephrine is in place in the school	Ensure implementation stock epinephrine policies and protocols where allowed by law	Ensure all nutrition service staff are trained by school health to recognize and know their role in the school ECP	If you determine schools identified without policies then collaborate with allergists to work toward policy implementation and supporting the school
		Support epinephrine administration training of school community	Encourage partnering with school health and being included in school-wide policies	
		Ensure that standing orders exist in the school and that there is a school physician. If not, consider becoming one and consider providing orders and protocols		
		Collaborate and work with the school physician		
		Encourage use of evidence-based protocols		
Advocacy	Encourage parent to know which school staff are caring for their child at school (is there a school nurse?)	Use local chapters and pediatric organizations to assist in policy creation and implementation	Work with school nutrition to support them especially with potential increased responsibilities	Work with allergist to encourage and advocate for school nurse presence
	If no available full-time school nurse, encourage discussion with administration and school board	If no available full-time school nurse, encourage discussion with administration and school board		
		Consider speaking at school board meeting to promote use of stock epinephrine		

Abbreviations: ECP, emergency care plan; IHP, individualized health care plan; RN, registered nurse; USDA, US Department of Agriculture.
Adapted with permission from Pistiner M, AllergyHome.org.

and the treating pediatrician and allergist provide essential medical documentation demonstrating the need for accommodations within the school setting. A 504 Plan requires a formal meeting with a 504 Coordinator, essential staff, and the family to create an official plan. Student are still responsible for general education curriculum, but the school provides various supports to their environment, and more targeted interventions for a longer periods but still in the least restrictive environment as required by the ADA. A 504 is legally binding. It may be useful for the pediatrician or allergist to encourage parents to request a 504 if building level adjustments are insufficient for any reason for the child with food allergy to receive an education.

Individualized education plan accommodations

In cases in which students have other disabilities that affect their education beyond food allergy, the highest level of support is an IEP. In that case, food allergy would be outlined under medical needs in the IEP. Typically, a child with a food allergy alone does not qualify for, or need, an IEP. Only a few students are eligible for an IEP based on categories of disability outlined in the ADA. An IEP is legally binding. It may be useful for pediatricians and allergists to encourage parents to request an IEP if the child presents with confirmed or suspected learning deficits, in addition to food allergy.

SUMMARY

Community pediatricians, working in consultation with allergists, create a medical home that is the central focus of care for the child with life-threatening food allergies. They participate in coordinating mutual and critical collaborations within schools that support families and children (**Table 3**). They can provide leadership and guidance to both families and schools to safeguard children and adolescents, thereby extending the medical home goals into the school setting. Physicians can serve as school physicians when possible and collaborate with those school health professionals employed and/or school health administrators or even board members. Ways to do this might include serving on school boards and school wellness councils and promoting the presence of a school physician in every district and a school nurse in every building. The pediatrician and allergist can also work to educate and set appropriate expectations for the family for management of food allergy in schools. They can especially assist families in situations when schools are struggling to implement management strategies, so that a child or adolescent is neither overly restricted or put at risk. Pediatricians and allergists can promote trust and encourage families on working in a positive, collaborative fashion with schools that will have the care for their child for years to come. The most effective management of life-threatening food allergies and anaphylaxis occurs when the medical home, the family home, and the educational home work together as a team for the benefit of the child or adolescent, ultimately affording the student the least restrictive environment with the greatest chance for safety and maximal opportunity to learn and thrive.

ACKNOWLEDGMENTS

Special thanks to our reviewers, Michael Young, MD; Julie Wang, MD; and Chuck Norlin, MD.

REFERENCES

1. Centers for Disease Control and Prevention. Voluntary guidelines for managing food allergies in schools and early care and education programs. Washington, DC: US Department of Health and Human Services; 2013. p. 49–51.

2. Young MC, Munoz-Furlong A, Sicherer SH. Management of food allergies in schools: a perspective for allergists. J Allergy Clin Immunol 2009;124:175–82, 182.e1–4; [quiz 83–4].

3. Sicherer SH, Mahr T. Management of food allergy in the school setting. Pediatrics 2010;126:1232–9.

4. Greenhawt MJ, Green T, Pistiner M, et al. Empathy, understanding, and objectivity need to prevail for students with food allergies. Ann Allergy Asthma Immunol 2011;107:93–4.

5. Pistiner M, Devore C. The role of pediatricians in school food allergy management. Pediatr Ann 2013;42(8):334–40. Available at: http://www.healio.com/pediatrics/journals/pedann/2013-8-42-8/%7B4d17b1a3-26c1-4ac3-932a-6152129b2eea%7D/the-role-of-pediatricians-in-school-food-allergy-management.

6. Boyce JA, Assa'ad A, Burks AW, et al. Guidelines for the diagnosis and management of food allergy in the United States: report of the NIAID-sponsored expert panel. J Allergy Clin Immunol 2010;126:S1–58.

7. Muñoz-Furlong A. Daily coping strategies for patients and their families. Pediatrics 2003;111(Suppl 3):1654–61.

8. McIntyre CL, Sheetz AH, Carroll CR, et al. Administration of epinephrine for life-threatening allergic reactions in school settings. Pediatrics 2005;116(5):1134–40.

9. Hefle SL, Furlong TJ, Niemann L, et al. Consumer attitudes and risks associated with packaged foods having advisory labeling regarding the presence of peanuts. J Allergy Clin Immunol 2007;120(1):171–6.

10. Maloney JM, Chapman MD, Sicherer SH. Peanut allergen exposure through saliva: assessment and interventions to reduce exposure. J Allergy Clin Immunol 2006;118(3):719–24.

11. Sampson MA, Munoz-Furlong A, Sicherer SH. Risk-taking and coping strategies of adolescents and young adults with food allergy. J Allergy Clin Immunol 2006;117(6):1440–5.

12. Monks H, Gowland MH, MacKenzie H, et al. How do teenagers manage their food allergies? Clin Exp Allergy 2010;40(10):1533–40.

13. Simonte SJ, Ma S, Mofidi S, et al. Relevance of casual contact with peanut butter in children with peanut allergy. J Allergy Clin Immunol 2003;112(1):180–2.

14. Wainstein BK, Yee A, Jelley D, et al. Combining skin prick, immediate skin application and specific-IgE testing in the diagnosis of peanut allergy in children. Pediatr Allergy Immunol 2007;18:231–9.

15. Perry TT, Conover-Walker MK, Pomés A, et al. J Allergy Clin Immunol 2004;113(5):973–6.

16. Tulve N, Suggs JC, McCurdy T, et al. Frequency of mouthing behavior in young children. J Expo Anal Environ Epidemiol 2002;12:259–64.

17. Nicas M, Best DJ. A study quantifying the hand-to-face contact rate and its potential application to predicting respiratory tract infection. J Occup Environ Hyg 2008;5(6):347–52.

18. Kim JS, Sicherer SH. Living with food allergy: allergen avoidance. Pediatr Clin North America 2011;58(2):459–70.

19. Roberts G, Golder N, Lack G. Bronchial challenges with aerosolized food in asthmatic, food-allergic children. Allergy 2002;57(8):713–7.

20. Simons FE, Clark S, Camargo C. Anaphylaxis in the community: learning from the survivors. J Allergy Clin Immunol 2009;124(2):301–6.

21. Sampson HA, Munoz-Furlong A, Campbell RL, et al. Second symposium on the definition and management of anaphylaxis: summary report–second National

Institute of Allergy and Infectious Disease/Food Allergy and Anaphylaxis Network symposium. J Allergy Clin Immunol 2006;117:391–7.

22. Simons FE, Gu X, Silver NA, et al. EpiPen Jr versus EpiPen in young children weighing 15 to 30 kg at risk for anaphylaxis. J Allergy Clin Immunol 2002;109:171–5.

23. Sheikh A, ten Broek VM, Brown SG, et al. H1-antihistamines for the treatment of anaphylaxis: Cochrane systematic review. Allergy 2007;62(8):830–7.

24. Sicherer SH, Simons FE, Section on Allergy and Immunology, American Academy of Pediatrics. Self-injectable epinephrine for first-aid management of anaphylaxis. Pediatrics 2007;119(3):638–46.

25. Oren E, Banerji A, Clark S, et al. Food-induced anaphylaxis and repeated epinephrine treatments. Ann Allergy Asthma Immunol 2007;99:429–32.

26. Rudders SA, Banerji A, Corel B, et al. Multicenter study of repeat epinephrine treatments for food-related anaphylaxis. Pediatrics 2010;125:e711–8.

27. Devore CD, Wheeler LS, Council on School Health, et al. Role of the school physician. Pediatrics 2013;131(1):178–82.

28. American Academy of Pediatrics Council on School Health, Magalnick H, Mazyck D. Role of the school nurse in providing school health services. Pediatrics 2008;121(5):1052–6. Accessed September 3, 2015.

29. National Association of School Nurses. Allergy/anaphylaxis management in the school setting. 2012. Available at: http://www.nasn.org/Portals/0/positions/2012psallergy.pdf. Accessed January 14, 2015.

30. National Association of School Nurses. Anaphylaxis: a collaborative approach. 2015. Available at: https://www.nasn.org/portals/0/resources/Comprehensive_Anaphylaxis_School_Policy.pdf. Accessed January 22, 2015.

31. Engelke M, Guttu M, Warren M, et al. School nurse case management for children with chronic illness: health, academic, and quality of life outcomes. J Sch Nurs 2008;24(4):205–14.

32. American Nurses Association (ANA). The nursing process. 2014. Available at: http://www.nursingworld.org/EspeciallyForYou/What-is-Nursing/Tools-You-Need/Thenursingprocess.html.

33. Herdman T, editor. NANDA international nursing diagnoses: definitions & classifications, 2012-2014. Oxford (United Kingdom): Wiley-Blackwell; 2012.

34. Stanford University. SMART Goals - template. 2012. Available at: http://hrg.stanford.edu/documents/SMARTGOALSTemplate2012.doc. Accessed September 4, 2015.

35. Wang LY, Vernon-Smiley M, Gapinski MA. Cost-benefit study of school nursing services. JAMA Pediatr 2014;168(7):642–8.

36. Bollinger ME, Dahlquist LM, Mudd K, et al. The impact of food allergy on the daily activities of children and their families. Ann Allergy Asthma Immunol 2006;96(3):415–21.

37. Avery NJ, King RM, Knight S, et al. Assessment of quality of life in children with peanut allergy. Pediatr Allergy Immunol 2003;14(5):378–82.

38. Marklund B, Ahlstedt S, Nordström G. Health-related quality of life in food hypersensitive school-children and their families: parents' perceptions. Health Qual Life Outcomes 2006;4:48.

39. Lieberman JA, Weiss C, Furlong TJ, et al. Bullying among pediatric patients with food allergy. Ann Allergy Asthma Immunol 2010;105(4):282–6.

40. National Association of School Nurses. Individualized healthcare plans for the school nurse. 2013. Available at: http://www.nasn.org/Portals/0/positions/2013psihp.pdf. Accessed January 22, 2015.

Why Does Australia Appear to Have the Highest Rates of Food Allergy?

Katrina J. Allen, MBBS, FRACP, PhD[a,b,c,d,e,*], Jennifer J. Koplin, PhD[a,d]

KEYWORDS

- Peanut allergy • Prevalence • Hygiene hypothesis • Microbial exposure • Migration
- Food allergy • Vitamin D

KEY POINTS

- Food allergy is on the rise in developed countries and has been well-described in Australia using challenge-proven outcomes. It is believed to be linked to the modern-day lifestyle.
- The 3 key hypotheses for the rise in food allergy in the 21st century are currently (1) the hygiene hypothesis (which includes microbial diversity); (2) the dual allergen exposure (or Lack) hypothesis, and (3) the vitamin D hypothesis. There are as yet few published data with regard to other factors pertaining to food allergy as an outcome, although there are many studies in progress.
- High rates of food allergy in infants of Asian migrants provide a unique opportunity to explore possible explanations for this modern day phenomenon.

INTRODUCTION

Food allergy appears to have risen in many developed countries around the world but none more so than in Australia.[1–4] We reported in 2011 that in a population cohort of more than 5000 1-year-old infants, more than 10% had evidence of challenge-proven food allergy.[1] Although there are now many hypotheses as to why food allergy appears to be rising worldwide, until recently there has been little direct evidence formally

Disclosure Statement: K.J. Allen has received speaker's honorarium from Danone, Nutricia, Nestle, Alphapharm, and Aspen. J.J. Koplin has nothing to declare.
a Centre of Food and Allergy Research, Murdoch Children's Research Institute, The Royal Children's Hospital, Melbourne 3052, Australia; b Department of Allergy and Clinical Immunology, The Royal Children's Hospital, Melbourne 3052, Australia; c Department of Gastroenterology and Clinical Nutrition, The Royal Children's Hospital, Melbourne 3052, Australia; d Department of Paediatrics, The Royal Children's Hospital, University of Melbourne, Melbourne 3052, Australia; e Institute of Inflammation and Repair, University of Manchester, Manchester, UK
* Corresponding author. Centre of Food and Allergy Research, Murdoch Children's Research Institute, The Royal Children's Hospital, Melbourne 3052, Australia.
E-mail address: katrina.allen@rch.org.au

Pediatr Clin N Am 62 (2015) 1441–1451
http://dx.doi.org/10.1016/j.pcl.2015.07.005
0031-3955/15/$ – see front matter © 2015 Elsevier Inc. All rights reserved.

pediatric.theclinics.com

evaluating risk factors in populations in which the rise has been demonstrated. The current leading hypotheses of postnatal modifiable factors for the rise in food allergy are (1) the "dual allergen exposure" or Lack hypothesis, (2) the vitamin D hypothesis, and (3) the hygiene hypothesis (which includes factors associated with microbial diversity and the modern lifestyle). This review will present insights from the one of the first large-scale studies, the Healthnuts study, to formally assess these hypotheses using challenge-confirmed food allergy undertaken in all food-sensitized infants. By reviewing the literature, particularly in reference to studies that use the gold standard of oral food challenge, this article aims to understand potential lifestyle and environmental factors that might be driving the Australian epidemic and reviews other potential hypotheses that are as yet unstudied but may also contribute to this perplexing phenomenon of the 21st century.

HOW CONVINCING IS THE EVIDENCE FOR A 10% PREVALENCE OF FOOD ALLERGY IN AUSTRALIA?

The Healthnuts study provided evidence of unexpectedly high rates of challenge-proven immunoglobulin (Ig)E-mediated food allergy in infants in Melbourne, Australia, an urban population in Australia's most southern mainland city.[1] These findings may not be generalizable to other more rural areas of the state of Victoria because of differences in distribution of potentially protective factors, such as microbial exposure linked to contact with livestock or other rural factors. However, the prevalence of peanut allergy in Healthnuts (3%) is similar to the overall Victorian prevalence reported in the Longitudinal Study of Australian Children of 2.9% parent-reported peanut allergy in a cohort of more than 4000 children aged 6 to 7 years.[5] Because peanut allergy is uncommonly outgrown and peanut allergy is invariably IgE-mediated, this similarity between the 2 Victorian-based cohorts is reassuring. Findings from Healthnuts are also not necessarily applicable to other Australian states because there is evidence of a latitude gradient of food allergy prevalence in Australia, as there is for North America and Chile, with those living farthest from the equator in the south of Australia (including Victoria) having higher rates than those living farther north.[5,6]

Although higher than initially expected when the study was mounted, the high prevalence of food allergy found in Australia is not particularly surprising when viewed in the context of Australian hospital admission figures for food-induced anaphylaxis, which have risen fivefold in young children from the mid-1990s to the mid-2000s,[7] with similar increases in allergy waiting lists, which are now more than 12 months for most specialty clinics around the country. To date, these observations are limited to young children with only modest increases of anaphylaxis admissions for older children and adults[7] and no formal reports of rising rates in the adult population. A high food allergy prevalence in Australian infants is also consistent with the country having one of the highest rates of asthma and eczema in the world, perhaps suggesting a second-wave epidemic of allergic disease.[8]

One last factor to consider is that the Healthnuts study used raw egg for its oral food challenges, which may have overestimated clinically relevant egg allergy, a large determinant of the high prevalence of positive challenges. Countering this, however, is the observation that a history of acute allergic reactions to egg were reported by 6.5% of those exposed to dietary egg by age 1 year (K.J. Allen and J.J. Koplin, personal communication, 2011). As Lack observed, the prevalence of baked egg allergy (the most severe egg allergy phenotype) was 2% in Healthnuts, which is much more in line with prevalence rates published of challenge-proven semicooked egg allergy in the United Kingdom.[9]

WHY ARE THE RATES OF FOOD ALLERGY SO HIGH IN AUSTRALIAN INFANTS?

There are a multitude of potential explanations for why food allergy may be on the rise. However, it is important to consider them in the context of lifestyle factors that have changed over the past 20 to 30 years, the time period in which the rise in food allergy in developed countries has been noted. At the general public health level, there has been a slow but persistent urbanization of cities with increasing use of asphalt, cleaner water supplies, cleaner food supplies, a more sedentary lifestyle, and increased intake of a Westernized diet. In addition, there has been parallel increase in obesity and wide-scale use of antibiotics in not only the human population, but also in feed lots for livestock at low levels to optimize growth, a significant decline in smoking, and a decreasing prevalence of *Helicobacter pylori* infection. In infants, there has been an increased uptake of immunization and altered infant feeding patterns. Although these factors all began to change before the epidemic of food allergy, only infant feeding patterns have been significantly temporally linked to the most recent rise in food allergy specifically as opposed to the rise in allergic disease in general. Last, potential factors that appear somewhat unique to Australia are rising rates of migration from Asia and rising rates of vitamin D insufficiency in both mothers and children. There has been a modest public health response to the latter, with proactive identification of maternal vitamin D insufficiency with antenatal supplementation. However, there are currently no general recommendations for vitamin D food chain fortification (other than margarine) or consideration of preventive infant supplementation in the absence of risk factors for vitamin D insufficiency.

The Dual Allergen Exposure Hypothesis (Lack Hypothesis)

This hypothesis proposes that allergic sensitization to foods may occur through exposure to low doses of allergen through the skin due to food allergens in the environment being absorbed through a damaged skin barrier (such as in eczema or presence of filaggrin loss-of-function mutations). Oral exposure to these allergens through consumption of allergenic foods early in infancy, before skin sensitization, leads to lasting oral tolerance and prevents the development of sensitization and allergy even with subsequent skin exposure.[9]

Mechanistic evidence supporting this hypothesis comes from mouse models showing that sensitization can be induced following application of allergen to damaged skin, and that this can be prevented by previous high-dose oral allergen exposure.[10] Recent studies suggest that the activation of innate immune pathways in the skin Through TSLP and Basophil Activation may play a key role in development of food allergy secondary to cutaneous sensitization in animal models.[11,12] Studies of human populations to date have primarily focused on peanut allergy, demonstrating that peanut allergens can be found in the household environment and that higher exposure to environmental peanut antigens appears to increase the risk of peanut allergy in children with either filaggrin loss-of-function mutations[13] or atopic dermatitis.[14]

This hypothesis is appealing in the Australian context because eczema is extremely common in infants in Australia, with up to 25% of Healthnuts infants having a history of doctor-diagnosed eczema or nurse-observed eczema at age 1 year.[15] As reported previously, eczema frequently coassociates with food allergy, with 50% of those with early-onset moderately severe eczema developing food allergy by age 1 year.[16] This, coupled with distinct changes to infant feeding guidelines in the late 1990s/early 2000s with recommendations to delay allergenic solids such as egg to 10 months and peanut until age 3 years, providing the correct temporal framework for this hypothesis to have had a potential effect on the epidemic.[17]

Adequate early-life skin barrier function

It is important to note that filaggrin loss-of-function mutations appear to be equally common among individuals with asymptomatic food sensitization and those with true food allergy,[18] suggesting that filaggrin confers a risk for food sensitization, the first step to food allergy, but not further for food allergy itself. Previous studies reporting an association with food allergy were not designed to untangle any differential effect between sensitized tolerant and sensitized allergic individuals.[19] Recent data from the Isle of Wight birth cohort used path analysis to demonstrate that the effect of filaggrin loss-of-function mutations on food allergy at age 10 occurred indirectly through an effect on eczema and food sensitization in early childhood.[20] Together these findings suggest that skin barrier function plays a role in sensitization status but not in the second step of food allergy versus tolerance development.

Two exciting new studies were recently published that both undertook randomized controlled trial of daily moisturizing from birth in an attempt to reduce infantile eczema and associated effects. The first demonstrated an impressive 50% reduction in eczema.[21] The second also examined egg sensitization as a secondary outcome. Although effective at preventing atopic dermatitis, there was no evidence of a reduction in sensitization to egg white in this relatively small study of 118 infants.[22] Follow-up results to these trials and larger studies will be intriguing. Currently there is little information about early infant bathing and moisturizing practices in Australia, although avoiding soap in the first few weeks of life is generally recommended. The Barwon Infant Study, a prospective prenatal birth cohort study of 1000 infants undertaken in Geelong, 80 km southwest of Melbourne, has gathered this information, which is likely to shed light on this question in Victoria, Australia.[23]

Timing of introduction of solids and infant feeding

The Lack hypothesis suggests the second factor in the 2 steps to food allergy is delayed oral allergen exposure. This is partially supported by data from the STAR trial, which randomized infants with eczema to egg avoidance or early regular egg consumption from age 4 months, finding a lower prevalence of egg allergy by 12 months in the intervention group (33% vs 51%, $P = .11$).[24] These findings suggest a potentially protective effect of early allergen introduction that requires investigation in larger studies, and we await further studies. The STAR trial results also indicate that egg sensitization and allergy (at least in infants with eczema) may already be present as early as 4 months; however, introduction of oral solids before 4 months is likely to be extremely controversial. The recently published landmark study by Du Toit and Colleagues[25] is the first RCT to Demonstrate a protective effect of early introduction of peanut with a dramatic reduction in development of peanut allergy if peanut was introduced between 4 and 11 months of age.

Early evidence, which requires further investigation, suggests that if a window of opportunity for promoting tolerance exists, it may be different for each food.[17] For example, the optimal timing of introduction of milk appears to be earlier compared with egg. In one observational study, infants introduced to milk at 4 to 6 months were more likely to be milk allergic compared with those introduced to milk later. Lower rates of cow's milk allergy among those who were exposed to cow's milk formula within the first 14 days of life suggest that very early exposure to cow's milk protein might promote tolerance, although this requires further investigation.[26]

Weaning practices in Australia coupled with high eczema rates may contribute to the high prevalence of food allergy. In Healthnuts, fewer than 5% of infants received solid foods before 3 months of age, compared with 27% in a United Kingdom–based birth cohort study,[27] with delayed introduction of solids likely to have a flow on effect in delaying the timing of oral exposure to potentially allergenic foods. High-quality evidence for an association between timing of introduction of allergenic foods remains sparse, but the studies published to date generally show a reduced risk of food allergy in those introduced to specific allergenic foods earlier in infancy.[26,28,29]

More recent attention has turned to diet diversity, which may be one factor change that coincides temporally with the rise in food allergy and could reflect changes that occur following migration to a new country. Several studies in the past year examined the role of diversity of early-life food exposures in the development of food sensitization and food allergy. A prospective birth cohort study of 856 children reported increased diversity of complementary foods introduced in the first year of life was associated with a reduced risk of food allergy.[30] In a prospective longitudinal study, dietary patterns in the first year of life consisting of more fresh fruit and vegetables and home-prepared meals were associated with less challenge-proven food allergy by the age of 2 years.[31]

At the population levels, changes in the timing of food introduction may contribute to but are unlikely to completely explain recent increases in the prevalence of food allergy. Recently we assessed the impact of changing guidelines on infant feeding practices in the general population in Healthnuts. Changing guidelines had some impact on timing of allergenic foods, with these introduced earlier after changes in guidelines, although changes were less pronounced among those with a family history of allergy and in families of lower socioeconomic status.[32] Despite this, there was no decrease in the overall prevalence of food allergy in the second half of the cohort (when timing of allergenic solids was less delayed) compared with the first half of the cohort (K.J. Allen and J.J. Koplin, personal communication, 2015) although analysis is ongoing to assess the impact of differential uptake of guideline changes among those at higher risk of food allergy on this finding.

Vitamin D Hypothesis

Recent hypotheses that low vitamin D may increase the risk of food allergy are supported by 2 lines of ecological enquiry. First, countries farther from the equator (and thus with lower ambient ultraviolet radiation) have recorded more pediatric admissions to hospital for food allergy–related events and more prescriptions of hypoallergenic formulas for the treatment of cow's milk allergy and adrenaline auto injectors for the treatment of anaphylaxis in children.[6,33–35] These findings appear to be independent of longitude, physician density, or socioeconomic status. Second, season of birth may play a role. For example, children attending emergency departments in Boston with a food-related acute allergic reaction were more likely to be born in autumn/winter, when vitamin D levels reach their nadir, than in spring/summer, and similar links of food allergy to birth seasonality were reported in the southern hemisphere.[36,37] As described previously, children residing in Australia's southerly state have twice the odds (95% confidence interval [CI] 1.2–5.0) of peanut allergy at age 4 to 5 years and 3 times (95% CI 1.0–9.0) the odds of egg allergy than those in the northern states.[5] Despite a sunny clime, Australia has high rates of vitamin D deficiency, including in infants, with a highly successful "slip, slop, slap, wrap" anti–skin cancer public health campaign (slip on a t-shirt, slop on sunscreen, slap on a hat, and wrap on sunglasses) and absence of fortification and universal supplementation presumably contributing to this.[38]

We recently described that infants with vitamin D insufficiency were 3 times more likely to have either peanut or egg allergy, the odds increasing to fourfold among those with 2 or more food allergies. Furthermore, among food-sensitized infants, those with vitamin D insufficiency were 6 times more likely to be food allergic than tolerant.[39] These effects were observed among infants with Australian-born parents but not those with parents born outside Australia. Investigation of genetic risk factors may help to explain these differences in associations between populations. Genetic polymorphisms contribute to variation in vitamin D–binding protein levels, explaining almost 80% of variation in levels. Binding protein levels in turn alter the biological availability of serum vitamin D, with lower levels increasing the availability of serum vitamin D (25OHD3). We recently found that polymorphisms resulting in lower binding protein levels appeared to compensate for adverse effects of low serum vitamin D on food allergy risk (JJ Koplin and colleagues, manuscript under review), presumably by increasing ability to utilize available vitamin D. As well as supporting a potentially causal link between vitamin D and food allergy, these findings suggest that reference ranges to define low levels of serum vitamin D with a detrimental effect on food allergy risk may need to take into account differences in binding protein level. Randomized controlled trials stratified by genetic, racial, or migratory status are required to determine whether correction of vitamin D status either prevents infantile food allergy or promotes the development of tolerance in food-allergic infants.

Hygiene Hypothesis

There is increasing evidence that the interaction between the host microbiome and the immune system is essential to the development of immune regulation and oral tolerance. The maturation of the mucosal immune system is prompted by exposure to microbes after birth. In searching for explanations for food allergy, attention has been turned to the composition and timing of exposure to gut microflora, and their possible role in disease development or prevention. One hypothesis to explain the increased incidence of sensitization to food allergens is that the reduction in early childhood infections (the hygiene hypothesis) or in exposure to microbial products (eg, endotoxin, microbial exposure) may impede the development of early immunoregulatory responses. This leaves the immune system more susceptible to inappropriate reactivity to innocuous antigens, resulting in an "allergic" reaction.

As described in the landmark paper by David Strachan in 1989,[40] the traditional concept of the "hygiene hypothesis" described a protective effect of an increasing number of siblings in a household on the risk of developing allergic rhinitis. This was thought to potentially relate to the shared exposure to common childhood infections transmitted through direct contact with older siblings or by maternal contact with her older children prenatally. Although a protective sibling effect has been confirmed for challenge-proven food allergy outcomes in our own infant cohort study (Healthnuts)[41] and by others for various food sensitization and allergy outcomes,[42] it is by no means clear as to the underlying mechanism of this phenomenon. Although the concept is interesting and reproducible, changes to postwar houses and sanitation, sizes of families, as well as the emergence of national immunization programs with high uptakes moderates our interpretation of the mechanisms underlying the protective effects of siblings. Further evidence of a protective effect of dog ownership on food allergy risk in Healthnuts may point to sharing of microbes or even parasites, the latter underpinning the "old friends hypothesis," which is predicated on the teleologic emergence of the IgE antibody immune mechanism as primary protection against parasite infestation. More generally speaking, there is some early evidence to suggest a difference between prevalence of food allergy in rural versus urban environments, which appears to be reflected in rising rates of food allergy described in cities in China (such as Chongquing) undergoing rapid urbanization.[43]

HOW DO THESE HYPOTHESES FIT WITH THE OBSERVED CHANGES IN FOOD ALLERGY FOLLOWING MIGRATION TO AUSTRALIA FROM ASIA?

In Healthnuts, challenge-confirmed peanut allergy was 3 times more common in infants with parents born in East Asia compared with those with parents born in

Australia.[44] Similar effects were seen for other food sensitizations and food allergies and for eczema. The increased risk of allergic disease in Australian-born infants of Asian-born parents appears to have occurred in a single generation, with the prevalence of reported allergic disease similar or even lower in Asian-born parents themselves compared with Australian-born parents. Furthermore, the increased risk of peanut allergy appeared to be specific to infants of Asian parents and was not seen among infants of parents born in the United Kingdom or Europe.

COULD REMOVAL OF THE PROTECTIVE ASIAN ENVIRONMENT INCREASE THE EXPRESSION OF GENETICALLY AT-RISK INFANTS?

Migration may be associated with changes to a number of factors (some of which were not measured in Healthnuts) that might be interrelated (**Fig. 1**). These include humidity (and its impact on skin barrier function), microbial exposure (hygiene hypothesis), dietary changes, and changes in latitude (vitamin D). For example, changes to the skin barrier function and risk of eczema as an early risk factor of food allergy may result from higher humidity in Asia than Australia but equally may result from differences in infant washing practices (types of soap and water composition) that occur in each country and may exert an effect through the hygiene hypothesis. Microbial exposure factors that differ not only include variations in the quality of water supply (and differences in risk of water-borne gastrointestinal infections) but differences in microbes that are a part of the food chain supply (for example in unwashed vegetables or higher use of antibiotics in the food chain supply of meat-producing animals), number of children in a family, and issues of crowding and exposure to pets, farm animals, and stray animals (which may have higher rates of parasites), as well as variations in overprescribing of antibiotics in each region. Dietary differences are multiple. These include higher use of herbicides and pesticides that might affect the microbial load of food and increased sterilization and use of plastic in developed countries. Foods may have allergenicity altered through cooking practices (eg, boiled vs roasted peanut). Last, vitamin D status is likely to differ between the 2 regions, not only from latitude

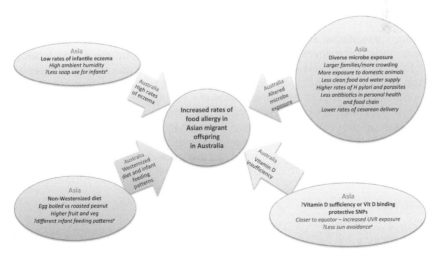

Fig. 1. Modifiable lifestyle risk factors that could explain the rise in food allergy risk in offspring of Asian migrants in Australia. [a]Potential differences between Asia and Australia but limited published evidence to date.

changes and UV exposure, but through variations in dietary intake and supplement/fortification programs, both antenatally and postnatally. Earlier observations from the United Kingdom of an overrepresentation of non-white children in pediatric allergy clinics suggests that this migration effect may also be present among children of Asian parents migrating to other developed countries and similar risk factors are likely to apply.[45]

THE ROLE OF GENE-ENVIRONMENT AND EPIGENETIC MODIFICATION

Because the rise in the prevalence of allergic diseases has occurred more rapidly than can be accounted for by population-based changes in genetic sequence, it is most likely due to environmental factors. However, the rising incidence may be primarily occurring in those genetically at risk. The continuous dialogue between the genome and the environment (GxE) is important for the pathogenesis of complex diseases that exhibit a heritable component but do not follow Mendel's laws. Food allergy, like other complex diseases, is presumed to be caused by a combination of subtle genetic and environmental factors. The GxE reflects how environmental exposures (including lifestyle and diet) interact with genetic predisposition to modify disease risk and/or outcome. An interaction is indicated when the simultaneous influence of 2 or more factors on a phenotype is not additive. Thus, the presence of one factor affects the influence (manifestation of risk) associated with a second. For example, the influence of the C-159 T polymorphism on the CD14 gene may depend on microbial stimulation from the environment,[46] with individuals carrying the TT genotype appearing to have increased protection from eczema with dog exposure.[47] Environmental factors that have commonly been considered in interaction with genetic risk factors include vitamin D (which has known direct genetic effects), smoking, air pollution, and microbial exposures. However, other environmental factors for which there is evidence of involvement in allergic diseases have not been considered in interaction with genetics. It also would be useful to consider factors such as diet and food supplements in relation to genetic risks such as FLG mutations.

SUMMARY

The recent rise in food allergy poses significant challenges to untangling its cause. It remains important to investigate potential mechanisms of food allergy using carefully characterized phenotypes. Confounding factors (both measured and unmeasured) remain important issues for observational studies and only randomized controlled trials will provide the highest level of evidence of causation. However multi-intervention randomized controlled trials are notoriously difficult to undertake, and genetic stratification may be required to ensure gene-environment interactions are taken into account. For the time being we remain dependent on single-effect randomized controlled trials to try to elucidate why food allergy is on the rise and whether there is anything that we can do to turn back the tide.

REFERENCES

1. Osborne NJ, Koplin JJ, Martin PE, et al. Prevalence of challenge-proven IgE-mediated food allergy using population-based sampling and predetermined challenge criteria in infants. J Allergy Clin Immunol 2011;127(3):668–76.
2. Prescott SL, Pawankar R, Allen KJ, et al. A global survey of changing patterns of food allergy burden in children. World Allergy Organ J 2013;6(1):21.

3. Rona RJ, Keil T, Summers C, et al. The prevalence of food allergy: a meta-analysis. J Allergy Clin Immunol 2007;120(3):638–46 [Systematic reviews].

4. Nwaru BI, Hickstein L, Panesar SS, et al. The epidemiology of food allergy in Europe: a systematic review and meta-analysis. Allergy 2014;69(1):62–75 [Systematic reviews].

5. Osborne NJ, Ukoumunne OC, Wake M, et al. Prevalence of eczema and food allergy is associated with latitude in Australia. J Allergy Clin Immunol 2012;129(3):865–7.

6. Mullins R, Clark S, Camargo CJ. Regional variation in EpiPen prescriptions in Australia: more evidence for the vitamin D-anaphylaxis hypothesis. Ann Allergy Asthma Immunol 2009;103(6):488–95.

7. Poulos LM, Waters AM, Correll PK, et al. Trends in hospitalizations for anaphylaxis, angioedema, and urticaria in Australia, 1993-1994 to 2004-2005. J Allergy Clin Immunol 2007;120(4):878–84.

8. Prescott S, Allen KJ. Food allergy: riding the second wave of the allergy epidemic. Pediatr Allergy Immunol 2011;22(2):155–60.

9. Lack G. Update on risk factors for food allergy. J Allergy Clin Immunol 2012; 129(5):1187–97.

10. Strid J, Hourihane J, Kimber I, et al. Epicutaneous exposure to peanut protein prevents oral tolerance and enhances allergic sensitization. Clin Exp Allergy 2005;35(6):757–66.

11. Noti M, Kim BS, Siracusa MC, et al. Exposure to food allergens through inflamed skin promotes intestinal food allergy through the thymic stromal lymphopoietin-basophil axis. J Allergy Clin Immunol 2014;133(5):1390–9.

12. Muto T, Fukuoka A, Kabashima K, et al. The role of basophils and proallergic cytokines, TSLP and IL-33, in cutaneously sensitized food allergy. Int Immunol 2014; 26(10):539–49.

13. Brough HA, Simpson A, Makinson K, et al. Peanut allergy: effect of environmental peanut exposure in children with filaggrin loss-of-function mutations. J Allergy Clin Immunol 2014;134(4):867–75.

14. Brough HA, Liu AH, Sicherer S, et al. Atopic dermatitis increases the effect of exposure to peanut antigen in dust on peanut sensitization and likely peanut allergy. J Allergy Clin Immunol 2015;135(1):164–70.

15. Martin PE, Koplin JJ, Eckert JK, et al. The prevalence and socio-demographic risk factors of clinical eczema in infancy: a population-based observational study. Clin Exp Allergy 2013;43(6):642–51.

16. Martin PE, Eckert JK, Koplin JJ, et al. Which infants with eczema are at risk of food allergy? Results from a population-based cohort. Clin Exp Allergy 2015; 45(1):255–64.

17. Koplin JJ, Allen KJ. Optimal timing for solids introduction—why are the guidelines always changing? Clin Exp Allergy 2013;43(8):826–34.

18. Tan HT, Ellis JA, Koplin JJ, et al. Filaggrin loss-of-function mutations do not predict food allergy over and above the risk of food sensitization among infants. J Allergy Clin Immunol 2012;130(5):1211–3.

19. Brown SJ, Asai Y, Cordell HJ, et al. Loss-of-function variants in the filaggrin gene are a significant risk factor for peanut allergy. J Allergy Clin Immunol 2011;127(3):661–7.

20. Venkataraman D, Soto-Ramirez N, Kurukulaaratchy RJ, et al. Filaggrin loss-of-function mutations are associated with food allergy in childhood and adolescence. J Allergy Clin Immunol 2014;134(4):876–82.

21. Simpson EL, Chalmers JR, Hanifin JM, et al. Emollient enhancement of the skin barrier from birth offers effective atopic dermatitis prevention. J Allergy Clin Immunol 2014;134(4):818–23.

22. Horimukai K, Morita K, Narita M, et al. Application of moisturizer to neonates prevents development of atopic dermatitis. J Allergy Clin Immunol 2014;134(4):824–30.

23. Vuillermin P, Saffery R, Allen KJ. Cohort Profile: The Barwon Infant Study. Int J Epidemiol 2015. [epub ahead of print].

24. Palmer DJ, Metcalfe J, Makrides M, et al. Early regular egg exposure in infants with eczema: a randomized controlled trial. J Allergy Clin Immunol 2013;132(2): 387–92.

25. Du Toit G, Roberts G, Sayre PH, et al. LEAP Study Team. Randomized trial of peanut consumption in infants at risk for peanut allergy. N Engl J Med 2015;372(9): 803–13.

26. Katz Y, Rajuan N, Goldberg MR, et al. Early exposure to cow's milk protein is protective against IgE-mediated cow's milk protein allergy. J Allergy Clin Immunol 2010;126(1):77–82.

27. Venter C, Pereira B, Voigt K, et al. Factors associated with maternal dietary intake, feeding and weaning practices, and the development of food hypersensitivity in the infant. Pediatr Allergy Immunol 2009;20(4):320–7.

28. Koplin JJ, Osborne NJ, Wake M, et al. Can early introduction of egg prevent egg allergy in infants? A population-based study. J Allergy Clin Immunol 2010;126(4): 807–13.

29. Du Toit G, Katz Y, Sasieni P, et al. Early consumption of peanuts in infancy is associated with a low prevalence of peanut allergy. J Allergy Clin Immunol 2008; 122(5):984–91.

30. Roduit C, Frei R, Depner M, et al. Increased food diversity in the first year of life is inversely associated with allergic diseases. J Allergy Clin Immunol 2014;133(4): 1056–64.

31. Grimshaw KE, Maskell J, Oliver EM, et al. Diet and food allergy development during infancy: birth cohort study findings using prospective food diary data. J Allergy Clin Immunol 2014;133(2):511–9.

32. Tey D, Allen KJ, Peters RL, et al. Population response to change in infant feeding guidelines for allergy prevention. J Allergy Clin Immunol 2014;133(2):476–84.

33. Camargo CA, Clark S, Kaplan MS, et al. Regional differences in EpiPen prescriptions in the United States: the potential role of vitamin D. J Allergy Clin Immunol 2007;120(1):131–6.

34. Mullins RJ, Clark S, Camargo CA Jr. Regional variation in infant hypoallergenic formula prescriptions in Australia. Pediatr Allergy Immunol 2010;21(2 Pt 2): e413–20.

35. Rudders SA, Espinola JA, Camargo CA Jr. North-south differences in US emergency department visits for acute allergic reactions. Ann Allergy Asthma Immunol 2010;104(5):413–6.

36. Vassallo MF, Banerji A, Rudders SA, et al. Season of birth and food-induced anaphylaxis in Boston. Allergy 2010;65(11):1492–3.

37. Mullins RJ, Clark S, Katelaris C, et al. Season of birth and childhood food allergy in Australia. Pediatr Allergy Immunol 2011;22(6):583–9.

38. Munns C, Zacharin MR, Rodda CP, et al. Prevention and treatment of infant and childhood vitamin D deficiency in Australia and New Zealand: a consensus statement. Med J Aust 2006;185(5):268–72.

39. Allen KJ, Koplin JJ, Ponsonby AL, et al. Vitamin D insufficiency is associated with challenge-proven food allergy in infants. J Allergy Clin Immunol 2013;131(4): 1109–16.

40. Strachan DP. Hay fever, hygiene, and household size. BMJ 1989;299(6710): 1259–60.

41. Koplin JJ, Dharmage SC, Ponsonby AL, et al. Environmental and demographic risk factors for egg allergy in a population-based study of infants. Allergy 2012; 67(11):1415–22.
42. Marrs T, Bruce KD, Logan K, et al. Is there an association between microbial exposure and food allergy? A systematic review. Pediatr Allergy Immunol 2013; 24(4):311–20 [Systematic reviews].
43. Hu Y, Chen J, Li H. Comparison of food allergy prevalence among Chinese infants in Chongqing, 2009 versus 1999. Pediatr Int 2010;52(5):820–4.
44. Koplin JJ, Peters RL, Ponsonby AL, et al. Increased risk of peanut allergy in infants of Asian-born parents compared to those of Australian-born parents. Allergy 2014;69(12):1639–47.
45. Dias RP, Summerfield A, Khakoo GA. Food hypersensitivity among Caucasian and non-Caucasian children. Pediatr Allergy Immunol 2008;19(1):86–9.
46. Lau MY, Dharmage SC, Burgess JA, et al. CD14 polymorphisms, microbial exposure and allergic diseases: a systematic review of gene-environment interactions. Allergy 2014;69(11):1440–53 [Systematic reviews].
47. Myers JMB, Ning W, Grace KL, et al. Genetic and environmental risk factors for childhood eczema development and allergic sensitization in the CCAAPS cohort. J Invest Dermatol 2010;130:430–67.

Quality of Life in Food Allergy Patients and Their Families

Madeline Walkner, BS[a], Christopher Warren, BA[b],
Ruchi S. Gupta, MD, MPH[a,b],*

KEYWORDS

- Childhood food allergy • Quality of life • Anxiety • Daily life • Caregivers

KEY POINTS

- Many factors can impact a child's food allergy-related quality of life, including their age, perceived food allergy severity, and reaction history.
- Daily activities such as grocery shopping, meal preparation, and eating at restaurants can place added emotional stress on parents of food-allergic children.
- Because food is involved in the majority of school and social activities, children with food allergy may feel singled out and are often the target of bullying.
- Constant vigilance associated with food allergen avoidance can put stress on children and their families.

INTRODUCTION

Food allergy affects an estimated 8% of US children,[1] and the rate is expected to continue to rise.[2] There is no curative treatment for food allergy, and effective management involves avoiding exposure to known food allergens or treatment of symptoms.[3,4] Allergen avoidance may place an emotional burden on food allergy patients and their caregivers. The looming threat of anaphylaxis has been found to strain relationships with family and friends, lead to concerns about stigmatization and isolation, as well as precipitate marital conflict.[5] Life outside of the home, in schools, and in restaurants, can also become challenging. Daily activities such as making dinner, packing lunch, and going to school can be difficult and emotionally taxing on families,[5,6] as

Disclosure Statement: Dr R.S. Gupta has received grants from Mylan LP and Food Allergy Research and Education.
[a] Ann & Robert H. Lurie Children's Hospital of Chicago, 225 E. Chicago Ave, Chicago, IL 60611, USA; [b] Northwestern University Feinberg School of Medicine, 6th Floor, 750 North Lake Shore Drive, Chicago, IL 60611, USA
* Corresponding author. Center for Community Health, 6th Floor, 750 North Lake Shore Drive, Chicago, IL 60614.
E-mail address: rgupta@northwestern.edu

Pediatr Clin N Am 62 (2015) 1453–1461
http://dx.doi.org/10.1016/j.pcl.2015.07.003
0031-3955/15/$ – see front matter
pediatric.theclinics.com

family members constantly anticipate the next reaction. Primary care providers are often the first to see patients with a suspected food allergy after a reaction, and are thus frequently tasked with ensuring that patients and families are educated and prepared in the event of a future reaction. Indeed, recent work has found that increasing preparedness and improving coping skills can significantly ease anxiety and improve quality of life among parents of children with food allergy.[7] The aim of this article is to describe the factors that affect quality of life in food allergy patients and their caregivers and to inform providers of strategies to help families improve their quality of life.

SOCIAL ACTIVITIES
Schools and Bullying

Social interactions play a pivotal role in child development, especially those taking place within the school context. However, growing evidence suggests that food allergy may make children more vulnerable in social situations to social ostracism or bullying in school.[8] A study by Shemesh and colleagues[9] found that 31.5% of children aged 8 to 17 years reported they were bullied specifically because of their food allergy. Similarly, work by Gupta and colleagues[10] reported that 43% of students with food allergy aged 14 to 22 years old reported they were bullied at school because of their food allergy. Furthermore, a recent Italian study found children aged 8 to 19 years with food allergy were twice as likely to be bullied as their nonfood-allergic peers.[11] In their study, Shemesh and colleagues[9] noted that 80% of children who were bullied because of a food allergy were bullied by a classmate. This is particularly alarming, because school classmates typically spend many hours each day together. In this case, bullying consisted mostly of threats with food and verbal teasing.[9] Children may not know that intentionally exposing a food-allergic child to their allergen could be dangerous and lead to a life-threatening reaction. As such, is important to make sure that an action plan is in place at school in the event of a reaction. Another study by Lieberman and colleagues[12] reported that 82% of bullying episodes occurred while at school and 21% of those who were bullied were bullied by teachers or school staff. Furthermore, Gupta and colleagues[10] also reported that 38% of respondents desired better support for their food allergy while at school. A longitudinal evaluation of food allergy-related bullying found that when parents initiated a dialogue with school personnel regarding their child's bullying, such bullying was less likely to recur.[13] However, if teachers and students are not aware of bullying or the potential severity of food allergy, food-allergy related bullying is likely to remain ignored or unaddressed. This can provoke unneeded stress and anxiety for the child and put him or her in a potentially dangerous situation.

Social Activities/Dining Out

Although school constitutes a key social environment for children, food allergy often impacts other activities outside of the home, such as sporting events and restaurant dining. A systematic review by Cummings and colleagues[6] outlined multiple ways in which having a child with food allergies in the household significantly impacts family activities. When outside the relatively controlled home environment, children must be vigilant in making sure foods do not contain their allergen(s), since roughly half of fatal reactions result from food consumed away from home.[14] A study by Avery and colleagues[15] investigated quality of life among children with peanut allergy compared to children with type 1 diabetes and found that anxiety was particularly elevated among children with peanut allergy at social events such as birthday parties, holiday parties, and on public transport. Remarkably, this study also found that when compared to children with type 1 diabetes, children with peanut allergy experienced significantly greater anxiety and impaired quality of life.

Multiple studies have found food allergy to particularly limit quality of life in the context of dining out. When asked about their dining habits, most children surveyed by Avery and colleagues[15] noted that they frequently visit the same restaurant, because they know their food allergy will be catered for, putting them at ease. For young children, caregivers are often the ones making decisions about what their child eats. In a study by Bollinger and colleagues,[16] it was reported that 16% of caregivers of food-allergic children avoided going to restaurants because of their child's food allergy. Other social activities impacted by food allergy were also recorded. Five percent of caregivers avoided family outings, and 6% avoided going out of town or on vacation because of food allergy.[16] Although 11% reported avoiding letting their child play at a friend's house, 11% avoided school parties and sports; 10% avoided letting their child go to birthday parties, and 26% avoided letting their child go to camp.[16] These missed social activities may put additional stress on the food-allergic child, and lead to increased feelings of isolation.

DAILY ACTIVITIES
Meals and Nutrition

Although there are many dangers when eating outside of the home with a food-allergic child, meal planning within the home also becomes more challenging and time-consuming. Caregivers must avoid using the allergen while cooking the meal, and this often means they must plan far in advance when going to the grocery store or visit specialty stores. The extra time it takes planning and picking out items for the meal can add time and stress to the caregiver's daily activities. Regarding meal preparation at home, Bollinger and colleagues[16] found that 76% of caregivers reported that a child's food allergies significantly impacted grocery shopping behaviors, while 60% of caregivers reported food allergies significantly impacted meal planning for their family. These researchers also found that 67% of respondents reported that food allergies significantly impacted meal preparation, and 76% reported that food allergies significantly impacted meals or snacks on the run.[16] Daily activities such as grocery shopping and meal preparation that are easy for most families can cause families with a food-allergic child to become overwhelmed and stressed. In addition to meal planning, another source of stress for caregivers is their child's diet. A study by Springston and colleagues[5] assessed food allergy-related quality of life among 1126 caregivers of food-allergic children. Twenty-nine percent of caregivers were extremely troubled by concerns for their child's health due to food allergy, while 22.3% were extremely troubled by concerns for their child's nutrition.[5] Because of the absence of curative treatment options for food allergy, many caregivers are told by their physician to have their child avoid the food. Particular concern may arise when children are allergic to more than one food or a food that is an ingredient found in many other foods. In these cases, parents may fear that avoiding the food(s) will lead to nutritional deficiencies in the child's diet, leading to additional parental concern about the degree to which their child is getting well-balanced meals.

Parental Emotions

Many studies have examined familial knowledge, attitudes, and beliefs toward food allergy, including how differences in parenting styles can lead to strained relationships between parents of children with food allergy. A study conducted by Gupta and colleagues[17] found that 25% of parents reported that their child's food allergy caused strain in their marriage or primary relationship. Mothers are often charged with preparing meals for the child in and out of the home. Some mothers even go as far as quitting their job to allow for more time to make sure their child is safe.[18] Mothers tend to have a more protective approach to food allergy and are more likely to be hypervigilant regarding allergen avoidance. It is within this context that a recent study found mothers to have impaired food allergy-related quality of life relative to fathers, despite reporting greater empowerment to care for their food-allergic child.[19] This was hypothesized to be because of increased fear among mothers of their child's potential exposure to allergens when outside of their immediate supervision (eg, at school, at a friend's house). To this point, a recent qualitative study found mothers of children with severe food allergies to experience significant distress as the child gained independence and mothers were forced to place trust in others to ensure their child's well-being.[20] Misunderstanding and perceived disregard for a child's food allergy is a major source of stress for parents.[18] Past work has also found that mothers can feel unfairly labeled by other family members as neurotic and overprotective when it comes to their child's food allergy[18] when they engage in efforts to prevent their child's exposure to food allergens. In fact, a recent study suggested that maternal quality of life is more strongly impacted by such social negativity regarding their child's food allergy than by the social support gleaned through social relationships.[21] As such, while children and their caregivers should be educated about food allergy management and preparedness, they must also be prepared to educate the people around them, including family and friends. Such efforts may help alleviate tension stemming from misunderstandings about the potential seriousness of a food-allergic reaction.

Raising a child with food allergy can not only result in relationship problems between parents, but can also adversely impact the emotional well-being of parents on a more individual level. A study by King and colleagues[22] reviewed the impact of peanut allergy on anxiety, stress, and quality of life in families in the United Kingdom. Mothers of food-allergic children rated their own physical and psychological quality of life worse than fathers.[22] It was also reported that fathers had lower scores of stress and anxiety then mothers did.[22] Furthermore, when asked to what degree having a peanut allergy adversely impacted their child's quality of life, mothers perceived their child's peanut allergy as having a more adverse impact on quality of life than did the child's father, siblings, or the food-allergic child him/herself.[22] A study by Warren and colleagues[19] reported that fathers generally reported increased food allergy caregiver quality of life when their children lacked a history of severe allergic reactions and when they felt that they had ample social support and resources to care for their child. Although each of these factors also served as significant predictors of increased quality of life among mothers, perceptions of ample social support and resources had a greater impact on maternal quality of life than on paternal quality of life, whereas the severity of a child's food allergy had a reduced impact on mothers relative to fathers.[19]

A child's food allergy type has been found to predict systematic differences in parental food allergy-related quality of life. Specifically, allergies to ubiquitous foods like milk and egg more negatively impact parental quality of life than allergies to more easily avoidable foods like fin fish.[19] These findings are consistent with work by Howe and colleagues,[23] which also found presence of multiple food allergies and history of severe reactions to be associated with decreased parental quality of life. A study by Annunziato and colleagues[24] of 454 caretakers assessed mental health needs and utilization by food allergy families. This study found that 32% of food allergy caretakers reported levels of distress above the predefined clinical threshold score, and 70% reported that mental health services would have been useful to them.[24] However, only 23% of caregivers sought mental health care for their distress from their child's food allergy.[24] These findings suggest that pediatricians should consider how they might more effectively connect caregivers of children with food allergy to mental health services when appropriate.

Child's Emotions

Food allergy has an impact on the emotional well-being of families and caregivers as well as on the affected child. A food allergy diagnosis requires children to constantly be aware of their surroundings at school, sporting events, family parties, and even in their own home. Without a proven treatment, children are forced to resort to strict allergen avoidance while also having a plan for accidental exposure in order to manage their food allergy. This places a large amount of stress on the child, especially in situations where the caregiver is not around and the child must decide for himself or herself what is safe to ingest. However, there can be some positive aspects to having a food allergy. For example, Gupta and colleagues[10] surveyed 14- to 22-years-olds on risk-taking behaviors and found that most adolescents surveyed reported that living with a food allergy made them more responsible, empathetic to others with special needs, and a better advocate for themselves and others.

Many factors, including gender and age, play a role in determining quality of life among individuals with food allergy. King and colleagues[22] reported that as compared with their female siblings, girls with peanut allergy reported significantly reduced overall quality of life as well as within multiple subdomains, including at school and relating to physical health. However, this study found that male students reported their peanut allergy only impacted their quality of life at school.[22] Interestingly, when a group of Swedish parents answered questionnaires assessing health-related quality of life among their children with food allergy, girls with food allergy were found to have poorer parent-reported mental health due to their food allergy, whereas boys had worse parent-reported physical functioning and general health-related quality of life due to their food allergy.[25] These findings suggest that further examination of such gender differences may inform future interventions targeting food allergy-related quality of life.

The age of a child can also have an effect on parental perspectives of the child's quality of life. Marklund and colleagues[25] found that in general, parents reported that a child's food allergy more negatively impacts everyday family activities at younger ages. Warren and colleagues[19] found that among mothers, quality of life increased from age 2 to age 13 and then declined thereafter, whereas child age had no effect on paternal quality of life. As children enter adolescence, they tend to become more educated and aware of their food allergy and in turn manage it more independently. However, recent cross-sectional work suggests that this transition may be accompanied by increased anxiety as adolescents assume greater self-management of their condition. Additional longitudinal studies are needed in order to more fully understand how quality of life may change across development among both children with food allergy and their caregivers.

Severity of reaction and reaction history can be important factors to consider when evaluating the quality of life of a food-allergic individual as well. Past work has found presence of a severe food allergy reaction history to have mixed effects on quality of life among children and their caregivers. One such study by Bollinger and colleagues[16] reported that a history of anaphylaxis had no impact on the quality of life of either the child or his or her caregivers. Another recent study of a European food allergy cohort found that although a child's anaphylaxis history was not predictive of his or her quality of life, his or her own perceptions of the severity of his or her food allergy were significantly associated with quality of life.[26] These findings are consistent with a qualitative study that found that if the child was too young at the time of an allergic reaction to remember it, then it was not likely to impact the child, whereas the occurrence of such reactions did substantially impact parental well-being.[27]

Experiencing or observing the symptoms of a severe anaphylactic reaction can be traumatic, and some have suggested that such events can lead to post-traumatic stress disorder.[28] There is a wide range of symptoms for allergic reactions, ranging from flushed face, to gastrointestinal distress, to loss of consciousness. One study by Marklund and colleagues[25] reported that parents of children who showed gastrointestinal distress during their allergic reaction were more emotionally impacted by the reaction then when other symptoms were present. On the other hand, parents reported a better sense of well-being regarding their child if the child's allergic reaction included symptoms that would be considered more severe such as anaphylaxis or trouble breathing.[25] Another recent paper found that increased reaction severity was a significant predictor of decreased parental quality of life for both mothers and fathers of children with food allergy.[19]

Recently, attention has been turned to teenagers and college-aged individuals who have food allergy due in part to their relatively high rates of fatal reactions relative to other age groups.[14] It has been reported that this age group tends to take the most risks when it comes to their food allergy.[29–33] A study by Greenhawt and colleagues[30] of 513 college students at the University of Michigan reported that only 39.7% of respondents with a food allergy regularly avoided their food allergen. What's more, only 6.6% of students reported that they always carry their epinephrine autoinjector with them.[30] This becomes dangerous in college, because many freshmen do not cook for themselves, instead eating most of their meals in the dining hall or at restaurants.[30] Greenhawt and colleagues[30] also found that dining halls themselves did not take adequate precautions, reporting that only 11.5% of surveyed students stated dining hall foods were always labeled for allergen content. Such inconsistencies can cause confusion for students trying to decipher whether a meal contains their allergen. Furthermore, most school dining hall staff are student employees who may not have proper knowledge about food allergy and cross-contamination. When students were asked why they engaged in risky behaviors, such as not always avoiding their food allergen, 37.6% mentioned they had no history of severe reactions.[30] However, research shows that fatal reactions are not always preceded by a severe reaction.[34] When asked about support preferences, the majority of students reported needing more public awareness about food allergy.[10] More research is needed on the impact this risk-taking behavior has on quality of life, especially as adolescents begin to live on their own.

Although quality of life has been repeatedly shown to be adversely affected by childhood food allergy, few interventions have been evaluated that aim to improve quality of life among families with food allergy. One such intervention provided parents of children with food allergy with 3 nurse-facilitated counseling sessions that promoted self-regulation for chronic disease management.[7] Researchers found that parental quality of life, including indicators of frustration, helplessness, anxiety, and confidence significantly improved after receiving the intervention.[7] Another study found a half-day group food allergy education and skills-training workshop for children with food allergy and their parents to be effective in improving parental quality of life and perceived competence in coping with food allergy.[35] Furthermore, a recent cross-sectional study assessing food allergy-related quality of life found that caregivers of children with food allergy who had undergone an oral food challenge had significantly increased quality of life compared with caregivers whose children had not undergone an oral food challenge.[36] Interestingly, quality of life did not differ among parents of children who underwent an oral food challenge and passed (eg, did not react) compared with parents of children who underwent an oral food challenge and did not pass (eg, did react).[36] Although prospective replication studies are needed, this suggests that confirmatory oral food challenge may not only be the gold standard for food allergy diagnosis, but also a useful intervention to improve caregiver quality of life. However, additional interventions should be evaluated in order to improve quality of life among both food-allergic children and their caregivers.

SUMMARY

It is clear that food allergy has an impact on the quality of life of affected individuals and their caregivers. Many factors can impact a child's food allergy-related quality of life, notably his or her age, food allergy severity, and reaction history. The importance of food allergy education should be emphasized, not only for the patient and his or her caregivers, but also for families and communities. Making sure patients and their caregivers understand how to manage their food allergy and have a clear action plan in the event of accidental exposure are keys to helping ease the stress added by a food allergy diagnosis. Ensuring that patients are sent home with a concise anaphylaxis action plan and the proper medication can help the child feel more at ease at school. Educating families on using self-regulation for chronic disease strategies, conducting confirmatory oral food challenges, and keeping them informed about how to manage their child's food allergy may be effective strategies to help increase the quality of life for patients and their caregivers.

REFERENCES

1. Gupta RS, Springston EE, Warrier MR, et al. The prevalence, severity, and distribution of childhood food allergy in the United States. Pediatrics 2011;128(1): e9–17.
2. Branum AM, Lukacs SL. Food allergy among children in the United States. Pediatrics 2009;124(6):1549–55.
3. Sampson HA. Food allergy. Part 2: diagnosis and management. J Allergy Clin Immunol 1999;103(6):981–9.
4. Panel N-SE. Guidelines for the diagnosis and management of food allergy in the United States: report of the NIAID-sponsored expert panel. J Allergy Clin Immunol 2010;126(6):S1–58.
5. Springston EE, Smith B, Shulruff J, et al. Variations in quality of life among caregivers of food allergic children. Ann Allergy Asthma Immunol 2010;105(4): 287–94. e283.
6. Cummings A, Knibb RC, King R, et al. The psychosocial impact of food allergy and food hypersensitivity in children, adolescents and their families: a review. Allergy 2010;65(8):933–45.
7. Baptist AP, Dever SI, Greenhawt MJ, et al. A self-regulation intervention can improve quality of life for families with food allergy. J Allergy Clin Immunol 2012;130(1):263–5.e6.
8. Lieberman JA, Sicherer SH. Quality of life in food allergy. Curr Opin Allergy Clin Immunol 2011;11(3):236–42.
9. Shemesh E, Annunziato RA, Ambrose MA, et al. Child and parental reports of bullying in a consecutive sample of children with food allergy. Pediatrics 2013; 131(1):e10–7.
10. Gupta RS, DA, Pence J, Dyer AA, et al. Adolescents with food allergy: the good, the bad, and the beautiful. The Pediatric Academic Societies Annual Meeting. San Diego (CA), April 27, 2015.

11. Muraro A, Polloni L, Lazzarotto F, et al. Comparison of bullying of food-allergic versus healthy schoolchildren in Italy. J Allergy Clin Immunol 2014;134(3):749–51.

12. Lieberman JA, Weiss C, Furlong TJ, et al. Bullying among pediatric patients with food allergy. Ann Allergy Asthma Immunol 2010;105(4):282–6.

13. Annunziato RA, Rubes M, Ambrose MA, et al. Longitudinal evaluation of food allergy-related bullying. J Allergy Clin Immunol Pract 2014;2(5):639–41.

14. Bock SA, Muñoz-Furlong A, Sampson HA. Further fatalities caused by anaphylactic reactions to food, 2001-2006. J Allergy Clin Immunol 2007;119(4):1016–8.

15. Avery NJ, King RM, Knight S, et al. Assessment of quality of life in children with peanut allergy. Pediatr Allergy Immunol 2003;14(5):378–82.

16. Bollinger ME, Dahlquist LM, Mudd K, et al. The impact of food allergy on the daily activities of children and their families. Ann Allergy Asthma Immunol 2006;96(3):415–21.

17. Gupta RS, Springston EE, Smith B, et al. Food allergy knowledge, attitudes, and beliefs of parents with food-allergic children in the United States. Pediatr Allergy Immunol 2010;21(6):927–34.

18. Gupta RS, Kim JS, Barnathan JA, et al. Food allergy knowledge, attitudes and beliefs: focus groups of parents, physicians and the general public. BMC Pediatr 2008;8(1):36.

19. Warren CM, Gupta RS, Sohn M-W, et al. Differences in empowerment and quality of life among parents of children with food allergy. Ann Allergy Asthma Immunol 2015;114(2):117–25. e113.

20. Rouf K, White L, Evans K. A qualitative investigation into the maternal experience of having a young child with severe food allergy. Clin Child Psychol Psychiatry 2011;17(1):49–64.

21. Williams NA, Hankey M. Support and negativity in interpersonal relationships impact caregivers' quality of life in pediatric food allergy. Qual Life Res 2014;24:1–10.

22. King R, Knibb RC, Hourihane JB. Impact of peanut allergy on quality of life, stress and anxiety in the family. Allergy 2009;64(3):461–8.

23. Howe L, Franxman T, Teich E, et al. What affects quality of life among caregivers of food-allergic children? Ann Allergy Asthma Immunol 2014;113(1):69–74.e2.

24. Annunziato RA, Shemesh E, Weiss CC, et al. An assessment of the mental health care needs and utilization by families of children with a food allergy. J Health Psychol 2013;18(11):1456–64.

25. Marklund B, Ahlstedt S, Nordström G. Health-related quality of life in food hypersensitive schoolchildren and their families: parents' perceptions. Health Qual Life Outcomes 2006;4(1):48.

26. Saleh-Langenberg J, Goossens N, Flokstra-de Blok B, et al. Predictors of health-related quality of life of European food-allergic patients. Allergy 2015;70(6):616–24.

27. Akeson N, Worth A, Sheikh A. The psychosocial impact of anaphylaxis on young people and their parents. Clin Exp Allergy 2007;37(8):1213–20.

28. Kelsay K. Psychological aspects of food allergy. Curr Allergy Asthma Rep 2003;3(1):41–6.

29. Youth Risk Behavior Surveillance: National College Health Risk Behavior Survey—United States, 1995. MMWR CDC Surveill Summ 1997;46(6):1–56.

30. Greenhawt MJ, Singer AM, Baptist AP. Food allergy and food allergy attitudes among college students. J Allergy Clin Immunol 2009;124(2):323–7.

31. Pumphrey RS, Gowland MH. Further fatal allergic reactions to food in the United Kingdom, 1999–2006. J Allergy Clin Immunol 2007;119(4):1018–9.

32. Rolison MR, Scherman A. Factors influencing adolescents' decisions to engage in risk-taking behavior. Adolescence 2002;37(147):585.

33. Sampson MA, Muñoz-Furlong A, Sicherer SH. Risk-taking and coping strategies of adolescents and young adults with food allergy. J Allergy Clin Immunol 2006; 117(6):1440–5.

34. Pumphrey R. Anaphylaxis: can we tell who is at risk of a fatal reaction? Curr Opin Allergy Clin Immunol 2004;4(4):285–90.

35. LeBovidge JS, Timmons K, Rich C, et al. Evaluation of a group intervention for children with food allergy and their parents. Ann Allergy Asthma Immunol 2008; 101(2):160–5.

36. Franxman TJ, Howe L, Teich E, et al. Oral food challenge and food allergy quality of life in caregivers of children with food allergy. J Allergy Clin Immunol Pract 2015;3(1):50–6.

Food Protein–Induced Enterocolitis Syndrome

Stephanie A. Leonard, MD[a], Anna Nowak-Węgrzyn, MD[b],*

KEYWORDS

- Non–IgE-mediated food allergy • Food protein–induced enterocolitis syndrome
- FPIES • Gastrointestinal food allergy

KEY POINTS

- Food protein–induced enterocolitis syndrome (FPIES) is a rare, non-immunoglobulin E–mediated gastrointestinal food allergy that continues to be misdiagnosed, contributing to delays in diagnosis and increased morbidity.
- Varied presentations of FPIES have been reported in different populations, however acute and repetitive vomiting remains the predominant feature.
- Although most cases are diagnosed in infants and resolve by school age, FPIES may present at any age and persist into teenage and adult years.
- Further study into the prevalence, pathophysiology, and natural course of FPIES is warranted.

INTRODUCTION

Food protein–induced enterocolitis syndrome (FPIES) is a rare, non–immunoglobulin E (IgE)-mediated gastrointestinal food allergy primarily diagnosed in infancy. Acute FPIES reactions typically present with delayed, repetitive vomiting, lethargy, and pallor within 1 to 4 hours of food ingestion. Chronic FPIES typically presents with protracted vomiting, diarrhea, or both, accompanied by weight loss or poor growth. Foods regularly included in the diet are thought to induce chronic symptoms, such as cow's milk (CM) or soy formula, while acute reactions are commonly reported after intermittent ingestion of the causative food. The pathophysiology of FPIES is unknown but is thought to be immunologic and cellular in nature.[1]

Owing to nonspecific symptoms and the lack of diagnostic testing, FPIES is often initially misdiagnosed, leading to a delay in diagnosis and increased morbidity from

The authors have nothing to disclose.

[a] Division of Pediatric Allergy & Immunology, Rady Children's Hospital San Diego, University of California, San Diego, 3020 Children's Way, MC 5114, San Diego, CA 92123, USA; [b] Division of Pediatric Allergy, Department of Pediatrics, Jaffe Food Allergy Institute, Icahn School of Medicine at Mount Sinai, Box 1198, One Gustave L. Levy Place, New York, NY 10029, USA
* Corresponding author.
E-mail address: anna.nowak-wegrzyn@mssm.edu

Pediatr Clin N Am 62 (2015) 1463–1477
http://dx.doi.org/10.1016/j.pcl.2015.07.011
0031-3955/15/$ – see front matter © 2015 Elsevier Inc. All rights reserved.

extensive workups and hospitalizations. Varying clinical manifestations of FPIES in different populations further complicate the picture. An understanding of the various presentations of FPIES along with increased awareness of the condition by general practitioners and emergency room providers will help to improve the management and quality of life of patients with FPIES.

EPIDEMIOLOGY

Large population studies to assess the overall prevalence of FPIES are lacking. In the only such study with more than 13,000 Israeli infants prospectively enrolled, the cumulative incidence of CM FPIES was reported at 0.34%.[2] IgE-mediated CM allergy, a condition considered more common than FPIES, was diagnosed in 0.5% of the same population.

Several studies have reported an increase in FPIES diagnosis, frequently attributed to increased awareness of the syndrome as separate from other food sensitivities. In an Italian cohort, a significant increase in the number of FPIES cases was noted in 2008, when the diagnostic criteria for FPIES were modified at one of its centers, with a constant level of cases reported thereafter.[3] Alternatively, in an Australian cohort, although the number of FPIES cases increased steadily over a 16-year period, the median number of prediagnosis FPIES reactions did not substantially change, suggesting that increased awareness did not play a role.[4] In a recent large United States cohort, no increase in the number of FPIES cases was observed over a 6 year period.[5]

Although FPIES develops primarily in infancy, reports in older children and adults indicate that it may develop at any age.[5–7] There does not seem to be a gender predilection in childhood, however a female predominance in a small cohort of adults with FPIES has been reported, similar to that seen in IgE-mediated food allergy.[7] In a large United States cohort, 65% of FPIES subjects were Caucasian, mirroring the referral population evaluated their allergy clinic.[5] In Israel, FPIES was more common in the Jewish population (P = .03).[4] Overall, FPIES has been reported across all races and ethnicities.[5,8]

Many FPIES patients have an atopic background. Eczema was reported in 9% to 57% of FPIES subjects, similar to or higher than the overall population.[3–6] Wheezing or asthma was reported in 3% to 25% of FPIES subjects, similar to or lower than overall population.[4–6] Allergic rhinitis was reported in 38% of FPIES subjects, IgE-mediated food allergy to other foods in 11% to 30%, and eosinophilic esophagitis in 1 FPIES subject.[4,6] A family history of allergic disease was reported in 20% to 77% of FPIES cases.[3,6] In one cohort, 34% of FPIES subjects had a family history of food allergy, and 6% (n = 10) had a family history of FPIES.[6]

CM FPIES in the Israeli cohort was not found to be associated with gestational age, birth weight, maternal age, number of siblings, dairy consumption by mother, or age of CM introduction.[2] However, infants with CM FPIES were more likely than healthy infants to have been born by cesarean section (27% vs 15%, respectively) (P = .003). Conversely, in a United States FPIES cohort, the rate of cesarean section was 29%, lower than the overall population.[6] In the Italian FPIES cohort, 95% were breastfed for a median duration of 4 months (range 0.5–12), whereas the breastfeeding rate in a large United States cohort was 47%, similar to the national rate.[3,5]

CLINICAL PRESENTATION

The rates of FPIES symptoms in different cohorts are presented in **Table 1**. Vomiting is the predominant FPIES symptom, while diarrhea is typically reported in 50% or fewer FPIES cases. Isolated vomiting and isolated diarrhea have been reported.[3] It has been

Table 1
Most common symptoms of FPIES in cohort studies (%)

	Mehr et al[4] (N = 35; 66 Episodes)	Katz et al[2] (N = 44 CM FPIES)	Sopo et al[3] (N = 66)	Ruiz-Garcia et al[11] (N = 16)	Tan & Smith[7] (N = 31 Adults)	Ludman et al[8] (n = 50 Acute, n = 4 Chronic)	Caubet et al[6] (N = 74 Positive OFCs)
Vomiting	100 (66)	100 (44)	98 (65)	100 (16)	71 (24)	81 (44)	96 (70)
Diarrhea	24 (16)	25 (11)	54 (36)	56 (9)	58 (18)	37 (20)	7 (5)
Lethargy	85 (55)	77 (34)	—	25 (4)	—	17 (9)[a]	7 (5)
Pallor	67 (44)	14 (6)	80 (53)	19 (3)	—	15 (8)[b]	—
Abdominal pain	—	—	—	—	77.4 (24)	6 (3)	80 (59)
Hypotension	—	—	77 (51)	—	—	—	19 (14)

Values are percent (no. of subjects).
Abbreviation: CM, cow's milk.
a "Listless".
b "Gray appearance".

suggested that diarrhea is likely associated with more severe cases, exacerbating fluid loss, and infancy.[4] In the study by Sopo and colleagues,[3] 47% versus 27% of acute reactions with and without diarrhea, respectively, required hospitalization and were treated with intravenous fluids (IVF). However, diarrhea was reported in only 7% of a large United States cohort of oral food challenges (OFCs), while hypotension was reported in 19%.[6]

Hypotension has been reported in 5% to 77% of different cohorts.[3,5,6] This large range is likely due to differences in methodology, whether blood pressure was measured, and the number of cases observed during OFCs or treated at a medical facility compared with symptoms reported by parents. Sopo and colleagues[3] reported that pallor and hypotension/lethargy never occurred alone. There was no mention of pallor or hypotension in the adult cohort, although these symptoms were reported in an adult case report of scallop FPIES.[9] In the adult cohort, abdominal pain was reported in 77% of cases, more so than vomiting (71%).[7]

Other reported presenting symptoms included dehydration, lethargy, irritability, loss of consciousness, clamminess, hypotonia, cyanosis, and other stool changes, including bloody diarrhea, melena, and malodorous, pale or sticky stools.[5,8,10] Mehr and colleagues[4] reported that 6 of 25 (24%) patients who had body temperature measured were hypothermic ($<36°C$). Weight loss and poor growth has been reported in chronic FPIES.[8]

The amount ingested that causes FPIES symptoms can be very low, as in the case of a 6-month-old diagnosed with rice FPIES who developed symptoms after chewing on a wrapper from a rice cake.[12] Similarly, Bansal and colleagues[13] reported 4 cases where increasingly smaller amounts were needed to trigger subsequent FPIES reactions. Conversely, Katz and colleagues[2] reported that 54% of subjects with CM FPIES tolerated 121 mL or more of CM before having symptoms during OFCs.

Although approximately 60% of FPIES cases occur on first exposure, many cases occur after a period of tolerance.[2,4] In the study by Mehr and colleagues,[4] 12% of the cohort developed FPIES symptoms on second exposure, 12% on third, and 15% on fourth. Katz and colleagues[2] reported that 16% of infants with CM FPIES tolerated CM for more than 4 days and 11% tolerated CM for 14 to 30 days before developing symptoms. FPIES in adults has been reported to be acquired after tolerating the trigger food previously.[7]

The appearance of symptoms after ingestion of trigger foods is typically delayed in comparison with IgE-mediated food allergy.[2,11] The median reported time from first dose to development of symptoms during OFCs in 2 cohorts was 1.5 to 2 hours, with a range of 0.5 to 4 hours.[3,4] This is similar to the findings of Katz and colleagues,[2] who reported a range of 30 minutes to 5.25 hours between ingestion and symptoms, with 60% occurring after 2 hours. In the fish-related FPIES cohort of Zapatero Remón and colleagues,[14] two patients reported symptoms within 5 to 10 minutes and one showed symptoms at 6 hours; during observed OFCs the range of time from ingestion to symptoms was between 30 minutes and 5 hours. The duration of symptoms has been reported to be between 2 and 48 hours.[3,14] During observed OFCs, the median time to recovery was 50 minutes (interquartile range [IQR] 13–95 minutes) in the cohort of Caubet and colleagues.[6]

The age at onset of FPIES seems to differ according to food trigger (**Table 2**). Likely because of delays in diagnosis, the overall median age at FPIES diagnosis was 15 months (IQR 9–24 months) in one cohort, and the overall mean age at diagnosis was 14 months in another cohort.[3,6] Several cohorts report CM or soy FPIES presenting earlier than solid food FPIES, mostly before 6 months of age.[2,3,5,6] Late-onset fish or shellfish FPIES was diagnosed after infancy in 7% of one cohort with a median age

Table 2
FPIES cohort studies

	Country, Location	Type of Study	No. of Patients; Gender	Age at Onset	No. of Foods
Mehr et al,[4] 2009	Sydney, Australia, tertiary	Retrospective, 16 y (1992–2007)	35; 57% male	Mean 5.5 ± 2.4 mo	83% to 1 food, 17% to 2 foods
Sopo et al,[3] 2012	Rome, Benevento, and Florence, Italy, tertiary	Retrospective, 7 y	66; 61% male	Overall mean 5.7 ± 5.1 mo; milk 3.5 ± 2.4 mo; other foods 10.6 ± 6.7 mo	85% to 1 food, 15% to multiple triggers
Hsu & Mehr,[21] 2013	Sydney, Australia, tertiary	Retrospective, 4 y (2008–2012)	38; 53% male	Mean 6 mo	66% to 1 food, 34% to multiple triggers
Ruffner et al,[5] 2013	Philadelphia, PA, USA, tertiary	Retrospective, 6 y	462; 60.4% male	Overall mean 9.7 ± 10.2 mo; milk/soy 7 ± 0.7 mo; solids 12.1 ± 1.1 mo	70% to 1 or 2 foods, 30% to ≥3 foods; 5% reacted to >6 foods
Ruiz-García et al,[11] 2014	Madrid, Spain, tertiary	Retrospective, 12 y	16; 10 boys, 6 girls	Median 6.5 mo (range, 1–30)	94% to 1 food, 1 (6%) to 2 foods
Ludman et al,[8] 2014	London, UK, tertiary	Retrospective, 3 y	54; 59% male	Median 8 mo (range, 0.75–60); milk/soy 6 mo (0.75–36); solid 8 mo (3–60); chronic 5 mo (0.75–12)	70% to 1 food, 30% to multiple triggers
Caubet et al,[6] 2014	New York, NY, USA, tertiary	Retrospective and prospective (51%), 11 y	160; 54% male	Milk/soy only: median 5 mo (IQR 2–10); solid food only: median 7 mo (IQR 6–12); milk/soy and solid food: median 4 mo (IQR 2–6)	65% to 1 food, 26% to 2 foods, 9% to ≥3 foods; median 3 foods (range, 3–10 foods)
Tan & Smith,[7] 2014	South Australia, Australia, private practice	Retrospective, 8 y	31; 23% male	Median 29 y (IQR 22–45.8)	84% to 1 food, 13% to 2 foods, 3% to 3 foods

at diagnosis of 30 months.[6] Zapatero Remón and colleagues[14] reported the age of onset of fish FPIES to be between 9 and 12 months.

Ruffner and colleagues[5] found no significant difference in age at FPIES presentation between breastfed and formula-fed infants. Caubet and colleagues[6] found that in solid food FPIES, formula was introduced later (median 1.5 months) and breastfeeding lasted longer (median 2.8 months) than in those with CM or soy FPIES, for whom formula was introduced and breastfeeding lasted a median 0.03 months ($P = .0002$). In this cohort, 62% of CM or soy FPIES infants were exposed to CM or soy formula in the first few weeks of life. In addition, most CM or soy FPIES presented with chronic symptoms, such as diarrhea, colitis, reflux, or failure to thrive, occurring shortly after CM or soy formula introduction, which resolved with avoidance. Subsequent acute episodes to CM or soy occurred at a mean age of 7 months (range, 0.3–60 months).[6]

Acute CM or soy FPIES in exclusively breastfed infants is rare.[3,15–17] Theories about breast milk being protective include the presence of protective immunoglobulin A, that the food is highly processed, or that the threshold dose may not be present in breast milk.[18] Three breastfed infants in one cohort (N = 160) had symptoms of chronic FPIES to CM in the maternal diet.[6] By contrast, in a parent survey (N = 263), a surprising proportion (42%) reported reactions through breast milk exposure.[19] This result may be affected by recall bias and may depend on the definition of FPIES symptoms.

The amount ingested that causes FPIES symptoms can be very low, as in the case of a 6-month-old diagnosed with rice FPIES who developed symptoms after chewing on a wrapper from a rice cake.[12] Similarly, Bansal and colleagues[13] reported 4 cases where increasingly smaller amounts were needed to trigger subsequent FPIES reactions. Conversely, Katz and colleagues[2] reported that 54% of subjects with CM FPIES tolerated 121 mL or more of CM before having symptoms during OFCs.

CAUSATIVE FOODS

Foods that have been reported in the literature to trigger FPIES are listed in **Table 3**.[3–14,20–23] The rates of the most common foods causing FPIES in cohorts are presented in **Table 4**. In the two large United States cohorts, CM, soy, rice, and oats are the most common foods.[5,6] In the study by Caubet and colleagues,[6] solid food–only FPIES was reported in 31% of subjects, CM only in 22%, soy only in 22%, CM and soy in 13%, and CM and/or soy plus solid food in 11%. In the cohorts from Australia, Israel, and Italy, soy FPIES was not common.[2–4] Ruffner and

Table 3	
Reported food triggers identified in the literature	
Liquids	Cow's milk, soy milk (also a legume), goat's milk
Grains	Rice, oat, barley, wheat
Vegetables	Sweet potatoes, squash, pumpkin, corn, carrots, white potato, spinach, cauliflower, cucumber
Legumes	Green pea, peanut, string bean, green bean, lentil, kidney bean
Fruits	Banana, orange, pineapple, apple, strawberry, blueberry, raspberry, mango, peach, pear, plum, apricot, grape, cherry, kiwi, watermelon, avocado, coconut, tomato
Animal protein	Egg, chicken, turkey, beef, lamb, pork, duck
Seafood	Fish, shellfish, mollusks
Other	Almond, other tree nuts, mushroom, quorn, probiotic *Saccharomyces boulardii*

Table 4
Most common food triggers of FPIES in cohort studies (%)

	Mehr et al[4] (N = 35)	Sopo et al[3] (N = 66)	Hsu and Mehr[21] (N = 38)	Ruffner et al[5] (N = 462)	Ruiz-Garcia et al[11] (N = 16)	Ludman et al[8] (N = 52)	Caubet et al[6] (N = 160)
Cow's milk	20 (7)	67 (44)	32 (12)	67 (309)	44 (7)	46 (25)	44 (70)
Soy	34 (12)	4 (3)	13 (5)	41 (189)	6 (1)	11 (6)	41 (66)
Rice	40 (14)	4 (3)	53 (20)	19 (88)	—	4 (2)	23 (36)
Oat	6 (2)	—	18 (7)	16 (74)	—	6 (3)	16 (26)
Wheat	—	—	—	10 (46)	6 (1)	11 (6)	1 (2)
Poultry	3 (1)	3 (2)	—	4.5 (21)	6 (1)	7 (4)	—
Fish	3 (1)	12 (8)	—	—	31 (5)	15 (8)	—
Egg	—	6 (4)	10 (4)	11 (51)	—	13 (7)	—
Peanut	—	—	—	1.9 (9)	—	—	—
Corn	—	2 (1)	—	8 (37)	—	—	—
Banana	3 (1)	—	—	3.5 (16)	—	6 (3)	—
Sweet potato	6 (2)	—	—	4.1 (19)	—	—	—

Values are percent (no. of subjects).

colleagues[5] reported that the most common fruit was banana (3.5%), while the most common vegetables were sweet potato (4.1%) and pea (3.2%).

Fish was the second most common FPIES trigger after CM in the Italian cohort, and was also reported in the cohorts from Spain.[3,11,14] Fish is introduced early into children's diets in Spain and Italy, however so is rice, which was not a common FPIES trigger in these populations. Similar to IgE-mediated fish allergy, while some subjects developed FPIES to multiple fish, others in the cohort of Sopo and colleagues[3] were able to tolerate some species of fish.

Egg is becoming a more frequently reported trigger of FPIES, for example in the British (13%) and Australian (10%) cohorts.[8,21] In an adult cohort, egg was the second most common trigger (16%) after seafood.[7] Whereas chronic FPIES in infants is typically seen with CM or soy, egg was reported as a chronic trigger in one cohort.[8] There is one case report of FPIES reaction to egg yolk, although challenge to egg white alone was not undertaken so it is not known whether the trigger was small amounts of egg white in the egg yolk.[24]

There have been reports of tolerance to baked or processed FPIES foods, as is common with IgE-mediated food allergy to CM and egg. Miceli Sopo and colleagues[25] reported that 4 of 7 patients with CM or egg FPIES tolerated baked CM or egg. Caution is warranted, as FPIES reactions to baked CM and egg have also been reported.[21,25] Yasutomi and colleagues[26] also reported the case of an 8-month-old female with atypical (detectable specific IgE) rice FPIES who tolerated highly processed retort rice, but developed symptoms with boiled rice. The patient's IgE was found to bind to boiled rice extract, but not the retort rice, on Western blot analysis.

Reactions to Multiple Foods

Reactions to multiple foods in different cohorts are listed in **Table 2**. In the United States cohorts, Ruffner and colleagues[5] and Caubet and colleagues[6] reported that 43.5% and 37% of CM FPIES, respectively, also reacted to soy. Caubet and colleagues[6] reported that 61.5% of CM and soy FPIES had reactions to both within 2 months of each other. These results differ from those in cohorts outside the United States, where most patients with CM FPIES tolerated soy or had no reported reactions to soy.[2–4] In the CM FPIES cohort of Katz and colleagues,[2] 35 of 44 tolerated soy milk, and 5 of the remaining 9 added soy to the diet after a negative soy OFC.

In the United States cohorts, most subjects with multiple FPIES triggers reacted to CM and/or soy and solid foods.[5,6] In these same cohorts, 40% to 50% of subjects with grain FPIES reacted to two or more grains. No solid food FPIES was reported in cases of CM FPIES in several cohorts outside the United States.[2,10,14] Caubet and colleagues[6] found no difference in FPIES to one, two or three or more foods and age at diagnosis, age at onset, detectable specific IgE, detectable specific IgE to other foods, family history of atopy, or family history of FPIES.

DIAGNOSIS

Diagnosis of FPIES is usually based on clinical criteria. Because most FPIES patients are young and have a limited diet, an in-depth history is usually enough to elicit the trigger food. Diagnostic OFCs were performed for 53% and 64% of patients in the Sopo and Katz cohorts,[2,3] respectively. In the study by Caubet and colleagues,[6] 180 OFCs were performed in 82 subjects, and 30% of the FPIES population had OFCs diagnostic of FPIES.

For most subjects, skin-prick testing (SPT) and specific IgE (sIgE) levels to FPIES trigger foods were negative.[2–5,8,14] In several cohorts, less than 10% of subjects tested had a positive SPT to trigger foods, and between 11% and 24% had detectable sIgE levels.[2–6,8] Most of the detectable sIgE levels were to common foods that cause IgE-mediated allergy, such as CM, soy, egg, peanut, and tree nuts, but a few were also positive to rice and oats.[5,6]

Subjects with detectable sIgE levels to trigger foods have been noted to have a protracted course. For example, no subjects with CM-sIgE levels in the cohort of Caubet and colleagues[6] had outgrown CM FPIES, whereas those with undetectable CM-sIgE levels had resolution of FPIES at a median age of 61 months. In addition, 33% of subjects (41% with CM FPIES) with detectable sIgE levels converted to an IgE-mediated phenotype. This transition has been noted in other cohorts.[2,3,27] Katz and colleagues[2] noted that transition from FPIES to IgE-mediated food allergy was not associated with average age of onset, mean dose-evoking response, median time from ingestion to response, or SPT results at time of FPIES presentation. There has been one reported case of a 4-month-old with a history of IgE-mediated CM allergy that shifted to FPIES.[28]

Atopy patch testing (APT) has been suggested as a diagnostic test for FPIES because it is presumably T-cell mediated, and delayed cutaneous responses are thought to represent a cellular mechanism. In a series of 19 FPIES patients, Fogg and colleagues[29] reported APT to have sensitivity of 100% and specificity of 71%. In a subsequent study by the same group with a larger cohort, APT was found to have a 45% false-negative rate and was determined not to be useful in the diagnosis of FPIES.[5] In addition, in a series by Järvinen and Nowak-Węgrzyn[30] of 25 FPIES patients, the sensitivity and specificity of APT was only 11.8% and 85.7%, respectively, with a positive predictive value of 40% and a negative predictive value of 54.5%. In a small series (n = 8) in yet another population, less than half of those with a positive APT reacted during OFCs.[14]

An increased absolute neutrophil count (ANC), typically peaking at 6 hours, is a common finding in acute FPIES reactions.[31] Caubet and colleagues[6] reported that the ANC after positive OFCs showed a median increase of 1850 cells/mm^3 and a mean increase of 3228 cells/mm^3 (IQR 825–4200) 5 to 8 hours after a positive challenge; this is slightly lower than the increase of 3500 cells/mm^3 proposed by Powell.[31] This finding could be confounded by intravenous steroids, which increase ANC. While helpful, an isolated increase in ANC is not enough to diagnosis FPIES and should not be used to exclude foods from the diet.[6]

Two cohorts noted a mild increase in platelets. Caubet and colleagues[6] reported a median increase of 19,000/mm^3 (range, −121,000 to 110,000). Mehr and colleagues[4] reported thrombocytosis (>500 × 10^9 cells/L) in 63% of FPIES episodes with a median increase of 588 × 10^9 cells/L (range, 515–777 × 10^9 cells/L). Other laboratory findings, depending on severity and chronicity, have included metabolic acidosis, methemoglobinemia, anemia, hypoalbuminemia, and eosinophilia.[1]

Stool studies showing leukocytes and eosinophils have been proposed to support a diagnosis of FPIES.[1] However, as diarrhea is not a major feature in most FPIES cohorts, this may not be useful. In addition, although gastric juice aspirates showing an increase in leukocytes greater than 10 per high-powered field has been associated with positive FPIES OFCs, such a test may not be practical for most patients.[32]

Diagnostic Criteria

An OFC remains the gold standard for diagnosis of FPIES; however, OFCs may not be necessary in cases of repeated reactions, especially severe ones with hypotension in young infants.[33] In light of the recent large cohorts from different populations, modifications to the current criteria used to diagnose FPIES may be warranted. The most commonly used criteria for diagnosing FPIES (Powell's criteria) and newly proposed criteria are listed in **Table 5**. Some researchers suggest that repetitive vomiting with pallor and lethargy are enough for diagnosis.[2,3] Given the possibility that older children and adults can develop FPIES, it has also been proposed that the criteria should not include an age limit for age of onset.[6] Although symptoms are typically delayed, data from OFCs indicate that vomiting may begin as early as 30 minutes, so a delay in symptoms should not be a requirement for diagnosis either. Minor criteria could include pallor, lethargy, hypotension (typically present only in a subpopulation), and positive stool studies, as diarrhea is not as common in acute FPIES as previously thought.[6]

Delay in Diagnosis

Delays in diagnosis were common in most cohorts, and awareness is still lacking.[2–6,8] In a recent survey of general pediatricians, 24% had never heard of FPIES.[34] The likely reasons for this are the: (1) absence of a diagnostic test; (2) delay in onset of symptoms; (3) absence of classic allergy symptoms, such as rash or respiratory distress; and (4) low index of suspicion for grains and vegetables, which are typically considered hypoallergenic.[6]

The median number of FPIES reactions before diagnosis in several cohorts was 2 to 3 (range, 1–10).[3,4,7,11,14] Unfortunately, the mean number of reactions before diagnosis did not change over 7 years in the cohort of Sopo and colleagues.[3] A median delay in diagnosis of 4 to 7 months has been reported.[6,8] In the study by Ludman and colleagues,[8] subjects presented a mean of 2 times (range, 1–10) before an allergy or gastrointestinal referral was made. Sopo and colleagues[3] reported that 60% of their subjects were self-referred, 30% were referred by a general pediatrician, and 10% were referred by a general practitioner.

Seventy-three percent of general pediatricians in the survey conducted by Menon and colleagues[34] reported having FPIES patients in their practice, and 39% reported managing FPIES by themselves. Management included oral steroids and oral rehydration at home followed by evaluation in the ED, while 29% prescribed an epinephrine autoinjector. Similarly, 11% of FPIES patients discharged from the ED in one cohort

Table 5
Proposed old and new FPIES diagnostic criteria for acute reactions

Powell Criteria[31]	New Proposed Criteria
<9 mo at initial reaction	Major Criteria
Exposure to food elicits repetitive vomiting and/or diarrhea within 4 h without any other cause for symptoms	1. Repetitive vomiting or diarrhea within 6 h of food ingestion
Symptoms are limited to gastrointestinal tract	2. Absence of cutaneous and respiratory symptoms suggestive of an IgE-mediated allergy
Avoidance of the offending protein from the diet results in resolution of symptoms	3. Removal of causative food results in resolution of symptoms
Reexposure or a food challenge elicits the typical symptoms	4. Reexposure or a food challenge elicits the typical symptoms
	Minor Criteria
	a. Hypotension
	b. Lethargy, pallor, or hypotonia
	c. Negative skin-prick test and undetectable specific IgE level
	d. Absence of fever or hypothermia (<36°C)

were prescribed epinephrine autoinjectors,[4] and in a parent survey by Green and colleagues,[19] 14% reported carrying epinephrine autoinjectors for FPIES.

Differential Diagnosis and Misdiagnosis

Patients presenting with FPIES symptoms are often misdiagnosed with IgE-mediated food allergy, surgical abnormalities (eg, intussusception, malrotation, obstruction, volvulus), viral gastroenteritis, or sepsis.[4,8] In the study by Mehr and colleagues,[4] only 2 of 19 patients presenting to the ED were correctly diagnosed with FPIES. Workups have included abdominal imaging (eg, radiography, barium, ultrasonography), septic evaluation (eg, complete blood count, blood culture, chest radiograph, lumbar puncture), surgical consult, electrocardiogram, echocardiogram, Holter monitoring, brain MRI, electroencephalography, and urine metabolic screening.[4] Some evaluations have even been invasive, such as intestinal biopsies and laparotomies.[4,11,35,36] The treatment of patients presenting to the ED with FPIES have included IVF, antibiotics, oxygen, air or barium enema, and intravenous epinephrine.[4]

TREATMENT AND MANAGEMENT

OFCs may be used to assess for disease resolution, if multiple foods were ingested and the trigger food is not known, or to assess whether a food can safely be introduced in light of the high rate of multiple triggers. To decrease the need for OFCs, Sopo and colleagues[3] proposed that patients with 2 or more severe reactions be diagnosed clinically. Although OFCs to foods that were being avoided by way of precaution may seem low risk, 11% were positive in one cohort.[6]

Several investigators recommend that OFCs to food triggers be done under medical supervision, regardless of food.[6] Up to 33% of positive OFCs may require emergency treatment.[14] Ruiz-García and colleagues[11] reported one FPIES patient who was treated in the intensive care unit for severe dehydration, hypotension, and loss of consciousness after a fish OFC. Caubet and colleagues[6] reported 14 severe reactions (19%) with hypotension during OFCs to CM, soy, oat, and wheat. These investigators also reported that 20% of subjects with positive OFCs reported a history of tolerating a small amount of the trigger food. Furthermore, severity of reactions did not correlate with severity of reported reactions, gender, age, food, previous hospitalization due to FPIES, detectable sIgE level to trigger food, or sIgE levels to other foods.[6]

By contrast, some investigators have reported successful oral hydration after positive OFCs without significant hypotension.[2,14] Sopo and colleagues[3] reported 9 subjects who were reintroduced to the food at home by parents at a median 20 months after last FPIES reaction (range, 19–24 months). Over three years of follow-up, Caubet and colleagues[6] reported 11 patients (32%) who successfully reintroduced foods at home. In a parent survey, more than half of the cohort (n = 263) underwent home challenge for initial reintroduction.[19]

Several protocols for FPIES OFCs exist at different centers.[2,3,6] It is recommended that full resuscitation facilities be available, particularly for rapid IVF repletion. Patients are typically treated with IVF; a single dose of intravenous methylprednisolone can be used for more severe reactions, based on the presumed inflammatory pathophysiology.[6] Monitoring for 3 to 4 hours after ingestion is warranted, owing to the delayed nature of symptoms.[5] The time to onset of symptoms after ingestion may vary with the amount ingested during OFCs, but usually vomiting starts within 1 to 4 hours.[2,6] Often two equal doses are given over 30 minutes, so it is difficult to know which dose was the eliciting dose.[2] Forty percent of subjects in one cohort with symptom onset of less than 120 minutes had detectable sIgE to the trigger food.[6] If patients have a positive

SPT or detectable sIgE to trigger foods, the OFC procedure should be modified to a more incremental and gradual administration of challenge doses, as per the protocol for IgE-mediated food allergy, and preparation for IgE-mediated reactions must also be considered.

Recently, ondansetron has been reported to successfully shorten the duration of FPIES reactions. Holbrook and colleagues[37] reported that the use of intravenous ondansetron for positive OFCs in patients older than 3 years resolved symptoms within 10 to 15 minutes. One patient received oral ondansetron initially with mild improvement, followed by an intravenous dose with complete resolution. A second case series has reported resolution of symptoms within 15 minutes with the use of intramuscular ondansetron in 5 patients (4 of whom were <3 years old).[3] Empirically, liquid oral ondansetron has been used for reactions at home, resulting in resolution of symptoms (Leonard, personal communication, 2014). It is still advised that patients seek medical attention for FPIES reactions, even if ondansetron is used.

Close follow-up of young children with FPIES is advised to monitor for additional reactions and to assess for tolerance. Most investigators suggest a minimum of 12 months since the last FPIES reaction before considering an OFC to check for resolution.[3,5,8,14] Ruffner and colleagues[5] report normally waiting 18 months. SPT and sIgE levels are recommended at diagnosis and follow-up because those with positive testing tend to have a more protracted course, and the possibility of IgE-mediated reactions should be assessed before an OFC is performed.

Anticipatory Guidance

Patients should be warned of the possibility of multiple triggers. Owing to the high rate of simultaneous CM and soy FPIES in United States cohorts, Ruffner and colleagues[5] and Caubet and colleagues[6] do not recommend that infants with CM FPIES ingest soy at home. Breastfeeding is encouraged in these cases, or the use of extensively hydrolyzed casein or elemental formula is recommended.[1,6] If needed, tolerance of soy formula in a child with CM FPIES should be assessed by OFC. Cohorts from Australia, Italy, and Israel report a much lower rate of simultaneous CM and soy FPIES in infants, suggesting that soy may be an alternative for patients with CM FPIES in these countries.[2–4]

Extended dietary restrictions have been suggested for infants with FPIES for higher-risk foods such as CM, soy, grains, legumes, and poultry.[38] The theory is that delaying other common FPIES triggers might avoid sensitization/reactions to additional foods during a possible period of developmental susceptibility during infancy.[6] Because of the high rate of FPIES to multiple grains in infants, Caubet and colleagues[6] recommend delaying other grains until 1 year of age. With data from larger cohorts showing low rates of solid food FPIES, some investigators do not recommend precautionary avoidance. Fewer than 25% of CM FPIES subjects reacted to other foods besides soy in the cohort of Ruffner and colleagues,[5] leading the investigators to suggest that other foods can be introduced. Sopo and colleagues[3] recommend OFCs for the initial introduction of CM, grains, legumes, and poultry only in infants with solid food FPIES; otherwise, no restrictions on solid foods in CM or soy FPIES were recommended. In general, dietary advice should take into consideration sufficient nutritional intake to maintain and ensure growth and development.[39]

Natural Course

The reported rates of FPIES resolution for different foods are listed in **Table 6**. The differences across populations are likely explained by having more subjects with positive IgE testing, the increased prevalence of other atopic diseases at major

Table 6
Rates of FPIES resolution by cohort population

Cow's Milk	Soy	Grains	Meat/Fish
South Korea[10]: >60% by 10 mo	South Korea[10]: >90% by 10 mo	Australia[4]: 80% rice by 3 y	USA[6]: 50% meat by 5 y
Italy[3]: 63% by 24 mo	Israel[4]: 83% by 3 y	USA[6]: 66% grain by 5 y	USA[6]: 0% fish by 5 y
Israel[2]: 94% by 3 y	USA[6]: 20% by 3 y		
USA[6]: 20% by 3 y			

referral centers, and differences in methodologies.[6] Resolution of solid food FPIES appears later in some cohorts, while other cohorts show no difference in resolution between CM/soy and solid food.[5,11] Sopo and colleagues[3] reported CM tolerance at a mean age of 24 months (±8 months) compared with solid food tolerance at a mean age of 53 months (±17 months). Alternatively, Caubet and colleagues[6] reported tolerance at a median age of 4.7 years for rice, 4 years for oats, 6.7 years for soy, and 5.1 years for CM (without detectable CM-sIgE level). No subjects with detectable CM-sIgE level became tolerant during the study. Ruffner and colleagues[5] reported an overall FPIES resolution of 85% by age 5 years, and in 2 subjects, FPIES persisted into adolescence. Adult FPIES seems to persist for many years. In the cohort of Tan and Smith,[7] no resolution was observed in patients who all continued to avoid their trigger foods, but many had accidental ingestions and reactions at intervals of up to 30 years.

SUMMARY

FPIES continues to be an underrecognized condition of food allergy. Repetitive vomiting after causative food ingestion remains the predominant feature. The addition of larger cohort descriptions has improved our understanding of varied presentations of FPIES, particularly with respect to food triggers. Milk, soy, rice, and oats are the most common FPIES triggers in United States cohorts, while fish and egg have been identified as common triggers in other cohorts. FPIES is most often diagnosed in infants and resolves by school age; however it may present at any age and persist into adolescence or adulthood. Further study into the prevalence, pathophysiology, and natural course of FPIES is still needed.

REFERENCES

1. Leonard SA, Nowak-Wegrzyn A. Clinical diagnosis and management of food protein-induced enterocolitis syndrome. Curr Opin Pediatr 2012;24:739–45.
2. Katz Y, Goldberg MR, Rajuan N, et al. The prevalence and natural course of food protein-induced enterocolitis syndrome to cow's milk: a large-scale, prospective population-based study. J Allergy Clin Immunol 2011;127:647–53.e1–3.
3. Sopo SM, Giorgio V, Dello Iacono I, et al. A multicentre retrospective study of 66 Italian children with food protein-induced enterocolitis syndrome: different management for different phenotypes. Clin Exp Allergy 2012;42:1257–65.
4. Mehr S, Kakakios A, Frith K, et al. Food protein-induced enterocolitis syndrome: 16-year experience. Pediatrics 2009;123:e459–64.
5. Ruffner MA, Ruymann K, Barni S, et al. Food protein-induced enterocolitis syndrome: insights from review of a large referral population. J Allergy Clin Immunol Pract 2013;1:343–9.

6. Caubet JC, Ford LS, Sickles L, et al. Clinical features and resolution of food protein-induced enterocolitis syndrome: 10-year experience. J Allergy Clin Immunol 2014;134:382–9.

7. Tan JA, Smith WB. Non-IgE-mediated gastrointestinal food hypersensitivity syndrome in adults. J Allergy Clin Immunol Pract 2014;2:355–7.e1.

8. Ludman S, Harmon M, Whiting D, et al. Clinical presentation and referral characteristics of food protein-induced enterocolitis syndrome in the United Kingdom. Ann Allergy Asthma Immunol 2014;113:290–4.

9. Fernandes BN, Boyle RJ, Gore C, et al. Food protein-induced enterocolitis syndrome can occur in adults. J Allergy Clin Immunol 2012;130:1199–200.

10. Hwang J-B, Sohn SM, Kim AS. Prospective follow-up oral food challenge in food protein-induced enterocolitis syndrome. Arch Dis Child 2009;94:425–8.

11. Ruiz-García M, Díez CE, García SS, et al. Diagnosis and natural history of food protein-induced enterocolitis syndrome in children from a tertiary hospital in central Spain. J Investig Allergol Clin Immunol 2014;24:354–6.

12. Mane S, Hollister M, Bahna SL. Food protein-induced enterocolitis syndrome to trivial oral mucosal contact. Eur J Pediatr 2014;173:1545–7.

13. Bansal AS, Bhaskaran S, Bansal RA. Four infants presenting with severe vomiting in solid food protein-induced enterocolitis syndrome: a case series. J Med Case Rep 2012;6:160.

14. Zapatero Remón L, Alonso Lebrero E, Martín Fernández E, et al. Food-protein-induced enterocolitis syndrome caused by fish. Allergol Immunopathol (Madr) 2005;33:312–6.

15. Monti G, Castagno E, Liguori SA, et al. Food protein-induced enterocolitis syndrome by cow's milk proteins passed through breast milk. J Allergy Clin Immunol 2011;127:679–80.

16. Nomura I, Morita H, Hosokawa S, et al. Four distinct subtypes of non-IgE-mediated gastrointestinal food allergies in neonates and infants, distinguished by their initial symptoms. J Allergy Clin Immunol 2011;127:685–8.e1–8.

17. Tan J, Campbell D, Mehr S. Food protein-induced enterocolitis syndrome in an exclusively breast-fed infant—an uncommon entity. J Allergy Clin Immunol 2012;129:873 [author reply: 4].

18. Lake AM. Food-induced eosinophilic proctocolitis. J Pediatr Gastroenterol Nutr 2000;30(Suppl I):S58–60.

19. Green TD, Greenhawt MJ, Jacobs TS, et al. Clinical features, diagnosis, management and natural history of food protein-induced enterocolitis syndrome in a national cohort. J Allergy Clin Immunol 2014;133:AB213.

20. Mehr S, Kakakios A, Kemp A. Rice: a common and severe cause of food protein-induced enterocolitis syndrome. Arch Dis Child 2009;94:220–3.

21. Hsu P, Mehr S. Egg: a frequent trigger of food protein-induced enterocolitis syndrome. J Allergy Clin Immunol 2013;131:241–2.

22. Federly TJ, Ryan P, Dinakar C. Food protein-induced enterocolitis syndrome triggered by orange juice. Ann Allergy Asthma Immunol 2012;109:472–3.

23. Serafini S, Bergmann MM, Nowak-Węgrzyn A, et al. A case of food protein-induced enterocolitis syndrome to mushrooms challenging currently used diagnostic criteria. J Allergy Clin Immunol Pract 2015;3(1):135–7.

24. Arik Yilmaz E, Cavkaytar O, Uysal Soyer O, et al. Egg yolk: an unusual trigger of food protein-induced enterocolitis syndrome. Pediatr Allergy Immunol 2013;25:296–7.

25. Miceli Sopo S, Buonsenso D, Monaco S, et al. Food protein-induced enterocolitis syndrome (FPIES) and well cooked foods: a working hypothesis. Allergol Immunopathol (Madr) 2013;41:346–8.

26. Yasutomi M, Kosaka T, Kawakita A, et al. Rice protein-induced enterocolitis syndrome with transient specific IgE to boiled rice but not to retort-processed rice. Pediatr Int 2014;56:110–2.
27. Onesimo R, Dello Iacono I, Giorgio V, et al. Can food protein induced enterocolitis syndrome shift to immediate gastrointestinal hypersensitivity? A report of two cases. Eur Ann Allergy Clin Immunol 2011;43:61–3.
28. Banzato C, Piacentini GL, Comberiati P, et al. Unusual shift from IgE-mediated milk allergy to food protein-induced enterocolitis syndrome. Eur Ann Allergy Clin Immunol 2013;45:209–11.
29. Fogg MI, Brown-Whitehorn TA, Pawlowski NA, et al. Atopy patch test for the diagnosis of food protein-induced enterocolitis syndrome. Pediatr Allergy Immunol 2006;17:351–5.
30. Järvinen KM, Nowak-Węgrzyn A. Food protein-induced enterocolitis syndrome (FPIES): current management strategies and review of the literature. J Allergy Clin Immunol Pract 2013;1:317–22.
31. Powell GK. Food protein-induced enterocolitis of infancy: differential diagnosis and management. Compr Ther 1986;12:28–37.
32. Hwang JB, Song JY, Kang YN, et al. The significance of gastric juice analysis for a positive challenge by a standard oral challenge test in typical cow's milk protein-induced enterocolitis. J Korean Med Sci 2008;23:251–5.
33. Boyce JA, Assa'ad A, Burks AW, et al. Guidelines for the diagnosis and management of food allergy in the United States: report of the NIAID-sponsored expert panel. J Allergy Clin Immunol 2010;126:S1–58.
34. Menon N, Feuille E, Huang F, et al. Knowledge of food protein-induced enterocolitis (FPIES) among general pediatricians. J Allergy Clin Immunol 2013;131: AB177.
35. Ikola RA. Severe intestinal reaction following ingestion of rice. Am J Dis Child 1963;105:281–4.
36. Jayasooriya S, Fox AT, Murch SH. Do not laparotomize food-protein-induced enterocolitis syndrome. Pediatr Emerg Care 2007;23:173–5.
37. Holbrook T, Keet CA, Frischmeyer-Guerrerio PA, et al. Use of ondansetron for food protein-induced enterocolitis syndrome. J Allergy Clin Immunol 2013;132: 1219–20.
38. Sicherer SH. Food protein-induced enterocolitis syndrome: case presentations and management lessons. J Allergy Clin Immunol 2005;115:149–56.
39. Venter C, Groetch M. Nutritional management of food protein-induced enterocolitis syndrome. Curr Opin Allergy Clin Immunol 2014;14(3):255–62.

Gut Microbiome and the Development of Food Allergy and Allergic Disease

 CrossMark

Benjamin T. Prince, MD[a,b], Mark J. Mandel, PhD[c],
Kari Nadeau, MD, PhD[d], Anne Marie Singh, MD[a,b,*]

KEYWORDS

- Microbiome • Gut microbiota • Commensal flora • Food allergy • Asthma
- Allergic rhinitis • Eczema • Allergic disease

KEY POINTS

- Early microbial colonization plays an important role in the development of the innate and the adaptive immune systems, and there are several proposed mechanisms to explain how alterations in microbiome could lead to the development of allergic disease.
- Although some studies have identified notable relationships between the gastrointestinal microbiota and the development of asthma, allergic rhinitis, and eczema, specific studies examining the microbiome in human food allergy are lacking.
- As technology and knowledge of the microbiome advances, discoveries in food allergy and atopic disease will likely provide insight into primary prevention and treatment strategies.

INTRODUCTION

Food allergy, defined as an adverse, immune-mediated reaction to a food that is reproducible on a subsequent exposure,[1] affects nearly 5% of all adults[2] and up to 8% of children in the United States.[3] Recent data from the US Centers for Disease Control and Prevention have found that the prevalence among children 0 to 17 years increased by 50% from 1999 to 2011.[4] Even before this increase in prevalence, food

Conflicts of Interest/Corporate Sponsors: None.
[a] Division of Allergy and Immunology, Department of Pediatrics, Ann & Robert H. Lurie Children's Hospital of Chicago, Northwestern University, 225 East Chicago Avenue, #60, Chicago, IL 60611, USA; [b] Division of Allergy and Immunology, Department of Medicine, Northwestern Feinberg School of Medicine, Northwestern University, 225 East Chicago Avenue, #60, Chicago, IL 60611, USA; [c] Department of Microbiology-Immunology, Northwestern Feinberg School of Medicine, Northwestern University, Searle Building 3-403, 320 E. Superior Street, Chicago, IL 60611, USA; [d] Division of Allergy, Immunology, and Rheumatology, Department of Pediatrics, Stanford University School of Medicine, 730 Welch Rd, Stanford, CA 94305, USA
* Corresponding author. Department of Allergy and Immunology, Ann & Robert H. Lurie Children's Hospital of Chicago, Northwestern University, 225 East Chicago Avenue, #60, Chicago, IL 60611.
E-mail address: anne-singh@northwestern.edu

Pediatr Clin N Am 62 (2015) 1479–1492
http://dx.doi.org/10.1016/j.pcl.2015.07.007
0031-3955/15/$ – see front matter © 2015 Elsevier Inc. All rights reserved.
pediatric.theclinics.com

allergies were the leading cause of anaphylaxis in patients presenting to the emergency department in the United States.[5] Studies have also shown that a diagnosis of food allergy results in a significantly lower quality of life.[6–8] Despite the increase in prevalence, the life-threatening potential, and the disease burden of food allergies, the cause of this epidemic remains elusive.

One of the leading theories to explain this modern day allergy epidemic was introduced by Strachan[9] in 1989 as the hygiene hypothesis. In his hypothesis, Strachan proposed that a larger family size was protective against allergic disease because of early life exposure to sibling infections.[9] However, since its introduction, others have revisited this idea, suggesting that changes in early life viral and bacterial exposures and intestinal colonization patterns in western countries have contributed to the failure to induce and maintain tolerance, a state of unresponsiveness to harmless antigens.[10,11]

THE HUMAN MICROBIOME

It has been estimated that the human gut is populated with up to 100 trillion microbes.[12] Rough estimates are that the microbiota (previously termed flora or microflora) contain on the order of 150-fold more genes than are encoded in the human genome.[13] The ancient symbiotic relationship between multicellular animals and resident microbes has shaped the evolution of the immune system into its present state.[14] Although the composition of the microbiota changes substantially from infancy to adulthood, most organisms come from the four phyla Actinobacteria, Bacteroidetes, Firmicutes, and Proteobacteria.[15]

The advent of high-throughput DNA deep sequencing technologies has revolutionized the ability to characterize microbial diversity and compare this diversity across organs and individuals. Sequencing of diagnostic regions of the 16S rRNA gene sequence provides a robust method to identify the bacteria present in a sample. Because clinical samples can be sequenced directly, organisms are identified even if they cannot yet be cultured, and the resulting 16S rRNA sequence provides a reference for known bacterial taxa (ie, species) and for novel ones.[16,17] This bacterial census provides information on specific taxa that are present; loss of specific taxa and alterations in the community structure are associated with disease progression (eg, infection by *Clostridium difficile*).[18] Beyond 16S data, genome sequencing from microbial communities (ie, metagenomics) can enable functional studies, identify gene categories that influence the host, and reveal conservation at the level of gene function even in cases where those genes are derived from unrelated organisms.[19,20] Much current work is aimed at extending these techniques to understand gene expression at the RNA (transcriptional profiling) and protein (proteomics) levels, and to understand how microbial communities affect the flux of metabolites (metabolomics) in the host.[21]

THE MICROBIOME AND IMMUNE DEVELOPMENT

Early microbial colonization plays an important role the development of the innate and the adaptive immune systems,[22] and there are several proposed mechanisms to explain how alterations in microbiome could lead to the development of allergic disease. Experimental, germ-free (gnotobiotic) mouse models have demonstrated that gut-associated lymphoid tissues fail to develop when microbial colonization is delayed, leading to a Th2 skewed immune response.[23] Secretory IgA produced by resident B cells in gut-associated lymphoid tissues may also promote oral tolerance by binding allergens in the gut and preventing their uptake.[24] Microbial colonization has been shown to be important in the development of Th1[25,26] and regulatory

T cells (Tregs),[27–31] which are necessary to maintain immunologic balance and promote tolerance. Microbiota may also influence epigenetic modifications of genes. It is known that various forms of epigenetic changes, such as DNA methylation and histone modifications, play an important role in immune development and regulation,[32] and microbial metabolites butyrate and propionate have been shown to have inhibitory effects on histone deacetylases that may promote the development of peripherally induced Tregs.[33,34] Lastly, the gut microbiota plays a significant role in the development and maintenance of barrier function[35,36] and it is thought that a breakdown of this epithelial barrier may lead to allergic sensitization.[37,38]

The impact of the microbiome on human development, nutritional needs, and even psychological variations has become evident with advances in the ability to study these complex communities of microorganisms.[39,40] There is also a growing appreciation for the role of the microbiome in immune regulation, and it is plausible that changes in the commensal microbiota may influence the development of food allergy and other allergic diseases.[36] When considering various determinants that may influence the unique bacterial families that constitute the microbiome, there are several factors to consider, including environmental setting, mode of delivery, birth order, antibiotic exposure, and diet.[41] This article explores the relationship between the gastrointestinal microbiota and IgE-mediated food allergy and other allergic diseases.

THE INFLUENCE OF THE MICROBIOME IN ALLERGIC DISEASE

The potential impact of the microbiome on allergic disease was first studied in Europe using cross-sectional surveys to examine the prevalence of allergic diseases in children. The authors found that children living in farming environments had a significantly decreased frequency of hay fever, asthma, and eczema compared with children living in urban areas.[42,43] This relationship was further explored in the GABRIELA and PARSIFAL cohorts, which confirmed previous observations that children living on farms had decreased rates of allergic disease compared with urban children.[44,45] Although most studies have focused on the impact of postnatal environmental exposure, there is increasing evidence that prenatal exposure may also be important.[46–48] Epidemiologic studies examining the effect of prenatal exposures on the development of allergic disease have shown that maternal exposure to farming environments during pregnancy is associated with decreased rates of asthma, allergic rhinitis, and eczema in their children.[49,50]

Animal Exposure

Recent studies suggest that the protective association between farming and the development of allergic disease may be caused by differences in microbial exposure. Using single-strand conformational polymorphism DNA analysis to examine house dust in the same GABRIELA and PARSIFAL cohorts, Ege and colleagues[51] found that the diversity of microbial exposure was inversely associated with the prevalence of asthma even after controlling for farming status. Moreover, investigators examining the gut microbiota in children using 16S rDNA sequencing have shown that decreased microbial diversity early in life is associated with the development of asthma,[52] allergic rhinitis,[53] and atopic dermatitis.[54] Similarly, pet ownership has also been shown to increase the diversity of the microbial composition of house dust[55] and infant fecal samples,[56] and early life pet ownership has been associated with a decreased risk for asthma and other atopic diseases.[57–59] Specifically, several studies have shown that infants who develop allergic disease later in life tended to have less bacteroides, bifidobacteria, and enterococci, but more clostridiae comprising their microbiome early in life (**Table 1**).[54,60–62] It seems that a diverse microbial exposure perinatally and early in life modifies the innate[49] and adaptive[63] immune system resulting in a significantly decreased risk of allergic disease.

Mode of Delivery

Another factor that has been implicated in altering the human microbiome is birth by cesarean section. Instead of traveling through the birth canal where colonization by maternal microbiota would typically occur, the baby is delivered through a sterile surface.[64] Subsequently, delivery by cesarean section has been shown to delay the development of the gut microbiota and shape its colonization to patterns similar to the maternal skin.[65] Studies examining the impact of this difference in microbiome and the development of allergic disease have found that children born by cesarean section had decreased microbial diversity and reduced Th1 responses during the first 2 years of life.[26] Other studies have shown an association between cesarean section delivery and the development of asthma, allergic rhinitis, and eczema.[62,66–68] Specifically, the microbiome of babies born by cesarean section showed a reduced abundance of *Bacteroides*, bifidobacteria, and *Escherichia coli* but increased amounts of *Klebsiella*, *Enterobacter*, *Enterococcus*, and clostridia (see **Table 1**).[26,62,69,70]

Birth Order and Family Size

An observation that infants with higher numbers of siblings had a decreased incidence of allergic disease was one driving principle behind Strachan's[9] proposal of the initial hygiene hypothesis. Since then, several studies have reproduced the inverse relationship between sibling number and asthma, allergic rhinitis, and eczema.[71] This association was initially thought to arise from an increased exposure to infections during childhood. There is now evidence that birth order and family size may also mediate their protective effects through alterations in the gut microbiome.[70] Penders and colleagues[70] showed that infants with an increased number of older siblings had

Table 1
Summary of various early life environmental exposures and specific gut microbiota associated with the development of allergic disease

Exposure	Bacteria	Risk
Less animal exposure	↓ Bacteroides, bifidobacteria, and enterococci ↑ Clostridiae	↑ Asthma, allergic rhinitis, and eczema +/− Food allergy
Delivery by cesarean section	↓ Bacteroides, bifidobacteria, and *Escherichia coli* ↑ *Klebsiella*, *Enterobacter*, *Enterococcus*	↑ Asthma, allergic rhinitis, and eczema +/− Food allergy
Decreased siblingship	↑ Clostridia, lactobacillus, and bacteroides	↑ Eczema (clostridia) ? Asthma, allergic rhinitis, and food allergy
Perinatal antibiotic use	↓ Bifidobacteria and lactobacillus ↑ Proteobacteria and Enterobacteriaceae	↑ Asthma and eczema +/− Food allergy − Allergic rhinitis
Bottle feeding	↓ Staphylococcus ↑ *Clostridium difficile*, bacteroides, enterococci, and Enterobacteriaceae	↑ Asthma and eczema (high-risk patients) +/− Food allergy and allergic rhinitis

decreased colonization rates of clostridia and increased rates of *Lactobacillus* and *Bacteroides*. Moreover, colonization with clostridia was associated with an increased risk of developing atopic dermatitis (see **Table 1**).

Antibiotic Exposure

It is well known that early life antibiotic exposure can influence an infant's microbiome. Data from a population-based study done by the Centers for Disease Control and Prevention from 2003 to 2004 reported that 32% of laboring women received intrapartum antibiotics for group B *Streptococcus* infection prevention, maternal pyrexia, prematurity, and other factors.[72] One of the most frequent reasons for early antibiotic use is prematurity, and it has been shown that bacterial microbiota colonization can be delayed in children who have a prolonged neonatal hospital course.[73] Studies using quantitative polymerase chain reaction and 16S rRNA sequencing to specifically examine microbiome changes in preterm infants as a result of perinatal antibiotic exposure have found that infants receiving antibiotics had a lower bacterial diversity and higher abundance of *Enterobacter*.[74,75] Similar studies on full-term infants receiving perinatal antibiotics also showed that antibiotic treatment as associated with less bacterial diversity along with higher proportions of Proteobacteria and Enterobacteriaceae and lower proportions of *Bifidobacterium* and *Lactobacillus* (see **Table 1**).[76,77] When considering the relationship between the development of allergic disease and early life antibiotic exposure, there seems to be an association between prenatal[78,79] and postnatal[79–81] antibiotic exposure and asthma. It should be noted, however, that many studies might be confounded by an increased treatment of respiratory infections at an early age when manifestations of asthma may be indistinguishable from infection.[82,83] There may also be an association between postnatal but not prenatal antibiotic exposure and the development of atopic dermatitis,[84] but a significant relationship between early life antibiotic use and allergic rhinitis has not been established.[85,86]

Diet

A final area that has been shown to have significant effects on the microbiome is diet.[87] One specific dietary aspect that has been extensively studied in regard to its effects on gut microbial composition and the development of allergic disease is bottle versus breastfeeding. It has been demonstrated that breast milk may contain small oligosaccharides that promote the colonization of beneficial bacteria, such as bifidobacteria.[88] Most studies over the last 30 years, however, have only shown minor differences in gut microbiota between breastfed and formula-fed infants.[69] One of the most reproducible differences between breastfed and formula-fed infants is that formula-fed infants have higher amounts of *C difficile* that make up their gut microbiome.[89–92] Some studies also suggest that bacteroides, enterococci, and Enterobacteriaceae may be more common in the microbiome of formula-fed infants, whereas staphylococci tend to be more prevalent in breastfed infants (see **Table 1**).[69] When evaluating the impact of breastfeeding on the development of allergic disease, breastfed infants seem to have a lower rate of early wheezing and asthma, but this affect seems to diminish with age.[93–96] Studies examining the association between breastfeeding and the development of allergic rhinitis and eczema have been inconclusive, although there may be a protective effect for eczema in high-risk infants.[95,97]

More generally, it is well known that westernized countries have a higher prevalence of allergic disease,[98] and modern western diets have been associated with differences in the gut microbiome.[87] Studies have also shown that differences in consumption of animal fat, carbohydrates, and fiber can cause changes in gut microbiota that can have profound affects on the immune system.[99,100] A recent study further demonstrated that microbial metabolism of dietary fiber and subsequent production of short-chain fatty acids influenced Th2 inflammation and allergic airway disease in mice.[101] Work directly addressing the influence of dietary factors and the development of allergic disease in humans, however, is lacking.

THE INFLUENCE OF THE MICROBIOME IN FOOD ALLERGY

In contrast to other allergic diseases, there is significantly less literature specifically evaluating the impact of the microbiome on the development of food allergy, and most studies have been done using mouse models. Gnotobiotic and antibiotic-treated mice that are reconstituted with well-characterized populations of gut microbiota can provide a particularly useful insight into the role that the microbiome plays in the maintenance of oral tolerance.[23,102,103]

Murine Models

One of the first studies investigating the impact of the gut microbiota on oral tolerance induction showed that gnotobiotic mice had Th2 skewing and increased interleukin (IL)-4 production with OVA challenge that was abrogated with intestinal microbiota reconstitution of the bacteria *Bifidobacterium infantis*.[23] The authors demonstrated that the *Bifidobacterium* reconstitution was only effective when performed during the neonatal period, but not in older mice suggesting that there may be a window of time during immune development when the commensal microbiota plays an important regulatory role.[23] In a similar gnotobiotic mouse model, antibiotic-treated mice were shown to have an increased susceptibility to peanut sensitization characterized by increased peanut-specific IgE and anaphylactic symptoms with peanut challenge.[102,103] Moreover, colonizing antibiotic-treated mice with a clostridia-enriched microbiota, which has been previously shown to induce colonic Tregs,[28,104] confers a food-allergy protective phenotype in an IL-22-dependent mechanism by affecting intestinal barrier function and reducing the amount of peanut allergen in the bloodstream after intragastric gavage.[103] Another study demonstrated that colonization of gnotobiotic mice with *Bifidobacterium* spp and *Bacteroides* spp from the fecal microbiota of healthy infants was protective in a mouse model of cow's milk allergy (CMA).[105] Commensal microbiota may also impact the development of food allergy through its activation of toll-like receptors (TLR) of intestinal epithelial cells.[106] TLR4-deficient mice have been shown to have a Th2 skewed immune response and an increased susceptibility to food allergy that is abrogated with a TLR9 ligand.[102] Furthermore, peripheral blood mononuclear cells from food-allergic patients were shown to have a negative effect on barrier function of intestinal epithelial cells in vitro that was prevented with TLR9 activation.[107] Finally, a specific microbiota signature was recently linked to mice carrying a gain-of-function mutation in the IL-4 receptor α chain that results in an increased susceptibility to oral allergic sensitization and anaphylaxis.[108] The authors demonstrate that germ-free, wild-type mice reconstituted with this microbiota rendered these animals more prone to developing food allergy.

Human Studies

There have been a few epidemiologic studies that have examined the relationship between environmental factors that are known to alter the gut microbiome and food allergy. One important aspect to consider in many of these studies is how the diagnosis of food allergy is established. Many studies rely on self-reported diagnosis of food allergy or evidence of IgE sensitization with either skin-prick testing or serology, which is notoriously inaccurate compared with the gold standard of oral food challenge (OFC).[109,110]

Mode of delivery has been the most widely studied environmental factor thought to contribute to the development of food allergy. Overall, there is evidence that cesarean section delivery increases the risk of developing IgE sensitization to food allergens,[111] but studies using OFC-proved food allergy have shown mixed results.[112–115] Although several studies have addressed the effect of farming environment and animal exposure on the development of other allergic diseases, far less have examined this environmental exposure and food allergy. In an Australian infant cohort of 5276 infants, Koplin and colleagues[115] found that the presence of a dog in the home was inversely associated with the diagnosis of egg allergy at 1 year of age (adjusted odds ratio, 0.72); however, this is the only study with OFC-confirmed food allergy and more research needs to be done.[116] The same authors used this infant cohort to also examine the influence of birth order on food allergy and found that children with older siblings had a significantly reduced risk of egg allergy at 1 year of age.[115] Similar results have been found in studies evaluating siblingship size and CMA.[114] Antibiotic exposure has shown conflicting results when assessed as a risk factor for developing food allergy. Although one study found that prenatal and postnatal antibiotic exposure was associated with an increased risk of CMA,[117] other studies have not demonstrated a statistically significant association.[112,115,118] A final area that has been evaluated in association with the development of food allergy is bottle versus breastfeeding. Aside from the fact that many studies that have examined this relationship rely on the presence of sensitization as a marker for food allergy, another obstacle in interpreting this literature is that the extent and duration of breastfeeding varies substantially between studies. Considering these limitations, there are insufficient data at this time to suggest whether breastfeeding is a protective factor in the development of food allergy.[95,119,120]

Only a few studies have assessed the specific microbiota within the human gut that have been associated with the development of food allergy. Using conventional culturing techniques, a Spanish cohort of 46 patients with CMA demonstrated a greater total bacterial count and more anaerobes in the feces of patients with allergy at diagnosis compared with matched control subjects, but no difference in the percentage of bacterial species.[121] In a follow-up study of the same patient cohort, the authors better characterize the fecal microbiota using 10 fluorescent in situ hybridization and find that CMA patients had significantly more *Clostridium coccoides* and *Atopobium* cluster species compared with control subject without allergy, but there were no differences in *Bifidobacteria*, *Lactobacillus*, or *Bacteroides* genera.[122] Using 16SrRNA sequencing, a separate study found increased levels of *Clostridium sensu stricto* and *Anaerobacter* but decreased levels of *Bacteroides* and *Clostridium* XVIII in the feces of 17 Chinese infants with IgE-mediated food allergy.[123] Finally, using 16S rRNA sequencing to examine the gut microbiota in a cohort of Canadian infants, Azad and colleagues[124] showed that the 12 infants with food sensitization on skin prick testing had increased amounts of Enterobacteriaceae and less Bacteroidaceae in their feces.

SUMMARY

Early microbial colonization plays an important role the development of the innate and the adaptive immune systems, and there are several proposed mechanisms to explain how alterations in microbiome could lead to the development of allergic disease. Although some studies have identified notable relationships between the gastrointestinal microbiota and the development of asthma, allergic rhinitis, and eczema, specific studies examining the microbiome in human food allergy are lacking. Animal models suggest that the microbiome, particularly early in life, may play a crucial role in the susceptibility to food sensitization and food allergy; however, more work is required to confirm these findings. As technology and knowledge of the microbiome advances, discoveries in food allergy and atopic disease will likely provide insight into primary prevention and treatment strategies.

REFERENCES

1. NIAID-Sponsored Expert Panel, Boyce JA, Assa'ad A, et al. Guidelines for the diagnosis and management of food allergy in the United States: report of the NIAID-sponsored expert panel. J Allergy Clin Immunol 2010;126:S1–58.
2. Sicherer SH, Sampson HA. Food allergy: epidemiology, pathogenesis, diagnosis, and treatment. J Allergy Clin Immunol 2014;133(2):291–307.e5.
3. Gupta RS, Springston EE, Warrier MR, et al. The prevalence, severity, and distribution of childhood food allergy in the United States. Pediatrics 2011;128(1): e9–17.
4. Jackson KD, Howie LD, Akinbami LJ. Trends in allergic conditions among children: United States, 1997-2011. NCHS Data Brief 2013;(121):1–8.
5. Yocum MW, Khan DA. Assessment of patients who have experienced anaphylaxis: a 3-year survey. Mayo Clin Proc 1994;69(1):16–23.
6. Lieberman JA, Sicherer SH. Quality of life in food allergy. Curr Opin Allergy Clin Immunol 2011;11(3):236–42.
7. Flokstra-de Blok BMJ, Dubois AEJ, Vlieg-Boerstra BJ, et al. Health-related quality of life of food allergic patients: comparison with the general population and other diseases. Allergy 2010;65(2):238–44.
8. Shemesh E, Annunziato RA, Ambrose MA, et al. Child and parental reports of bullying in a consecutive sample of children with food allergy. Pediatrics 2013;131(1):e10–7.
9. Strachan DP. Hay fever, hygiene, and household size. BMJ 1989;299(6710): 1259–60.
10. Wold AE. The hygiene hypoteslis revised: is the rising frequency of allergy due to changes in the intestinal flora? Allergy 1998;53(Suppl 46):20–5.
11. Mutius von E. Allergies, infections and the hygiene hypothesis: the epidemiological evidence. Immunobiology 2007;212(6):433–9.
12. Ley RE, Peterson DA, Gordon JI. Ecological and evolutionary forces shaping microbial diversity in the human intestine. Cell 2006;124(4):837–48.
13. Qin J, Li R, Raes J, et al. A human gut microbial gene catalogue established by metagenomic sequencing. Nature 2010;464(7285):59–65.
14. McFall-Ngai M, Hadfield MG, Bosch TC, et al. Animals in a bacterial world, a new imperative for the life sciences. Proc Natl Acad Sci 2013;110(9):3229–36.
15. Wopereis H, Oozeer R, Knipping K, et al. The first thousand days - intestinal microbiology of early life: establishing a symbiosis. Pediatr Allergy Immunol 2014;25(5):428–38.
16. Morgan XC, Huttenhower C. Human microbiome analysis. PLoS Comput Biol 2012;8(12):e1002808.
17. Ivanov II, Atarashi K, Manel N, et al. Induction of intestinal Th17 cells by segmented filamentous bacteria. Cell 2009;139(3):485–98.
18. Schubert AM, Rogers MAM, Ring C, et al. Microbiome data distinguish patients with *Clostridium difficile* infection and non-*C. difficile*-associated diarrhea from healthy controls. MBio 2014;5(3):e01021–010214.

19. Turnbaugh PJ, Hamady M, Yatsunenko T, et al. A core gut microbiome in obese and lean twins. Nature 2009;457(7228):480–4.
20. Hehemann J-H, Correc G, Barbeyron T, et al. Transfer of carbohydrate-active enzymes from marine bacteria to Japanese gut microbiota. Nature 2010; 464(7290):908–12.
21. Waldram A, Holmes E, Wang Y, et al. Top-down systems biology modeling of host metabotype-microbiome associations in obese rodents. J Proteome Res 2009;8(5):2361–75.
22. Renz H, Brandtzaeg P, Hornef M. The impact of perinatal immune development on mucosal homeostasis and chronic inflammation. Nat Rev Immunol 2012; 12(1):9–23.
23. Sudo N, Sawamura S, Tanaka K, et al. The requirement of intestinal bacterial flora for the development of an IgE production system fully susceptible to oral tolerance induction. J Immunol 1997;159(4):1739–45.
24. Berin MC. Mucosal antibodies in the regulation of tolerance and allergy to foods. Semin Immunopathol 2012;34(5):633–42.
25. Mazmanian SK, Liu CH, Tzianabos AO, et al. An immunomodulatory molecule of symbiotic bacteria directs maturation of the host immune system. Cell 2005; 122(1):107–18.
26. Jakobsson HE, Abrahamsson TR, Jenmalm MC, et al. Decreased gut microbiota diversity, delayed Bacteroidetes colonisation and reduced Th1 responses in infants delivered by caesarean section. Gut 2014;63(4):559–66.
27. Round JL, Mazmanian SK. Inducible Foxp3+ regulatory T-cell development by a commensal bacterium of the intestinal microbiota. Proc Natl Acad Sci 2010; 107(27):12204–9.
28. Atarashi K, Tanoue T, Shima T, et al. Induction of colonic regulatory T cells by indigenous *Clostridium* species. Science 2011;331(6015):337–41.
29. Geuking MB, Cahenzli J, Lawson MAE, et al. Intestinal bacterial colonization induces mutualistic regulatory T cell responses. Immunity 2011;34(5):794–806.
30. Lochner M, Bérard M, Sawa S, et al. Restricted microbiota and absence of cognate TCR antigen leads to an unbalanced generation of Th17 cells. J Immunol 2011;186(3):1531–7.
31. Smith PM, Howitt MR, Panikov N, et al. The microbial metabolites, short-chain fatty acids, regulate colonic Treg cell homeostasis. Science 2013;341(6145):569–73.
32. Obata Y, Furusawa Y, Hase K. Epigenetic modifications of the immune system in health and disease. Immunol Cell Biol 2015;93(3):226–32.
33. Arpaia N, Campbell C, Fan X, et al. Metabolites produced by commensal bacteria promote peripheral regulatory T-cell generation. Nature 2013;504(7480): 451–5.
34. Furusawa Y, Obata Y, Fukuda S, et al. Commensal microbe-derived butyrate induces the differentiation of colonic regulatory T cells. Nature 2013;504(7480): 446–50.
35. Kabat AM, Srinivasan N, Maloy KJ. Modulation of immune development and function by intestinal microbiota. Trends Immunol 2014;35(11):507–17.
36. Hooper LV, Littman DR, Macpherson AJ. Interactions between the microbiota and the immune system. Science 2012;336(6086):1268–73.
37. Kalliomäki M, Isolauri E. Role of intestinal flora in the development of allergy. Curr Opin Allergy Clin Immunol 2003;3(1):15–20.
38. Chahine BG, Bahna SL. The role of the gut mucosal immunity in the development of tolerance versus development of allergy to food. Curr Opin Allergy Clin Immunol 2010;10(4):394–9.

39. Yatsunenko T, Rey FE, Manary MJ, et al. Human gut microbiome viewed across age and geography. Nature 2012;486(7402):222–7.

40. Diaz Heijtz R, Wang S, Anuar F, et al. Normal gut microbiota modulates brain development and behavior. Proc Natl Acad Sci U S A 2011;108(7):3047–52.

41. Rook GAW, Raison CL, Lowry CA. Microbial "old friends," immunoregulation and socioeconomic status. Clin Exp Immunol 2014;177(1):1–12.

42. Ehrenstein Von OS, Mutius von E, Illi S, et al. Reduced risk of hay fever and asthma among children of farmers. Clin Exp Allergy 2000;30(2):187–93.

43. Riedler J, Braun-Fahrlander C, Eder W, et al. Exposure to farming in early life and development of asthma and allergy: a cross-sectional survey. Lancet 2001;358(9288):1129–33.

44. Alfven T, Braun-Fahrlander C, Brunekreef B, et al. Allergic diseases and atopic sensitization in children related to farming and anthroposophic lifestyle: the PARSIFAL study. Allergy 2006;61(4):414–21.

45. Genuneit J, Strachan DP, Büchele G, et al. The combined effects of family size and farm exposure on childhood hay fever and atopy. Pediatr Allergy Immunol 2013;24(3):293–8.

46. Jiménez E, Marín ML, Martín R, et al. Is meconium from healthy newborns actually sterile? Res Microbiol 2008;159(3):187–93.

47. DiGiulio DB, Romero R, Amogan HP, et al. Microbial prevalence, diversity and abundance in amniotic fluid during preterm labor: a molecular and culture-based investigation. PLoS One 2008;3(8):e3056.

48. Gosalbes MJ, Llop S, Vallès Y, et al. Meconium microbiota types dominated by lactic acid or enteric bacteria are differentially associated with maternal eczema and respiratory problems in infants. Clin Exp Allergy 2013;43(2):198–211.

49. Ege MJ, Bieli C, Frei R, et al. Prenatal farm exposure is related to the expression of receptors of the innate immunity and to atopic sensitization in school-age children. J Allergy Clin Immunol 2006;117(4):817–23.

50. Douwes J, Cheng S, Travier N, et al. Farm exposure in utero may protect against asthma, hay fever and eczema. Eur Respir J 2008;32(3):603–11.

51. Ege MJ, Mayer M, Normand AC, et al. Exposure to environmental microorganisms and childhood asthma. N Engl J Med 2011;364:701–9.

52. Abrahamsson TR, Jakobsson HE, Andersson AF, et al. Low gut microbiota diversity in early infancy precedes asthma at school age. Clin Exp Allergy 2014;44(6):842–50.

53. Bisgaard H, Li N, Bonnelykke K, et al. Reduced diversity of the intestinal microbiota during infancy is associated with increased risk of allergic disease at school age. J Allergy Clin Immunol 2011;128(3):646–52.e1–5.

54. Abrahamsson TR, Jakobsson HE, Andersson AF, et al. Low diversity of the gut microbiota in infants with atopic eczema. J Allergy Clin Immunol 2012;129(2):434–40, 440.e1–2.

55. Fujimura KE, Johnson CC, Ownby DR, et al. Man's best friend? The effect of pet ownership on house dust microbial communities. J Allergy Clin Immunol 2010;126(2):410–2, 412.e1–3.

56. Azad MB, Konya T, Maughan H, et al. Infant gut microbiota and the hygiene hypothesis of allergic disease: impact of household pets and siblings on microbiota composition and diversity. Allergy Asthma Clin Immunol 2013;9(1):15.

57. Ownby DR, Johnson CC, Peterson EL. Exposure to dogs and cats in the first year of life and risk of allergic sensitization at 6 to 7 years of age. JAMA 2002;288(8):963–72.

58. Litonjua AA, Milton DK, Celedón JC, et al. A longitudinal analysis of wheezing in young children: the independent effects of early life exposure to house dust endotoxin, allergens, and pets. J Allergy Clin Immunol 2002;110(5):736–42.

59. Wegienka G, Johnson CC, Havstad S, et al. Lifetime dog and cat exposure and dog- and cat-specific sensitization at age 18 years. Clin Exp Allergy 2011;41(7): 979–86.

60. Kalliomäki M, Kirjavainen P, Eerola E, et al. Distinct patterns of neonatal gut microflora in infants in whom atopy was and was not developing. J Allergy Clin Immunol 2001;107(1):129–34.

61. Bjorksten B, Sepp E, Julge K, et al. Allergy development and the intestinal microflora during the first year of life. J Allergy Clin Immunol 2001;108(4):516–20.

62. van Nimwegen FA, Penders J, Stobberingh EE, et al. Mode and place of delivery, gastrointestinal microbiota, and their influence on asthma and atopy. J Allergy Clin Immunol 2011;128(5):948–55.e1–3.

63. Stern DA, Riedler J, Nowak D, et al. Exposure to a farming environment has allergen-specific protective effects on TH2-dependent isotype switching in response to common inhalants. J Allergy Clin Immunol 2007;119(2):351–8.

64. Biasucci G, Rubini M, Riboni S, et al. Mode of delivery affects the bacterial community in the newborn gut. Early Hum Dev 2010;86(Suppl 1):13–5.

65. Dominguez-Bello MG, Costello EK, Contreras M, et al. Delivery mode shapes the acquisition and structure of the initial microbiota across multiple body habitats in newborns. Proc Natl Acad Sci 2010;107(26):11971–5.

66. Thavagnanam S, Fleming J, Bromley A, et al. A meta-analysis of the association between caesarean section and childhood asthma. Clin Exp Allergy 2008;38(4): 629–33.

67. Guibas GV, Moschonis G, Xepapadaki P, et al. Conception via in vitro fertilization and delivery by caesarean section are associated with paediatric asthma incidence. Clin Exp Allergy 2013;43(9):1058–66.

68. Pistiner M, Gold DR, Abdulkerim H, et al. Birth by cesarean section, allergic rhinitis, and allergic sensitization among children with a parental history of atopy. J Allergy Clin Immunol 2008;122(2):274–9.

69. Adlerberth I, Wold AE. Establishment of the gut microbiota in Western infants. Acta Paediatr 2009;98(2):229–38.

70. Penders J, Gerhold K, Stobberingh EE, et al. Establishment of the intestinal microbiota and its role for atopic dermatitis in early childhood. J Allergy Clin Immunol 2013;132(3):601–7.e8.

71. Karmaus W, Botezan C. Does a higher number of siblings protect against the development of allergy and asthma? A review. J Epidemiol Community Health 2002;56(3):209–17.

72. Verani JR, McGee L, Schrag SJ. Division of Bacterial Diseases, National Center for Immunization and Respiratory Diseases, Centers for Disease Control and Prevention (CDC). Prevention of perinatal group B streptococcal disease–revised guidelines from CDC, 2010. MMWR Recomm Rep 2010;59(RR-10):1–36.

73. Bennet R, Eriksson M, Nord CE, et al. Fecal bacterial microflora of newborn infants during intensive care management and treatment with five antibiotic regimens. Pediatr Infect Dis 1986;5(5):533–9.

74. Greenwood C, Morrow AL, Lagomarcino AJ, et al. Early empiric antibiotic use in preterm infants is associated with lower bacterial diversity and higher relative abundance of Enterobacter. J Pediatr 2014;165(1):23–9.

75. Arboleya S, Sánchez B, Milani C, et al. Intestinal microbiota development in preterm neonates and effect of perinatal antibiotics. J Pediatr 2015;166(3):538–44.

76. Fouhy F, Guinane CM, Hussey S, et al. High-throughput sequencing reveals the incomplete, short-term recovery of infant gut microbiota following parenteral antibiotic treatment with ampicillin and gentamicin. Antimicrob Agents Chemother 2012;56(11):5811–20.

77. Tanaka S, Kobayashi T, Songjinda P, et al. Influence of antibiotic exposure in the early postnatal period on the development of intestinal microbiota. FEMS Immunol Med Microbiol 2009;56(1):80–7.

78. Stensballe LG, Simonsen J, Jensen SM, et al. Use of antibiotics during pregnancy increases the risk of asthma in early childhood. J Pediatr 2013;162(4): 832–8.e3.

79. Murk W, Risnes KR, Bracken MB. Prenatal or early-life exposure to antibiotics and risk of childhood asthma: a systematic review. Pediatrics 2011;127(6): 1125–38.

80. Ong M-S, Umetsu DT, Mandl KD. Consequences of antibiotics and infections in infancy: bugs, drugs, and wheezing. Ann Allergy Asthma Immunol 2014;112(5): 441–5.e1.

81. Sun W, Svendsen ER, Karmaus WJJ, et al. Early-life antibiotic use is associated with wheezing among children with high atopic risk: a prospective European study. J Asthma 2015;1–6.

82. Wickens K, Ingham T, Epton M, et al. The association of early life exposure to antibiotics and the development of asthma, eczema and atopy in a birth cohort: confounding or causality? Clin Exp Allergy 2008;38(8):1318–24.

83. Cullinan P, Harris J, Mills P, et al. Early prescriptions of antibiotics and the risk of allergic disease in adults: a cohort study. Thorax 2004;59(1):11–5.

84. Tsakok T, McKeever TM, Yeo L, et al. Does early life exposure to antibiotics increase the risk of eczema? A systematic review. Br J Dermatol 2013;169(5): 983–91.

85. Harris JM, Mills P, White C, et al. Recorded infections and antibiotics in early life: associations with allergy in UK children and their parents. Thorax 2007;62(7): 631–7.

86. Kummeling I, Stelma FF, Dagnelie PC, et al. Early life exposure to antibiotics and the subsequent development of eczema, wheeze, and allergic sensitization in the first 2 years of life: the KOALA Birth Cohort Study. Pediatrics 2007;119(1):e225–31.

87. Maslowski KM, Mackay CR. Diet, gut microbiota and immune responses. Nat Immunol 2011;12(1):5–9.

88. Zivkovic AM, German JB, Lebrilla CB, et al. Human milk glycobiome and its impact on the infant gastrointestinal microbiota. Proc Natl Acad Sci U S A 2011;108(Suppl 1):4653–8.

89. Benno Y, Sawada K, Mitsuoka T. The intestinal microflora of infants: composition of fecal flora in breast-fed and bottle-fed infants. Microbiol Immunol 1984;28(9): 975–86.

90. Tullus K, Aronsson B, Marcus S, et al. Intestinal colonization with *Clostridium difficile* in infants up to 18 months of age. Eur J Clin Microbiol Infect Dis 1989; 8(5):390–3.

91. Penders J, Thijs C, Vink C, et al. Factors influencing the composition of the intestinal microbiota in early infancy. Pediatrics 2006;118(2):511–21.

92. Azad MB, Konya T, Maughan H, et al. Gut microbiota of healthy Canadian infants: profiles by mode of delivery and infant diet at 4 months. Can Med Assoc J 2013;185(5):385–94.

93. Silvers KM, Frampton CM, Wickens K, et al. Breastfeeding protects against current asthma up to 6 years of age. J Pediatr 2012;160(6):991–6.e1.

94. Guibas GV, Xepapadaki P, Moschonis G, et al. Breastfeeding and wheeze prevalence in pre-schoolers and pre-adolescents: the Genesis and Healthy Growth studies. Pediatr Allergy Immunol 2013;24(8):772–81.

95. Matheson MC, Allen KJ, Tang MLK. Understanding the evidence for and against the role of breastfeeding in allergy prevention. Clin Exp Allergy 2012;42(6):827–51.

96. Dogaru CM, Nyffenegger D, Pescatore AM, et al. Breastfeeding and childhood asthma: systematic review and meta-analysis. Am J Epidemiol 2014;179(10): 1153–67.

97. Blattner CM, Murase JE. A practice gap in pediatric dermatology: does breastfeeding prevent the development of infantile atopic dermatitis? J Am Acad Dermatol 2014;71(2):405–6.

98. Devereux G. The increase in the prevalence of asthma and allergy: food for thought. Nat Rev Immunol 2006;6(11):869–74.

99. Wu GD, Chen J, Hoffmann C, et al. Linking long-term dietary patterns with gut microbial enterotypes. Science 2011;334(6052):105–8.

100. Thorburn AN, Macia L, Mackay CR. Diet, metabolites, and "western-lifestyle" inflammatory diseases. Immunity 2014;40(6):833–42.

101. Trompette A, Gollwitzer ES, Yadava K, et al. Gut microbiota metabolism of dietary fiber influences allergic airway disease and hematopoiesis. Nat Med 2014; 20(2):159–66.

102. Bashir MEH, Louie S, Shi HN, et al. Toll-like receptor 4 signaling by intestinal microbes influences susceptibility to food allergy. J Immunol 2004;172(11): 6978–87.

103. Stefka AT, Feehley T, Tripathi P, et al. Commensal bacteria protect against food allergen sensitization. Proc Natl Acad Sci U S A 2014;111(36):13145–50.

104. Atarashi K, Tanoue T, Oshima K, et al. Treg induction by a rationally selected mixture of Clostridia strains from the human microbiota. Nature 2013; 500(7461):232–6.

105. Rodriguez B, Prioult G, Hacini-Rachinel F, et al. Infant gut microbiota is protective against cow's milk allergy in mice despite immature ileal T-cell response. FEMS Microbiol Ecol 2012;79(1):192–202.

106. de Kivit S, Tobin MC, Forsyth CB, et al. Regulation of intestinal immune responses through TLR activation: implications for pro- and prebiotics. Front Immunol 2014;5:60.

107. de Kivit S, Tobin MC, DeMeo MT, et al. In vitro evaluation of intestinal epithelial TLR activation in preventing food allergic responses. Clin Immunol 2014;154(2): 91–9.

108. Noval Rivas M, Burton OT, Wise P, et al. A microbiota signature associated with experimental food allergy promotes allergic sensitization and anaphylaxis. J Allergy Clin Immunol 2013;131(1):201–12.

109. McGowan EC, Keet CA. Prevalence of self-reported food allergy in the National Health and Nutrition Examination Survey (NHANES) 2007-2010. J Allergy Clin Immunol 2013;132(5):1216–9.e5.

110. Keet CA, Wood RA, Matsui EC. Limitations of reliance on specific IgE for epidemiologic surveillance of food allergy. J Allergy Clin Immunol 2012;130(5): 1207–9.e10.

111. Koplin J, Allen K, Gurrin L, et al. Is caesarean delivery associated with sensitization to food allergens and IgE-mediated food allergy: a systematic review. Pediatr Allergy Immunol 2008;19(8):682–7.

112. Eggesbø M, Botten G, Stigum H, et al. Is delivery by cesarean section a risk factor for food allergy? J Allergy Clin Immunol 2003;112(2):420–6.

113. Eggesbo M, Botten G, Stigum H, et al. Cesarean delivery and cow milk allergy/intolerance. Allergy 2005;60(9):1172–3.

114. Metsälä J, Lundqvist A, Kaila M, et al. Maternal and perinatal characteristics and the risk of cow's milk allergy in infants up to 2 years of age: a case-control study nested in the Finnish population. Am J Epidemiol 2010;171(12):1310–6.

115. Koplin JJ, Dharmage SC, Ponsonby AL, et al. Environmental and demographic risk factors for egg allergy in a population-based study of infants. Allergy 2012; 67(11):1415–22.

116. Campbell BE, Lodge CJ, Lowe AJ, et al. Exposure to "farming" and objective markers of atopy: a systematic review and meta-analysis. Clin Exp Allergy 2015;45(4):744–57.

117. Metsälä J, Lundqvist A, Virta LJ, et al. Mother's and offspring's use of antibiotics and infant allergy to cow's milk. Epidemiology 2013;24(2):303–9.

118. Mai XM, Kull I, Wickman M, et al. Antibiotic use in early life and development of allergic diseases: respiratory infection as the explanation. Clin Exp Allergy 2010; 40(8):1230–7.

119. Luccioli S, Zhang Y, Verrill L, et al. Infant feeding practices and reported food allergies at 6 years of age. Pediatrics 2014;134(Suppl 1):S21–8.

120. McGowan EC, Bloomberg GR, Gergen PJ, et al. Influence of early-life exposures on food sensitization and food allergy in an inner-city birth cohort. J Allergy Clin Immunol 2015;135(1):171–8.

121. Thompson-Chagoyan OC, Vieites JM, Maldonado J, et al. Changes in faecal microbiota of infants with cow's milk protein allergy: a Spanish prospective case-control 6-month follow-up study. Pediatr Allergy Immunol 2010;21(2 Pt 2): e394–400.

122. Thompson-Chagoyan OC, Fallani M, Maldonado J, et al. Faecal microbiota and short-chain fatty acid levels in faeces from infants with cow's milk protein allergy. Int Arch Allergy Immunol 2011;156(3):325–32.

123. Ling Z, Li Z, Liu X, et al. Altered fecal microbiota composition associated with food allergy in infants. Appl Environ Microbiol 2014;80(8):2546–54.

124. Azad MB, Konya T, Guttman DS, et al. Infant gut microbiota and food sensitization: associations in the first year of life. Clin Exp Allergy 2015;45(3):632–43.

Breast Milk and Food Allergy

Connections and Current Recommendations

Alice E.W. Hoyt, MD[a], Tegan Medico, MS, MPH, RDN[a],
Scott P. Commins, MD, PhD[b],*

KEYWORDS

- Breast milk • Breast feed • Newborn immune system • Food allergy

KEY POINTS

- Breast milk has important effects on the developing newborn and infant immune and gastrointestinal systems.
- The role of breast milk in the development of an infant's immunoglobulin E response is uncertain.
- Whether maternal dietary antigens appear in breast milk is the subject of ongoing research.

INTRODUCTION

Breast milk, the most natural source of nutrition for babies, is recommended by the American Academy of Pediatrics (AAP), who in 2012 reaffirmed its recommendation of "exclusive breastfeeding for about 6 months, followed by continued breastfeeding as complementary foods are introduced, with continuation of breastfeeding for 1 year or longer as mutually desired by mother and infant."[1] Breastfeeding rates are on the increase in the United States. In 2011, 79% of newborn infants started to breastfeed, 49% were breastfeeding at 6 months, and 27% at 12 months.[2] The incidence of food allergies is also on the increase: between 1997 and 2007, the incidence of food allergy increased by 18% in children younger than 18 years.[3] In 2011, 8% of children had food allergies.[4] Moreover, 29% of patients with food allergies also reported other atopic conditions such as asthma and eczema, compared with only 12% of children without

Disclosures: A.E.W. Hoyt and T. Medico: none. S.P. Commins: NIH grant support (K08 AI085109); UpToDate author.
[a] University of Virginia, PO Box 801355, 409 Lane Road MR-4 Building, Room 5051, Charlottesville, VA 22908, USA; [b] University of North Carolina School of Medicine, Department of Medicine, Division of Rheumatology, Allergy and Immunology, 3300 Thurston Building, CB 7280, Chapel Hill, NC 27599-7280, USA
* Corresponding author.
E-mail address: aw2nc@virginia.edu

Pediatr Clin N Am 62 (2015) 1493–1507
http://dx.doi.org/10.1016/j.pcl.2015.07.014
0031-3955/15/$ – see front matter © 2015 Elsevier Inc. All rights reserved.

food allergies.[3] The driving force, or forces, behind the increase in allergies is unknown, and the subject of wide discussions and research.

The objective of this article is to review the composition of human breast milk and its role in food allergy by exploring the nutrition and immunology of breast milk, including the effects of a mother's diet and contemporary means of storage of breast milk. The current literature on breast milk and food allergy is also reviewed.

THE PHYSIOLOGY OF BREAST MILK

Human breast milk is synthesized to match the developmentally appropriate nutritional needs of the baby. The processes and structures needed to create human milk begin when the woman herself is in her mother's womb. As reviewed by Creasy,[5] the milk streak is present at the fourth week of gestation, and the mammary gland is formed at the sixth week of gestation. Proliferation of milk ducts continues throughout embryogenesis, and breast buds are present at birth but, as maternal hormones diminish in the baby's circulation, the buds regress, growing proportionally to body growth until puberty.

Prepubertal changes in hormonal circulation induce the first phase of mammogenesis. Ductal growth is stimulated by estrogen production, which is generally unopposed in the first 1 to 2 years of menstrual cycles, creating type I lobules, which are alveolar buds clustered around a duct; upon cyclical changes in hormones, the types of lobules differentiate into type II lobules, which are more complex lobules that contain more alveoli.[6] This process continues throughout puberty, completing mature breast development.

The second phase of mammogenesis occurs when a woman becomes pregnant so that breast milk may be produced by lactocytes, which use 5 transport mechanisms to create breast milk (**Table 1**).[7] During the first half of pregnancy, lobules further differentiate into types III and IV, which have increased numbers of alveoli per lobule, thus establishing the milk-producing and milk-secreting framework.[6] During the second half of pregnancy, protein synthetic structures, such as the rough endoplasmic reticulum, mitochondria, and Golgi apparatus, begin to increase within the alveoli, and complex protein, milk fat, and lactose synthetic pathways are activated.[6] Regarding hormonal regulation, the initiation of human lactation involves (1) secretory differentiation, whereby mammary epithelial cells differentiate into lactocytes in the presence of progesterone, estrogen, and prolactin, and (2) secretory activation,

Table 1
Methods of transport within the mammary gland

Method of Transport	Transported Components
Exocytosis	Milk proteins Lactose Calcium Other components of the aqueous phase of milk
Lipid synthesis	Fat secretion with formation of cytoplasmic lipid droplets Secreted as a membrane-bound milk fat globule
Apical membrane transport	Monovalent ions Water Glucose
Transcytosis	Proteins such as immunoglobulins
Paracellular transport	Components of the interstitial space

whereby lactocytes secrete copious amounts of milk in the presence of prolactin, insulin, and cortisol when progesterone levels drop.[7] This ability to synthesize and secrete milk is termed lactogenesis. Lactogenesis I occurs about 12 weeks before parturition as acini produce colostrum while progesterone inhibits the production of milk. Lactogenesis II occurs around 2 to 3 days after delivery, when the sudden drop in progesterone causes changes in the mammary epithelium, resulting in the beginning of mature milk production. Lactogenesis III is the establishment of mature milk production, occurring about 10 days after delivery, and was formerly called galactopoiesis.[8]

NUTRITION OF EXPRESSED BREAST MILK

Regarded by the World Health Organization (WHO) and AAP as the optimum first food for infants, human milk is sufficient to meet the nutrition needs of the developing infant exclusively through the first 6 months of life and is the standard to which infant formulas are designed. The AAP recommends breastfeeding duration of 1 year minimum or as long as preferred by mother and child, and the WHO recommends breastfeeding continue through age 2 years so that breast milk may continue to provide a substantial proportion of toddlers' nutrition needs.[9,10]

Although human milk is the standard for infant nutrition, its exact profile of nutritive substances is fairly dynamic. On average, a deciliter of mature human milk provides 65 to 70 kilocalories, 0.9 to 1.2 g of protein, 3.2 to 3.6 g of lipid, and 6.7 to 7.8 g of lactose.[11] In reality, the composition of human milk varies diurnally, within feedings, and individually from mother to mother; furthermore, compared with mature milk, the nutrient profiles of breast milk differ greatly among colostrum, transitional milk, and preterm milk.[10,11]

MACRONUTRIENTS
Protein

The total protein concentration of human milk is relatively low in comparison with other mammalian milks, but the makeup is uniquely suited to provide both nutritive and nonnutritive benefits related to tolerance, development, and immune function. The relatively high proportion of whey compared with casein, the 2 main protein fractions, allows for greater solubility in gastric acid and faster gastric emptying in comparison with bovine proteins. Whey proteins of human milk include serum proteins (eg, α-lactalbumin, lactoferrin), enzymes (eg, lysozyme), and immunoglobulins (eg, secretory immunoglobulin A [IgA]). Lactoferrin, lysozyme, and secretory IgA are resistant to proteolysis and impart initial immune defense in the gastrointestinal tract. Casein phosphopeptides, intermediates of casein digestion, maintain the solubility of calcium, thereby aiding in absorption. In addition, free amino acids taurine and glutamine may stimulate intestinal growth, and nonprotein nitrogen from urea and nucleotides is used for the synthesis of nonessential amino acids, hormones, growth factors, and nucleic acids.[10–12]

Lipid

Human milk is lipid rich. Half of the total energy in human milk is provided by its lipid fraction, and its globule structure, which contains bile salt-stimulating lipase, promotes efficient digestion. Lipid concentrations are lower at the start of feed (foremilk) and rich toward the end of a feed (hindmilk). Breast milk is also high in cholesterol, which contributes to cell membrane construction of the rapidly growing infant.[10–12]

Unlike its protein and carbohydrate constituents, the fatty acid profile of human milk is affected directly by maternal diet, making it the most variable macronutrient. Despite this element of variability, breast milk remains higher in the polyunsaturated fatty acids arachidonic acid and docohexaenoic acid (DHA) in comparison with bovine milk. DHA is integral to visual and neurologic function.[10]

Carbohydrate

Lactose is the major carbohydrate source in breast milk, followed by oligosaccharides. Lactose facilitates calcium absorption and may contribute to the soft stools generally observed in breastfed infants. Oligosaccharides serve as prebiotics, aiding in the proliferation of beneficial bifidobacteria and lactobacilli in the gut. Because they structurally resemble bacterial antigen receptors, they also impede bacteria from attaching to the gut mucosa.[10–14]

MICRONUTRIENTS
Vitamins

The vitamin content of breast milk is partly reflective of maternal diet and, in the case of fat-soluble vitamins, the overall fat content of the milk. An appropriately growing, healthy infant of a mother with a nutritionally adequate diet generally will meet his or her micronutrient requirements with the exceptions of vitamins K and D. Because of the low production of vitamin K by infant intestinal flora, infants are provided a single dose of vitamin K at birth to prevent deficiency-associated hemorrhagic disease of the newborn. The vitamin D content of breast milk can be improved by maternal diet and sun exposure, but average levels are generally insufficient to meet the infant recommended dietary allowance, necessitating routine supplementation.[10–12]

Minerals

Mineral content of breast milk decreases gradually over the first 4 months of infant life, but this decline does not affect infant growth and may be kidney protective.[10] Human milk is notable for having lower amounts of calcium and phosphorus in comparison with bovine milk, but these are more bioavailable, as are magnesium, iron, and zinc. Nearly half of the iron content of breast milk is absorbed, compared with 10% in bovine milk and bovine milk–based infant formulas.[10,11] Maternal diet does not greatly affect the mineral content of breast milk.[15]

IMMUNOLOGY OF BREAST MILK
Neonatal Immune System

To better understand how immune development may go amiss (eg, the development of food allergy) and how breast milk is immunologically beneficial, a basic comprehension of a baby's immune system is beneficial. The ultimate goal of a newborn baby's immune system is to possess both innate and adaptive systems of protection with complement bridging these 2 arms of immunity. The innate immune system identifies and combats immediate defense concerns while also signaling the development and recruitment of the adaptive immune system. Because both the innate and the adaptive immune systems take time to develop, babies benefit from exogenous sources of immune protection, specifically in the form of breast milk.

Though immunologically immature, the innate immune system, composed primarily of complement, natural killer cells, polymorphonuclear cells, monocytes, and macrophages, provides more immune protection to the neonate than does the more immature adaptive immune system, which is composed of T lymphocytes, B lymphocytes, and immunoglobulins.[16] The 4 major categories of immunity are impaired in babies: phagocytosis, cell-mediated immunity, humoral immunity, and complement activity (**Table 2**).[17] Collectively the diffuse immaturity in these individual areas of immunity results in great susceptibility to infection, and the immunologic foundation developed during infancy in the presence of breast milk may contribute to tolerance more than is currently recognized.

Breast Milk Immunology

Breast milk is composed not only of macronutrients and micronutrients but also of living cells, antibodies, and other immunologically active agents, some of which fill immunologic gaps of the immature immune system. Breast milk composition is dynamic, changing as the baby develops and even altering with clinical changes, such as in the face of infection.[18] Although breast milk generally contains a repertoire of components, mothers produce milk with different defense functionality profiles.[19]

Antimicrobial, anti-inflammatory, and immunomodulatory factors that are underdeveloped in the neonatal immune system are found in human breast milk, playing a substitute role for those immune agents until the baby has developed them.[20] Secretory IgA, lactoferrin, complement C3, and lysozyme are just a few of the antimicrobial factors found in expressed breast milk. Secretory IgA provides antimicrobial protection not by activating complement but by immune exclusion, which is the prevention of bacteria traversing the gut epithelium, and possibly immune inclusion, which is the maintenance of protective gut biofilms.[21,22]

Lactoferrin is an iron-binding glycoprotein secreted in breast milk. Its highest total amounts are found in colostrum.[23] The amount decreases as milk matures; however, the percentage of total protein that is lactoferrin starts at 27% in colostrum, dips to 19% by day 28, then increases to 30% by day 84,[24] the timing of which correlates with the iron-deficiency anemia found in some exclusively breastfed babies. High levels of lactoferrin, such as those found in colostrum, stimulate intestinal proliferation, whereas low levels stimulate intestinal differentiation, both of which elucidate the critical role of lactoferrin as a first line of defense against pathogens invading the

---

Table 2
Four major categories of immunity in babies

Major Mechanism of Immune Activity	Status in the Neonate and Explanation
Phagocytosis: process of ingesting and killing microbes[77]	*Immature*: neutrophil chemotaxis is limited as is the presence of signaling molecules that participate in phagocytosis, such as immunoglobulins and complement[28]
Cell-mediated immunity: the protection against intracellular pathogens provided by T cells and macrophages[78]	*Immature*: neutrophils, monocytes, and antigen-presenting cells all hold both quantitative and qualitative defects[79]
Humoral immunity: the antibody-mediated protection against extracellular microbes and microbial toxins[80]	*Immature*: neutrophils, monocytes, and antigen-presenting cells all hold both quantitative and qualitative defects[79]
Complement activity: 1. Activates the inflammatory response 2. Opsonizes pathogens for phagocytosis and killing 3. Lyses susceptible organisms[81]	*Immature*: complement proteins are found in limited amounts in neonate and, thus, also convey less protection[82,83]

gastrointestinal tract.[25,26] Lactoferrin also takes up iron, preventing it from being used by bacteria and fungi, which thereby diminishes pathogen proliferation.[20]

Components of the complement system, such as complement C3, are present in human milk. Although small concentrations are present, such opsonins supplement the neonate's slowly developing complement system and aids in pathogen protection.[27,28]

Secretory IgA, lactoferrin, and complement C3 (and secretory component, the chaperone of IgA from mammary gland into the gut) vary greatly among lactating mothers; however, the proteins decrease between weeks 2 and 5, seemingly decreasing as the baby's immune system is expanding.[19] Lysozyme is another important immunologic protein in breast milk. This enzyme disrupts glycosidic linkages of some bacteria, a process aided by lactoferrin damaging bacterial outer membranes, creating a synergistic bacterial killing process.[29] From 6 weeks to 6 months, levels of secretory IgA, lactoferrin, lysozyme, and total protein vary greatly while playing important roles in neonatal immunity.[30] Of note, lactoferrin and lysozyme play roles against inflammation, as do platelet-activating factor acetylhydrolase and interleukin (IL)-10.[20]

Immunomodulatory factors are underdeveloped in the neonatal immune system, and the complete roster of factors present in breast milk continues to grow: humoral immunity is enhanced by IL-4 and IL-10; cellular immunity is enhanced by IL-12, tumor necrosis factor α, and interferon-γ; growth is enhanced by granulocyte-colony stimulating factor; and chemokine activity is enhanced by RANTES,[20] which plays a role in macrophage recruitment.[31]

Cells found in expressed breast milk include immune cells (leukocytes, such as granulocytes and mononuclear leukocytes including lymphocytes, monocytes, and macrophages), mammary epithelial cells, and stem cells.[32] Whereas the roles of mammary epithelial cells and breast milk stem cells in the neonatal immune system are not fully understood, immune cells play a vital role in neonatal protection, increasing in maternal and infant infections.[33]

Bacteria are also present in human breast milk. Although the sources of some of these microorganisms are thought to include maternal skin, infant mouth and skin, and the environment, maternal dendritic macrophages can transport bacteria from the maternal gut through the lymphatic system and into the mammary gland, where the bacteria are transferred into the breast milk.[34] This process was further demonstrated in breastfeeding mothers who consumed the probiotic *Lactobacillus*, after which the same strain of *Lactobacillus* was found in the feces of both the mothers their babies.[35] This mechanism is similar to the development of secretory IgA, which is produced by the mother when her enteric mucosa recognizes antigen and stimulates B-cell production of IgA; these B cells travel to the mammary glands, where the IgA is glycosylated and secreted into the breast milk.[36] In addition, oligosaccharides are present in breast milk and serve an important role in the development of infant gut microbiota (see later discussion).[37]

EFFECTS OF STORAGE ON BREAST MILK

Cultural trends affecting infant feeding and the recognition of the importance of breast milk in the care of hospitalized infants have made feeding human milk apart from the breast increasingly a reality.[38] The AAP and the Academy of Breastfeeding Medicine have published guidelines for the storage of breast milk to ensure not only safe infant feeding but also that the integrity of breast milk's bactericidal and nutritional properties is preserved. Among these guidelines are parameters related to refrigeration, freezing and thawing, and storage containers.

Refrigeration

Fresh breast milk that is not used within 4 to 6 hours should be refrigerated for up to 5 days. During this time nutrients may degrade at variable rates, with vitamin C noted to degrade rapidly.[11,38] The cream component of breast milk will separate during refrigeration but will blend easily with agitation on thawing; this does not affect the fat composition.

Freezing and Thawing

Breast milk that will not be used within 72 to 120 hours of expression should be frozen. Freezing preserves its nutritional and immunologic properties for up to 3 to 4 months in a refrigerator-freezer compartment or for up to 6 months in a deep freezer. It is recommended that thawed milk should be used within 24 hours and not be refrozen. Heating breast milk will reduce the content and bioactivity of heat-labile vitamins and proteins.[11,38]

Containers

Glass and hard plastic containers with airtight seals are the ideal storage containers for breast milk. For short-term (<72 hours) storage, plastic bags designed for human milk storage are appropriate. Longer storage increases the adherence of milk components to the plastic, thus affecting the nutritional quality of the milk.[38]

MOTHER AND HER DIET

The nutrient composition of breast milk remains relatively stable despite day-to-day fluctuations in maternal dietary intake and even during limited periods of dietary inadequacy. Chronic nutrient deprivation, however, can diminish the quality of human milk. Nutrients that are most vulnerable to maternal intake levels can vary.[11]

Macronutrients

The macronutrient concentrations in breast milk are largely unaffected by maternal diet, although the types of fatty acids present mimic maternal intake. Protein levels are affected more by infant age than maternal protein intake, with colostrum and preterm milk being highest in protein in comparison with transitional and mature milk; however, women who consume high-protein diets have been found to have higher concentrations of total nitrogen in their milk because of higher levels of urea and free amino acids. Carbohydrate concentration and type is not affected by maternal diet.[10,11]

Micronutrients

Mature milk may be affected by maternal diet, depending on the nutrient. Vitamin concentrations decline when mothers are in deficiency states, and these concentrations respond to therapeutic supplementation. Upper thresholds for vitamin levels, particularly water-soluble vitamins, are regulated. In contrast to vitamins, minerals are not as susceptible to maternal intake. The exceptions are selenium and iodine, which correlate with maternal plasma levels.[11]

FOOD ALLERGY AND BREAST MILK
Epidemiology and Developmental Pathophysiology of Food Allergies

Although the exact incidence of food allergy has yet to be established,[39] a recent prospective, observational study found that 9.9% of children developed food allergies by the age of 5 years.[40] This finding in an inner-city American cohort is similar to the greater than 10% of 1-year-old children found to have food allergies in Melbourne,

Australia.[41] What does seem certain is that the incidence of food allergy is increasing in westernized countries and in countries where food allergy was not previously considered to be a major issue, such as South Africa.[42]

The pathophysiology of childhood food allergy is not understood and is likely a complex interaction of prenatal, neonatal, early childhood, and maternal immunity, specifically interacting with the environment. Sicherer and Sampson[43] recently reviewed the possible mechanisms of the pathogenesis of food allergy, which include (1) gene-environment interaction, (2) the microbiome, (3) the route of sensitization (gut, skin, inhalation), (4) alteration of food preparation, such as heating/roasting, and (5) innate properties of the foods. The timing of when a food is introduced to a baby's diet may also play a role in the development of food allergy. To better understand how such timing affects food allergy, 2 studies are currently under way: the EAT study and the LEAP study.[44,45] The EAT Study, Enquiring About Tolerance, involves an early-introduction protocol of the most commonly allergenic foods with the goal of answering the question "does early exposure promote or prevent sensitization?"[44] Similarly, in the LEAP Study, Learning Early About Peanut Allergy, one arm of study participants avoids peanut in infancy while the other arm of infants consumes a measured, repeated amount of peanut-containing food.[45] The recently reported results showed an 11% - 25% risk reduction of developing peanut allergy, depending on whether subjects had a positive or negative skin test at study enrollment, supporting early peanut introduction between 4 and 11 months of age rather than peanut avoidance until age 5 years.[46] Moreover, interactions of breastfeeding, genes, and the environment were highlighted in the study by Hong and colleagues[47] in 2011. This study followed 970 children since birth, and found that children who were ever breastfed were at higher risk of food sensitization. This risk was further increased in children with variations in IL-12 receptor, toll-like receptor (TLR)-9, and thymic stromal lymphopoietin genes.

The gut microbiome, an area of active research in food allergy, may have modifiable effects on breast milk that could be enhanced by probiotics and prebiotics. *Lactobacillus reuteri* was supplemented in breastfeeding mothers and was then found in the feces of 82% of those babies but only in 20% of the nonsupplemented mothers' children's feces, and *L reuteri* was detected in more breast milk samples from the supplemented mothers than from the nonsupplemented mothers.[35] Human breast milk contains prebiotics in the form of oligosaccharides, which are nondigestible to babies but are secreted in milk and feed the microbiota of the baby's gut, characteristics shared with prebiotics.[37] Oligosaccharides also serve to prevent pathogen invasion of the gut mucosa.[44]

Breast milk may also have a role in preventing certain infections, an additional factor that may influence the development of food allergy. As proposed by Strachan[48] in 1989, the hygiene hypothesis proposed that allergic disease is the result of increased cleanliness. This theory has been further studied, and currently includes the proposal that early-life exposure of microbial components induces Th1-type responses as opposed to Th2-type responses.[49] Such exposure involves immune mediators such as TLRs. CD14 is a soluble component of TLR-4, which binds lipopolysaccharides of gram-negative bacteria, thereby causing an immune response. Although newborns initially have low levels of CD14, breast milk contains CD14 and is likely one of many breast milk constituents that influence allergy.[50]

History of Breastfeeding with Food Allergy

Recently, breastfeeding has been added to the list of theories behind the increase in food allergies, a change from its previously protective reputation. The protective role was observed in a 1995 study published in the *Lancet*, in which breastfeeding was associated with a decrease in food allergy.[51] In 2004, Muraro and colleagues[52] completed a thorough review of literature and concluded the following. In prospective observational studies, breastfeeding for at least 3 to 6 months and late introduction of solid foods (after 4–6 months) is associated with a decreased risk of cow's milk protein allergy/food allergy and atopic eczema up to 3 years of age and recurrent wheeze/asthma up to 6 to 17 years of age. As such, exclusively breastfeeding for the first 6 months of life as recommended by the WHO should be attempted in all infants and also recommended as an allergy-preventive measure. However, another study noted that components of breast milk can both enhance and suppress the immune response and participate in antigen exclusion, depending on the balance of such components.[53] Recent mouse models have supported the theory that breast milk reduces allergies. A 2011 study showed that the transfer of antigen and antibody in breast milk led to tolerance,[54] the results of which were similar to those of a 2010 study showing oral tolerance in pups of aerosol-sensitized mothers exposed to allergen.[55] A 2012 review further supported breast milk as being protective against allergy.[50]

In contrast to studies suggesting that breast milk protects against atopy, some work does suggest that breast milk is not protective against food allergy and may actually play a role in both food sensitization and allergy. A 2005 rostrum by Friedman and Zeiger[56] indicated that it could not be definitively determined that breast milk prevented sensitization to allergens. In keeping with the lack of a protective role, a follow-up study showed that breastfeeding did not protect against atopy and may have increased the risk of atopy.[57] More recently, a study of inner-city children of atopic parents showed that breastfeeding of any duration was significantly associated with food allergies.[40]

Review of the Literature on Food Allergies and Expressed Breast Milk

Understanding the relationship of food allergy and breast milk may create a new paradigm in allergy prevention research.[58] This area of allergy is already the focus of multiple studies including the content of allergen in breast milk and the immune factors in breast milk. Bernard and colleagues[59] identified peanut antigen that had been transferred through breast milk of 2 nonatopic mothers, and showed that immunoglobulin E (IgE)-mediated mast cell degranulation occurred in the presence of such antigen in mice, further arguing that such an antigen can cause sensitization. Macchiaverni and colleagues[60] identified Der p 1 (a major allergen from house dust mite) in human breast milk, and argued that it strongly promotes sensitization. Palmer and colleagues[61] found that the presence of egg ovalbumin in human milk was related to maternal egg intake but that excretion into breast milk varied among women, and that some women did not secrete ovalbumin into their milk.

The atopic status of a mother may affect her breast milk immunology. IL-4 has been shown to be higher in the breast milk of allergic mothers, with similar trends in IL-5 and IL-13, compared with nonallergic mothers.[62] Atopic mothers have been found to have decreased levels of IgA in breast milk, but this was not associated with whether her child developed allergies.[63] Low levels of breast milk transforming growth factor (TGF)-β2 have been associated with maternal allergy. In fact, TGF-β in breast milk may play an important role in immune tolerance.[64] TGF-β and IL-10 are tolerogenic cytokines found in breast milk.[50] In 2008, TGF-β was shown to play a significant role in breast milk–induced tolerance, mediating CD4$^+$ lymphocytes.[65] TGF-β1, along with IL-1β, IL-6, and IL-10, were recently associated with tolerance to cow's milk.[66] Conversely, TGF-β1 has been shown to be not associated with atopy.[67] As previously mentioned, low levels have been found in the milk of atopic mothers[68]; however, immune factors in breast milk that are related to milk allergy have been found to be independent of maternal atopy.[66]

IgA is the major antibody found in breast milk and is inversely related to atopic dermatitis.[67] Atopic mothers have lower levels of IgA than nonatopic mothers, but these levels have been found to be not associated with food allergy in children.[63] Higher levels of IgA in breast milk were associated with positive skin-prick testing at 6 months but not at 2 or 5 years of age.[30] Interestingly, and suggestive that some protein in breast milk may be associated with atopy in the first 2 years of life, the total protein in breast milk was higher in mothers with atopic babies than in mothers with nonatopic babies.[30]

Although proteins are generally considered the immunologic compounds of breast milk, fatty acids may also play a role in food allergy. The increase in food allergy in westernized societies has been accompanied by increased consumption of saturated and ω-6 fats along with a concomitant decrease in ω-3 consumption, each of which may play a role in the development of allergy.[69] Thijs and colleagues[70] recently explored this hypothesis in the context of fat content of human breast milk, and found that the sensitization at 1 year was inversely associated with breast milk concentrations of ω-3 fatty acids and rumenic fatty acids, which also had an impact on total IgE. No differences in breast milk fatty acids or ratios were found between atopic and nonatopic mothers.[70]

Current Recommendations on Breastfeeding and Food Allergy

The role of breast milk in food allergy is comprehensively unclear, although it does reduce cow's milk allergy in the first 2 years of life.[71] In 2008, Greer and colleagues[72] published 9 recommendations regarding atopy prevention. In 2014, the AAP included in its 2014 *Pediatrics Supplement: Best Articles Relevant to Pediatric Allergy and Immunology* McGowan's systematic review of the literature regarding primary prevention of food allergy, which concluded that the only intervention for which there is evidence of preventing the development of food allergy is for children at high risk to avoid cow's milk during the first 4 months of life.[73] Some recommendations commonly agreed on are found in the National Institute of Allergy and Infectious Diseases

---

Box 1
American Academy of Allergy, Asthma and Immunology recommendations from the food allergies practice parameter update, 2014

Recommendations to Prevent Food Allergies

1. Encourage exclusive breastfeeding for the first 4 to 6 months

2. For infants with a family history of atopy, consider a partially or extensively hydrolyzed infant formula for possible prevention of atopic dermatitis and infant cow's milk allergy if exclusive breastfeeding is not possible

3. Do not recommend allergen avoidance or avoidance of specific complementary foods at weaning because these approaches have not proved effective for primary prevention of atopic disease

4. Do not routinely recommend supplementation of the maternal or infant diet with probiotics or prebiotics as a means to prevent food allergy because there is insufficient evidence to support a beneficial effect

Adapted from Sampson HA, Aceves S, Bock SA, et al. Food allergy: a practice parameter update—2014. J Allergy Clin Immunol 2014;134(5):1025e15; with permission.

guidelines in food allergy published in 2010 by Boyce and colleagues,[74] which included (1) the recommendation against maternal diet restriction during pregnancy and lactation, (2) the recommendation supporting exclusive breastfeeding until 4 to 6 months of age, and (3) the suggestion that high-risk infants consume hydrolyzed formula when exclusive breastfeeding is unavailable ("high-risk" being defined as babies with biological parents or siblings with existing or a history of food allergy, atopic dermatitis, allergic rhinitis, or asthma). A 2012 update of risk factors published in the *Journal of Allergy and Clinical Immunology* further explores this topic.[75] A Cochrane review from 2014 also recommended against maternal dietary avoidance of antigens during pregnancy or lactation regarding decreasing atopy.[76] In 2014 the American Academy of Allergy, Asthma and Immunology published "Food allergy: a practice parameter update—2014," which included recommendations regarding the prevention of food allergy (**Box 1**).

SUMMARY

Breast milk is a complex immunologic liquid. In addition to the nutritional growth it provides, it plays a dynamic role in the neonatal immune system, contributing to both defense and apparent hyperdefense in the form of allergy. The body of literature regarding breast milk and food allergy continues to grow, and research to date indicates that this is just the beginning of understanding how breast milk affects the development of food allergy.

REFERENCES

1. Section on Breastfeeding. Breastfeeding and the use of human milk. Pediatrics 2012;129(3):e827–41.
2. Centers for Disease Control and Prevention. Breastfeeding report card. 2014:8.
3. Jackson KD, Howie LD, Akinbami LJ. Trends in allergic conditions among children: United States, 1997-2011. NCHS Data Brief 2013;(121):1–8.
4. Gupta RS, Springston EE, Warrier MR, et al. The prevalence, severity, and distribution of childhood food allergy in the United States. Pediatrics 2011;128(1): e9–17.
5. Creasy R. Creasy and Resnik's maternal-fetal medicine: principles and practice. 7th edition. Philadelphia: Saunders; 2014.
6. Bland K. Breast: comprehensive management of benign and malignant diseases. 4th edition. Philadelphia: Saunders; 2009.
7. Pang WW, Hartmann PE. Initiation of human lactation: secretory differentiation and secretory activation. J Mammary Gland Biol Neoplasia 2007;12(4):211–21.
8. Lawrence R. Breastfeeding. 7th edition. Maryland Heights (MO): Mosby; 2011.
9. Breastfeeding. 2014. Available at: http://www.who.int/maternal_child_adolescent/topics/child/nutrition/breastfeeding/en/. Accessed December 2, 2014.
10. Kleinman R. Pediatric nutrition handbook. 6th edition. Elk Grove Village (IL): American Academy of Pediatrics; 2009.
11. Ballard O, Morrow AL. Human milk composition: nutrients and bioactive factors. Pediatr Clin North Am 2013;60(1):49–74.
12. Rodriguez-Palmero M, Koletzko B, Kunz C, et al. Nutritional and biochemical properties of human milk: II. Lipids, micronutrients, and bioactive factors. Clin Perinatol 1999;26(2):335–59.
13. Boehm G, Lidestri M, Casetta P, et al. Supplementation of a bovine milk formula with an oligosaccharide mixture increases counts of faecal bifidobacteria in preterm infants. Arch Dis Child Fetal Neonatal Ed 2002;86(3):F178–81.

14. Kunz C, Rudloff S. Biological functions of oligosaccharides in human milk. Acta Paediatr 1993;82(11):903–12.
15. Prentice A. Calcium supplementation during breast-feeding. N Engl J Med 1997; 337(8):558–9.
16. Krishnan S, Craven M, Welliver RC, et al. Differences in participation of innate and adaptive immunity to respiratory syncytial virus in adults and neonates. J Infect Dis 2003;188(3):433–9.
17. Lawrence RM, Pane CA. Human breast milk: current concepts of immunology and infectious diseases. Curr Probl Pediatr Adolesc Health Care 2007;37(1): 7–36.
18. Riskin A, Almog M, Peri R, et al. Changes in immunomodulatory constituents of human milk in response to active infection in the nursing infant. Pediatr Res 2012;71(2):220–5.
19. Broadhurst M, Beddis K, Black J, et al. Effect of gestation length on the levels of five innate defence proteins in human milk. Early Hum Dev 2014;91(1):7–11.
20. Goldman A, Chheda S, Keeney S, et al. Immunology of human milk and host immunity. Fetal and neonatal physiology. 4th edition. Philadelphia: Saunders; 2008.
21. Mantis NJ, Rol N, Corthésy B. Secretory IgA's complex roles in immunity and mucosal homeostasis in the gut. Mucosal Immunol 2011;4(6):603–11.
22. Everett ML, Palestrant D, Miller S, et al. Immune exclusion and immune inclusion: a new model of host-bacterial interactions in the gut. Clin Appl Immunol Rev 2004;4:321–32.
23. Rai D, Adelman AS, Zhuang W, et al. Longitudinal changes in lactoferrin concentrations in human milk: a global systematic review. Crit Rev Food Sci Nutr 2014; 54(12):1539–47.
24. Montagne P, Cuillière ML, Molé C, et al. Changes in lactoferrin and lysozyme levels in human milk during the first twelve weeks of lactation. Adv Exp Med Biol 2001;501:241–7.
25. Jiang R, Du X, Lönnerdal B. Comparison of bioactivities of talactoferrin and lactoferrins from human and bovine milk. J Pediatr Gastroenterol Nutr 2014;59(5): 642–52.
26. Buccigrossi V, de Marco G, Bruzzese E, et al. Lactoferrin induces concentration-dependent functional modulation of intestinal proliferation and differentiation. Pediatr Res 2007;61(4):410–4.
27. Ogundele MO. Activation and deposition of human breast-milk complement C3 opsonins on serum sensitive *Escherichia coli* 0111. J Reprod Immunol 2000; 48(2):99–105.
28. Henneke P, Berner R. Interaction of neonatal phagocytes with group B streptococcus: recognition and response. Infect Immun 2006;74(6):3085–95.
29. Ellison RT, Giehl TJ. Killing of gram-negative bacteria by lactoferrin and lysozyme. J Clin Invest 1991;88(4):1080–91.
30. Zhang G, Lai CT, Hartmann P, et al. Anti-infective proteins in breast milk and asthma-associated phenotypes during early childhood. Pediatr Allergy Immunol 2014;25(6):544–51.
31. Chatterton DE, Nguyen DN, Bering SB, et al. Anti-inflammatory mechanisms of bioactive milk proteins in the intestine of newborns. Int J Biochem Cell Biol 2013;45(8):1730–47.
32. Hassiotou F, Geddes DT, Hartmann PE. Cells in human milk: state of the science. J Hum Lact 2013;29(2):171–82.
33. Bode L, McGuire M, Rodriguez JM, et al. It's alive: microbes and cells in human milk and their potential benefits to mother and infant. Adv Nutr 2014;5(5):571–3.

34. Rodríguez JM. The origin of human milk bacteria: is there a bacterial entero-mammary pathway during late pregnancy and lactation? Adv Nutr 2014;5(6): 779–84.

35. Abrahamsson TR, Sinkiewicz G, Jakobsson T, et al. Probiotic lactobacilli in breast milk and infant stool in relation to oral intake during the first year of life. J Pediatr Gastroenterol Nutr 2009;49(3):349–54.

36. Newburg DS. Innate immunity and human milk. J Nutr 2005;135(5):1308–12.

37. Coppa GV, Bruni S, Morelli L, et al. The first prebiotics in humans: human milk oligosaccharides. J Clin Gastroenterol 2004;38(6 Suppl I):S80–3.

38. Eglash A, Academy of Breastfeeding Medicine Protocol Committee. ABM clinical protocol #8: human milk storage information for home use for full-term infants (original protocol March 2004; revision #1 March 2010). Breastfeed Med 2010;5(3):127–30.

39. Longo G, Berti I, Burks AW, et al. IgE-mediated food allergy in children. Lancet 2013;382(9905):1656–64.

40. McGowan EC, Bloomberg GR, Gergen PJ, et al. Influence of early-life exposures on food sensitization and food allergy in an inner-city birth cohort. J Allergy Clin Immunol 2015;135(1):171–8.

41. Osborne NJ, Koplin JJ, Martin PE, et al. Prevalence of challenge-proven IgE-mediated food allergy using population-based sampling and predetermined challenge criteria in infants. J Allergy Clin Immunol 2011;127(3):668–76.e1-2.

42. Botha M, Levin M. Prevalence of IgE-mediated food sensitisation and food allergy in unselected 12-36 month old South African children. J Allergy Clin Immunol 2014;133:1A–4A.

43. Sicherer SH, Sampson HA. Food allergy: epidemiology, pathogenesis, diagnosis, and treatment. J Allergy Clin Immunol 2014;133(2):291–307 [quiz: 308].

44. EAT: enquiring about tolerance. Available at: http://www.eatstudy.co.uk/wp-content/uploads/2010/10/EATSummaryv1.022.pdf. Accessed January 5, 2015.

45. LEAP: learning early about peanut allergy. Available at: http://www.leapstudy.co.uk/LEAP.html. Accessed January 5, 2015.

46. Du Toit G, Roberts G, Sayre PH, et al. Randomized Trial of Peanut Consumption in Infants at Risk for Peanut Allergy. N Engl J Med 2015;372:803–13.

47. Hong X, Wang G, Liu X, et al. Gene polymorphisms, breast-feeding, and development of food sensitization in early childhood. J Allergy Clin Immunol 2011; 128(2):374–81.e372.

48. Strachan DP. Family size, infection and atopy: the first decade of the "hygiene hypothesis". Thorax 2000;55(Suppl 1):S2–10.

49. Land BVT, Boehm G, Garssen J. Breast milk: components with immune modulating potential and their possible role in immune mediated disease resistance. In: Watson, Ross R, Zibadi, et al, editors. Dietary components and immune function. New York: Springer Science+Business Media; 2010. p. 25–41.

50. Iyengar SR, Walker WA. Immune factors in breast milk and the development of atopic disease. J Pediatr Gastroenterol Nutr 2012;55(6):641–7.

51. Saarinen UM, Kajosaari M. Breastfeeding as prophylaxis against atopic disease: prospective follow-up study until 17 years old. Lancet 1995;346(8982):1065–9.

52. Muraro A, Dreborg S, Halken S, et al. Dietary prevention of allergic diseases in infants and small children. Part III: critical review of published peer-reviewed observational and interventional studies and final recommendations. Pediatr Allergy Immunol 2004;15(4):291–307.

53. Muraro A, Dreborg S, Halken S, et al. Dietary prevention of allergic diseases in infants and small children. Part I: immunologic background and criteria for hypoallergenicity. Pediatr Allergy Immunol 2004;15(2):103–11.

54. Yamamoto T, Tsubota Y, Kodama T, et al. Oral tolerance induced by transfer of food antigens via breast milk of allergic mothers prevents offspring from developing allergic symptoms in a mouse food allergy model. Clin Dev Immunol 2012;2012: 721085.

55. Mosconi E, Rekima A, Seitz-Polski B, et al. Breast milk immune complexes are potent inducers of oral tolerance in neonates and prevent asthma development. Mucosal Immunol 2010;3(5):461–74.

56. Friedman NJ, Zeiger RS. The role of breast-feeding in the development of allergies and asthma. J Allergy Clin Immunol 2005;115(6):1238–48.

57. Sears MR, Greene JM, Willan AR, et al. Long-term relation between breastfeeding and development of atopy and asthma in children and young adults: a longitudinal study. Lancet 2002;360(9337):901–7.

58. Munblit D, Boyle RJ. Modulating breast milk composition—the key to allergy prevention? Int Arch Allergy Immunol 2012;159(2):107–8.

59. Bernard H, Ah-Leung S, Drumare MF, et al. Peanut allergens are rapidly transferred in human breast milk and can prevent sensitization in mice. Allergy 2014;69(7):888–97.

60. Macchiaverni P, Rekima A, Turfkruyer M, et al. Respiratory allergen from house dust mite is present in human milk and primes for allergic sensitization in a mouse model of asthma. Allergy 2014;69(3):395–8.

61. Palmer DJ, Gold MS, Makrides M. Effect of maternal egg consumption on breast milk ovalbumin concentration. Clin Exp Allergy 2008;38(7):1186–91.

62. Böttcher MF, Jenmalm MC, Garofalo RP, et al. Cytokines in breast milk from allergic and nonallergic mothers. Pediatr Res 2000;47(1):157–62.

63. Hogendorf A, Stańczyk-Przyłuska A, Sieniwicz-Luzeńczyk K, et al. Is there any association between secretory IgA and lactoferrin concentration in mature human milk and food allergy in breastfed children. Med Wieku Rozwoj 2013;17(1):47–52.

64. Vickery BP, Scurlock AM, Jones SM, et al. Mechanisms of immune tolerance relevant to food allergy. J Allergy Clin Immunol 2011;127(3):576–84 [quiz: 585–6].

65. Verhasselt V, Milcent V, Cazareth J, et al. Breast milk-mediated transfer of an antigen induces tolerance and protection from allergic asthma. Nat Med 2008;14(2): 170–5.

66. Järvinen KM, Suárez-Fariñas M, Savilahti E, et al. Immune factors in breast milk related to infant milk allergy are independent of maternal atopy. J Allergy Clin Immunol 2014;135:1390–3.e1-6.

67. Orivuori L, Loss G, Roduit C, et al. Soluble immunoglobulin A in breast milk is inversely associated with atopic dermatitis at early age: the PASTURE cohort study. Clin Exp Allergy 2014;44(1):102–12.

68. Kuitunen M, Kukkonen AK, Savilahti E. Impact of maternal allergy and use of probiotics during pregnancy on breast milk cytokines and food antibodies and development of allergy in children until 5 years. Int Arch Allergy Immunol 2012; 159(2):162–70.

69. Black PN, Sharpe S. Dietary fat and asthma: is there a connection? Eur Respir J 1997;10(1):6–12.

70. Thijs C, Müller A, Rist L, et al. Fatty acids in breast milk and development of atopic eczema and allergic sensitisation in infancy. Allergy 2011;66(1):58–67.

71. Fleischer DM, Spergel JM, Assa'ad AH, et al. Primary prevention of allergic disease through nutritional interventions. J Allergy Clin Immunol Pract 2013;1(1): 29–36.

72. Greer FR, Sicherer SH, Burks AW, American Academy of Pediatrics Committee on Nutrition, American Academy of Pediatrics Section on Allergy and

Immunology. Effects of early nutritional interventions on the development of atopic disease in infants and children: the role of maternal dietary restriction, breastfeeding, timing of introduction of complementary foods, and hydrolyzed formulas. Pediatrics 2008;121(1):183–91.

73. McGowan EC, Keet CA. Primary prevention of food allergy in children and adults: systematic review. Pediatrics 2014;134(Suppl 3):S138.

74. Boyce JA, Assa'ad A, Burks AW, et al. Guidelines for the diagnosis and management of food allergy in the United States: report of the NIAID-sponsored expert panel. J Allergy Clin Immunol 2010;126(6 Suppl):S1–58.

75. Lack G. Update on risk factors for food allergy. J Allergy Clin Immunol 2012; 129(5):1187–97.

76. Kramer MS, Kakuma R. Cochrane in context: maternal dietary antigen avoidance during pregnancy or lactation, or both, for preventing or treating atopic disease in the child. Evid Based Child Health 2014;9(2):484–5.

77. Abbas A, Lichtman A, Pilla S. Basic immunology: functions and disorders of the immune system. 4th edition. Philadelphia: Saunders; 2014.

78. Nairn R, Helbert M. Immunology for medical students. 2nd edition. New York: Mosby; 2007.

79. Levy O. Innate immunity of the newborn: basic mechanisms and clinical correlates. Nat Rev Immunol 2007;7(5):379–90.

80. Abbas A, Lichtman A, Pillai S. Cellular and molecular immunology. 8th edition. Philadelphia: Saunders; 2015.

81. Rich R, Fleisher T, Shearer W, et al. Clinical immunology. 4th edition. London: Elsevier Limited; 2013.

82. Pettengill MA, van Haren SD, Levy O. Soluble mediators regulating immunity in early life. Front Immunol 2014;5:457.

83. McGreal EP, Hearne K, Spiller OB. Off to a slow start: under-development of the complement system in term newborns is more substantial following premature birth. Immunobiology 2012;217(2):176–86.

The Learning Early About Peanut Allergy Study

The Benefits of Early Peanut Introduction, and a New Horizon in Fighting the Food Allergy Epidemic

Matthew Greenhawt, MD, MBA, MSc[a,b],*

KEYWORDS

- Peanut allergy • Primary prevention • Food sensitization • Skin-prick testing
- LEAP study • Oral food challenge • Food allergy • Anaphylaxis

KEY POINTS

- Prior to 2008, peanut introduction was actively recommended to be delayed in high-risk infants to help prevent peanut allergy development.
- Emerging data in the past 10 years has suggested that early complementary food introduction of high-risk allergens may be protective of food allergy development.
- The LEAP study clearly shows that early, frequent peanut introduction is associated with both primary and secondary peanut allergy prevention in high-risk infants compared to delayed introduction.
- New interim guidance, supported by multiple international organizations, supports early, frequent peanut introduction in high-risk infants, and re-enforces prior guidance that no longer actively recommends delay in any complementary food introduction past 4–6 months in standard-risk infants.

Food allergy is major public health disorder affecting nearly 15 million Americans, including 8% of United States children, at a cost of $24.8 billion annually.[1–3] Allergic reactions may occur on initial food exposure and range from mild to highly severe (eg, anaphylaxis, and possible fatality), with poor predictability. Several promising treatments are under development, although none presently exist beyond allergen

[a] Division of Allergy and Clinical Immunology, Department of Internal Medicine, University of Michigan Medical School, 24 Frank Lloyd Wright Drive, Lobby H-2100, Box 442, Ann Arbor, MI 48106, USA; [b] Child Health Evaluation and Research Unit, Department of Pediatrics, University of Michigan Medical School, 24 Frank Lloyd Wright Drive, Lobby H-2100, Box 442, Ann Arbor, MI 48106, USA
* Child Health Evaluation and Research Unit, Division of Allergy and Clinical Immunology, Department of Pediatrics, University of Michigan Medical School, 24 Frank Lloyd Wright Drive, Lobby H-2100, Box 442, Ann Arbor, MI 48106.
E-mail address: mgreenha@med.umich.edu

Pediatr Clin N Am 62 (2015) 1509–1521
http://dx.doi.org/10.1016/j.pcl.2015.07.010
0031-3955/15/$ – see front matter © 2015 Elsevier Inc. All rights reserved.

avoidance.[2] Food allergy is associated with anxiety and poor child health-related quality of life (HRQL), poor parent HRQL as a proxy for their child's experience, and poor parent HRQL as a spillover effect of a perpetual fear of the child reacting from an accidental exposure—something that treatment could prevent.[4–18] Thus, finding ways to treat food allergy, reduce the risk of a severe reaction occurring, or possibly prevent food allergy from developing are highly desirable. Oral immunotherapy (OIT) and epicutaneous immunotherapy (EPIT) currently offer the most promise as treatment options for those with existing food allergy.[19–24] Trials of both EPIT and OIT immunotherapy are ongoing, although success rates, treatment duration, and long-term benefits of this experimental therapy are unclear. Moreover, OIT itself carries high risks for inducing allergic reactions and developing secondary illnesses (eosinophilic esophagitis).[25–29]

Although both OIT and EPIT are highly promising, these strategies could be preempted by efforts to reduce overall rates of food allergy occurrence through primary prevention. Several studies have suggested that nutritional interventions may be associated with reduced odds of developing asthma, eczema, and food allergy.[30–33] More recently, several studies have been launched focusing on the relationship between early introduction of certain foods and primary prevention of food allergy. Observational studies have explored associations between timing of peanut, egg, and milk introduction and food allergy development, noting significant associations with reduced respective rates of milk, egg, and peanut allergy associated with earlier timing of introduction.[34–36] Interventional studies developed to more definitively explore these outcomes have been published for egg and peanut, and are ongoing for multiple other allergens. One small trial of egg introduction at 4 months has been published, showing a nonsignificant but lower rate of egg allergy in the early introduction group, balanced by a surprisingly high rate of egg sensitization among previously egg-naïve infants at the start of study.[37] Other studies of egg and other high-risk allergens are ongoing. This review focuses on the recent publication regarding the Learning Early About Peanut Allergy (LEAP) study, its highly favorable results, the policy implications of its findings, and the horizon for primary prevention as a realistic strategy to prevent food allergy.[38]

PEANUT ALLERGY: AN EPIDEMIC OUT OF CONTROL?

Peanut allergy affects approximately 1% to 3% of children in westernized nations (United States, United Kingdom, Western Europe, Australia, Canada), and is a growing public health concern. In other parts of the world, peanut allergy is far less of a problem.[39–44] Reasons for this discrepancy are poorly understood, but there are several hypotheses to explain the differential rates, including timing of introduction of peanut into the diet of infants, genetics, form and preparation of peanut, cultural practices, and the multiple hygiene hypothesis arguments. In the United States, United Kingdom, and Australia, peanut allergy is occurring at nearly 100,000 cases annually. Rates in the United States, measured by parental report in a 3-part phone survey, have tripled during the last decade, although peanut allergy is still not as prevalent as milk or egg allergy.[39,41,42] The exact prevalence of peanut allergy is difficult to determine without use of prospective, challenge-based cohorts, a strategy not readily used, although few allergists would argue that peanut allergy has not been increasing.[40]

Food allergy has no cure or treatment beyond allergen avoidance and carriage of emergency medications for treatment in the event of an unwanted/unintended exposure.[19] Parents live with a perpetual burden of illness, resulting from a fear that the child will have an unintended allergen ingestion and potentially fatal reaction, and concern for safe accommodation for the child to avoid unintended ingestion.[4-16] Peanut allergy in particular is problematic, given that it is sometimes associated with severe reactions on initial ingestion in susceptible individuals, occurring with potentially small quantities, and is very unlikely to be outgrown (<20% of cases resolve). Furthermore, peanut allergy has been associated with fatal reactions and reactions occurring from cross-contact/contaminations. Thus, compared with allergens such as milk or egg, which are typically outgrown in childhood, a treatment or cure for peanut allergy would be of particular use because of its protracted nature.[19] Multiple treatments for peanut allergy are under development and can be reviewed elsewhere, including OIT, OIT with preadministration of anti–immunoglobulin E (IgE), EPIT, peanut vaccines, and a hypoallergenic peanut.[20-25] There is also particularly high interest in developing strategies to prevent peanut allergy from developing, as opposed to treating it once it has occurred.

Prevention of peanut allergy can be thought of in 2 respects. Primary allergy prevention refers to measures or interventions that would prevent a person from developing peanut allergy or any manifestation of an allergic response, such as allergen sensitization (eg, the development of IgE antibodies specific for a particular food, noted on either a positive skin test or serum-specific IgE test). Secondary prevention refers to a cessation or arrest of an allergic process under development, most specifically referring to an already allergen-sensitized individual remaining nonreactive to ingesting that item (eg, the individual has a positive test but does not react when the food is ingested).[30-33] In the strictest sense, IgE against peanut cannot be formed without prior exposure, but how such exposure occurs in these children is not understood because it seems unintended. A leading hypothesis for how such children become sensitized is that this occurs through environmental exposures (eg, ambient dust that accumulates in the household, nonoral exposures through lotions containing peanut).[45] Such preventative strategies represent potentially cost-effective and widely applicable solutions that may not require a large burden of health service utilization to achieve benefit at a population level, as opposed to treating someone who has already developed allergy.

PREVENTING PEANUT ALLERGY THROUGH TIMING OF INTRODUCTION
A Historical Shift of Opinion

In 2000, the American Academy of Pediatrics (AAP) issued guidance on the introduction of complementary foods into the diet of infants to prevent development of allergic disease. In particular, the AAP strongly recommended that peanut introduction be delayed until age 3 years in children at high risk for the development of allergic disease (defined as children with a biparental, parental, or sibling family history of allergy), that nursing mothers should eliminate peanut (and other foods such as milk, egg, and fish) from their diet while nursing, and that pregnant mothers should consider removing peanut from their diet.[46] Clinical guidelines from the United Kingdom in 1998 issued similar recommendations, although the European Society for Pediatric Allergology and Clinical Immunology/European Society for Pediatric Gastroenterology, Hepatology and Nutrition did not recommend these timelines.[47-49] However, newer recommendations by the AAP in 2008 stated that "the documented benefits of nutritional intervention that may prevent or delay the onset of atopic disease are largely limited to infants at high risk of developing allergy," nor did evidence support any maternal dietary restriction of foods during pregnancy or breastfeeding or delay of any introduction of complementary foods past 4 to 6 months of life to protect against development of atopic disease in non–high-risk infants.[50] This sentiment was echoed by the American Academy of Allergy, Asthma, and Immunology (AAAAI) in 2013.[31] These AAP and AAAAI guidelines are in line with present recommendations of other international organizations. The Australioasian Society of Allergy and Clinical Immunology, Israeli Association of Allergy and Clinical Immunology, Canadian Society of Allergy and Clinical Immunology, and the European Academy of Allergy and Clinical Immunology make no recommendations advocating delay of introduction of any complementary foods (including high-risk allergens such as peanut), or for pregnant or nursing mothers to avoid any high-risk foods as means of prevention of allergic disease.[30–33,51,52]

Association Study Evidence Supporting Early Peanut Introduction as Protective Against Peanut Allergy

In 2008, Du Toit and colleagues[34] published a provocative and innovative observational study conducted in Tel Aviv, Israel and London, England. This study compared reported societal rates of peanut allergy and timing of peanut introduction. It had been observed that peanut allergy rates were not as extensive in Israel as they were in Western nations. Reasons for this were poorly understood, although culturally it had been noted that in areas where peanut consumption was high during infancy (eg, Middle East, Asia, Africa), peanut allergy was not readily reported.[53] Using validated questionnaire-based responses in 2 cohorts, parents of 5171 United Kingdom and 5625 Israeli Ashkenazi (Eastern European heritage) Jewish children were surveyed about any development of food allergy in the child, other comorbid atopic disease, general demographics, and a food frequency questionnaire asking about maternal prenatal and maternal/child postnatal feeding habits.[34]

Comparatively, peanut allergy prevalence was 1.85% in the United Kingdom versus 0.17% in Israel, with an adjusted relative risk for peanut allergy in the United Kingdom of 5.8 (9.8 among elementary school children). The prevalence of peanut allergy remained significantly higher in the United Kingdom cohort even among just the high-risk groups, such as children with eczema (6.46% vs 0.79%). Similar differences in prevalence were seen for tree nut allergy and sesame allergy, but not milk or egg allergy (although these trended toward significance). After statistical adjustment, the only significant factor associated with the difference in peanut allergy prevalence was timing of peanut introduction, for which 69% of Israeli children had reported peanut introduction by 9 months compared with just 10% of the children in the United Kingdom. The Israeli children consumed up to a median of 7.1 g of peanut protein in the first year of life approximately 8 times per month, versus a median of 0 g of peanut in the United Kingdom. Moreover, significantly fewer mothers in the United Kingdom reported consuming peanut while breastfeeding. The investigators concluded that the reduced rate of peanut allergy in Israel was most likely associated with the timing of introduction (and not explained by differences in baseline atopy, sociodemographics, genetics, or allergenicity of commonly consumed peanut-containing products). However, despite this strong association, these data were observational and could not imply any causality. Other observational data regarding early peanut introduction has been restricted to sensitization rates only. In an inner-city observational birth cohort, Joseph and colleagues[54] noted that early reported peanut introduction (by 4 months) was protective against developing peanut sensitization in children with a family history of allergic disease, whereas delay until 1 year of age was associated with a 4.3-fold increased odds of sensitization.

A New Hope in Preventing the Onset of Peanut Allergy

Given the fairly strong association noted in their study between Tel Aviv and London, the same United Kingdom team conducted an innovative study, the LEAP trial.[38,53] LEAP was a single-center, open-label, randomized, controlled interventional study conducted in infants at high risk for developing allergic disease, to definitively test the effect of timing of peanut introduction on the rate of peanut allergy development. Over a 3-year period, 834 United Kingdom children between the ages of 4 and 11 months with severe eczema egg allergy, or both (**Box 1**) were screened for enrollment, with 118 excluded because of lack of severe eczema. All remaining children underwent further screening with peanut skin-prick testing (SPT), and were then stratified into 2 groups based on the test size. Those with negative (0 mm) tests comprised one group, and those with minimally positive tests (1–4 mm) comprised the second. A total of 76 children with SPT of 5 mm or larger were excluded from randomization on the suspicion that they were highly likely to be peanut allergic. The remaining 640 children were then randomized, within the SPT-positive and SPT-negative groups, respectively, to either begin immediate peanut introduction and consumption of up to 6 g of peanut protein thrice weekly, continued through age 5 years, or to not have any peanut exposure until age 5. All children randomized to early introduction had their initial feeding performed in the office under observation. A total of 7 children reacted to this initial feeding and were instructed to avoid peanut. All children in the study were then followed over the next 4 years at set intervals. Their families filled out detailed dietary frequency questionnaires and symptom questionnaires, and selected families agreed to household dust surveillance to determine ambient environmental peanut levels.[38,45,53]

At age 5 years, both groups underwent peanut challenge. By the time of this challenge, 12 children had withdrawn from the SPT-negative group, compared with none from the SPT-positive group. The challenge results show clear protective benefit for early introduction in comparison with delayed introduction. In the intention-to-treat analysis (eg, all children were analyzed according to the group to which they were randomized for treatment assignment, irrespective of their adherence to the treatment or withdrawal), 17.2% of the avoidance group developed peanut allergy compared with just 3.2% of the early introduction group, for an absolute risk reduction (ARR) of 14% and a number needed to treat (NNT: number of subjects needed to receive an intervention for 1 to gain benefit) of 7.1. In the per-protocol analysis (eg, those who completed their treatment assignment without protocol violation), the trend was

---

Box 1
Inclusion criteria for the LEAP study

1. Age 4 to 11 months at screening, having either or both
   a. Severe eczema—self-defined by questionnaire

      i. Frequent need for topical steroids or calcineurin inhibitors

      ii. Parental description of "a very bad rash in joints and creases" or "a very bad itchy, dry, oozing, or crusted rash"

      iii. SCORAD grade ($\geq$40)
   b. Egg allergy: skin-prick test 6 mm or larger in a person without a history of known egg ingestion, or skin-prick test 3 mm or larger in an infant with a history of egg ingestion and subsequent development of allergic symptoms

2. Screening peanut allergy skin test: wheal smaller than 5 mm

better: 17.3% in the avoidance group developed allergy compared with 0.3% in the consumption group, for an ARR of 17 and an NNT of 5.9. Looking more closely, an interesting finding is revealed when the effect within the SPT-positive and SPT-negative strata is examined. Within the SPT-negative stratum, 13.7% in the avoidance group versus 1.9% in the early introduction group developed peanut allergy, an ARR of 11.8% and NNT of 8.5. However, within the SPT-positive stratum, this effect was more dramatic: 35.3% of those in the avoidance group versus 10.6% in the early introduction group developed peanut allergy, an ARR of 24.8% and NNT of 4 (**Fig. 1**). This finding demonstrates a fairly dramatic heterogeneity of treatment effect exists, and that secondary prevention was actually more effective than primary

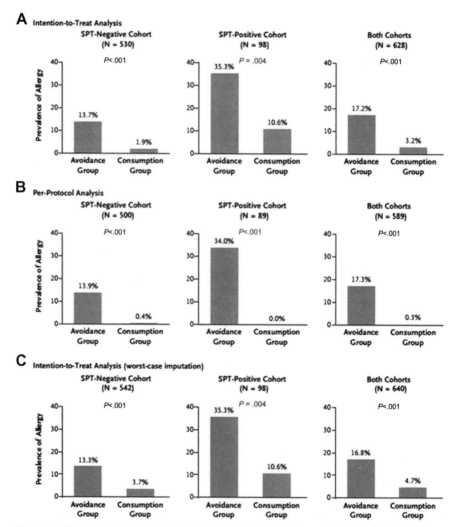

Fig. 1. (A–C) Results of the LEAP study. SPT, skin-prick test. (*From* Du Toit G, Roberts G, Sayre PH, et al. Randomized trial of peanut consumption in infants at risk for peanut allergy. N Engl J Med 2015;372(9):808. Copyright © 2015 Massachusetts Medical Society. Reprinted with permission from Massachusetts Medical Society.)

prevention. Unfortunately, the study did not explore effects within children with higher SPT sensitization (≥ 5 mm). These important findings show that there is a high value for the intervention in children with a positive skin test, and that providers should not necessarily fear peanut sensitization as too much of a risk factor, given that these children arguably benefited more than those without evidence of skin-test sensitization. Other important comparisons showed no difference in benefit based on race or ethnicity, and no difference in overall rates of adverse events based on peanut sensitization.[38]

Although the intervention conferred a high degree of benefit, it did not unequivocally prevent peanut allergy from developing. Rather, early introduction dramatically reduced the risk of developing peanut allergy, an important point to understand. In exploring rates of adverse reactions, 7 children reacted to the initial challenge, an additional 57 failed challenge at age 5 years (although 48 of these were from the avoidance group), and 9 children initially tolerated peanut consumption but then discontinued consumption after development of adverse events. Overall, only 9 children required epinephrine for a severe reaction. There were small differences in the risk of developing urticaria or gastrointestinal and upper respiratory infection symptoms in the consumption group ($P<.01$), and for anaphylaxis and infected eczema in the consumption group ($P<.05$). Overall retention of subjects over the 5 years was very high: 96% of the originally randomized participants underwent challenge at 5 years, and the investigators did note that this could represent a retention bias atypical for a randomized controlled trial (RCT) of this duration.

Criticisms of the study include that it was conducted at a single tertiary specialty referral center for food allergy, that the oral food challenges were not blinded, and that there was very high retention/adherence to protocol. These factors may have contributed to some participation bias. There are also some issues regarding how "high-risk" these patients were. There was an arbitrary SPT cutoff used to exclude participants, many of whom should not automatically be assumed to have been already peanut allergic per se, introducing some bias toward the effect sizes noted. Moreover, somewhat subjective entry criteria were used for both the rating of eczema severity (parental report of a severe rash being a poorly objective criteria, as is frequency of use of topical steroid) and egg allergy (children never exposed to egg, but having large egg skin tests, were considered "allergic").[38,53]

POLICY IMPLICATIONS OF THIS RESEARCH
Applicability of the Findings to the High-Risk and Standard-Risk Populations

The LEAP study demonstrates strong benefit conferred through early peanut introduction.[38] The burning question is how to position these findings in terms of policy. The study was a well conducted, randomized, controlled interventional trial, a considerable strength. Nonetheless this was a small-sized, single study conducted in a referral population within the United Kingdom, which may limit the generalizability of the findings. Moreover, the screening performed and the inclusion/exclusion criteria further limit the extent to which these findings can be broadly applied and replicated in practice. Multiple study outcomes were somewhat arbitrarily chosen, such as the amount of peanut protein the children consumed, the age at which consumption began, the duration of consumption, the optimal cutoff for exclusion of the peanut skin test (or the necessity of performing skin testing), the effect of short-term versus long-term discontinuation of consumption, and the effects of early consumption versus avoidance within children with lesser or no risk criteria. Thus, the degrees to which some of these decision points could vary and the effect of early introduction remain to be determined in future research. Determining these answers, however, may be difficult. There are strong arguments against replicating the study; as a delay in introduction is clearly associated with harm, repeating the study with an avoidance arm may not be ethical.

Considerations on an Implementation Strategy

Gruchalla and Sampson,[55] in an accompanying *New England Journal of Medicine* editorial for the LEAP study, recommended that all children between 4 and 8 months with moderate to severe eczema or egg allergy, as defined in the LEAP study, should be referred to a specialist skilled in the evaluation of food allergy for peanut skin testing, given the strong benefit of early introduction of peanut. Based on the skin testing, they recommended the following:

1. If the skin testing was negative (0 mm), the child should start consuming peanut thrice weekly, up to a total of 6 g.
2. If the skin test was 1 to 4 mm, a peanut challenge should be conducted in the office, and if passed, the child should begin a similar regimen.
3. If the skin test was 5 mm or greater, the child should not start peanut consumption.

In an accompanying correspondence to this editorial, this approach was criticized as being infeasible considering the small supply of providers skilled in food allergy skin testing and assessment in the United States and Canada, compared with the potential 20% of children younger than 1 year who may have eczema, and that the justification of such utilization of the health care service has not been shown to be cost-effective or logistically possible.[56] Prior research by the AAAAI has shown that fewer than 50% of all practicing allergists perform oral challenges, and of those 50% or so who do perform oral food challenges, approximately 80% perform only 1 challenge per week.[57] There are no data examining provider attitudes toward performing oral food challenge to peanut in infants, let alone infants with some degree of peanut sensitization. In fact, the LEAP study is actually the first large study exploring the feasibility of routine skin testing and challenge in such a young age group.[38] Provider comfort and experience with challenging children younger than 1 year may require further study, as does parent parental comfort and attitudes toward potentially invasive preevaluation. In particular, understanding parental goals and desires is highly important, given that their input and acceptance of a policy would be crucial to its success. Therefore, study of the feasibility of implementing any policy could greatly facilitate understanding the effects of early peanut introduction on overall pediatric and allergy health care.

Balancing the editorial recommendation is the practical experience from Israel and Australia, 2 nations where peanut is recommended to be introduced in the first 6 months of life without any prescreening measures or risk stratification. No data exist that show any rate of harm secondary to high rates of anaphylaxis attributable to early introduction at home, nor are there published rates of fatality associated with this practice.[52,53,58] In Australia, existing data show that there has been a significant increase in compliance with introduction of peanut before age 12 months between comparing responses pre-2009 (when Australian guidance on the subject was changed) with post-2009 responses.[58] However, the investigators noted that families were less likely to delay peanut introduction beyond 7 months in families without a history of food allergy and in families with higher socioeconomic status, demonstrating some barriers to implementation. United States data from a study conducted between 2005 and 2007 note that only approximately 25% of children younger than 1 year had been introduced to peanut, and are reflective of a potentially high barrier to changing existing complementary feeding practices in the United States.[59]

> **Box 2**
> **Summary of consensus interim recommendations**
>
> - There is now scientific evidence (level 1 evidence from a randomized controlled trial) that health care providers should recommend introducing peanut-containing products into the diet of "high-risk" infants early on in life (4–11 months of age) in countries where peanut allergy is prevalent, as delaying the introduction of peanut may be associated with an increased risk of developing peanut allergy.
> - Infants with early-onset atopic disease, such as severe eczema, or egg allergy in the first 4 to 6 months of life, may benefit from evaluation by an allergist or physician trained in management of allergic diseases in this age group to diagnose any food allergy and assist in implementing these suggestions regarding the appropriateness of early peanut introduction. Evaluation of such patients may consist of performing peanut skin testing and/ or in-office observed peanut ingestion, as deemed appropriate following discussion with the family. The clinician may perform an observed peanut challenge for those with evidence of a positive peanut skin test to determine whether they are clinically reactive, before initiating peanut introduction at home. Both such strategies were used in the LEAP study protocol.
> - Adherence in the LEAP trial was excellent (92%), with infants randomized to consume peanut ingesting a median of 7.7 g of peanut protein (interquartile range: 6.7–8.8 g) per week during the first 2 years of the trial compared with a median of 0 g in the avoidance group. While the outcome of the LEAP regimen was excellent, the study does not address use of alternative doses of peanut protein, minimal length of treatment necessary to induce the tolerogenic effect, or potential risks of premature discontinuation or sporadic feeding of peanut.

Current Interim Recommendations

A multinational task force comprising pediatric, dermatology, and multiple allergy organizations have reviewed the LEAP study data and have recently published interim consensus recommendations to help guide provider decision making (**Box 2**).[60] These guidelines do not make any specific recommendation for screening/skin testing or cutoffs for exclusion of early peanut introduction, however, and strongly advocate that the LEAP study provides further substantiation in support of early versus delayed peanut introduction, consistent with multiple existing guidelines on the subject. These recommendations also do not comment on feasibility of implementation, cost-effectiveness or other value-based care related to early peanut introduction, or comment on introduction of other foods beyond peanut. The National Institutes of Allergy and Infectious Diseases (NIAID) has convened an expert panel tasked with making more formal policy recommendations, which are anticipated for early 2016.

SUMMARY

The LEAP study therefore represents a milestone in that it was an RCT-based interventional study, tackling a very important question of the optimal time to introduce peanut into the diet of a child to help prevent peanut allergy. The conclusions provide level 1 evidence that give us pause to consider what is the most effective infant feeding strategy to help deter allergy and, more importantly, that such a strategy does exist. Although LEAP is only a single-center study, it does provide conclusive evidence of a beneficial effect for early peanut introduction. This effect is sufficiently strong that numerous allergy, pediatric, and dermatology societies and academies have provided a clear, consensus opinion that the findings should be implemented immediately to begin providing benefit. While awaiting the final expert opinion expected to be forwarded by the NIAID panel by early 2016, it is momentous that there now appears to be a bona fide and widely available strategy that should make a noticeable difference in lowering the rate of peanut allergy. At present there are insufficient available data to issue any policy statements regarding the optimal timing of introduction of other foods, but studies of other foods are under way and recommendations should be available in the near future.

REFERENCES

1. Gupta RS, Springston EE, Warrier MR, et al. The prevalence, severity, and distribution of childhood food allergy in the United States. Pediatrics 2011;128:e9–17.
2. Boyce JA, Assa'ad A, Burks AW, et al. Guidelines for the diagnosis and management of food allergy in the United States: report of the NIAID-sponsored expert panel. J Allergy Clin Immunol 2010;126:S1–58.
3. Gupta R, Holdford D, Bilaver L, et al. The economic impact of childhood food allergy in the United States. JAMA Pediatr 2013;167:1026–31.
4. Cohen BL, Noone S, Munoz-Furlong A, et al. Development of a questionnaire to measure quality of life in families with a child with food allergy. J Allergy Clin Immunol 2004;114:1159–63.
5. Sicherer SH, Noone SA, Munoz-Furlong A. The impact of childhood food allergy on quality of life. Ann Allergy Asthma Immunol 2001;87:461–4.
6. Primeau MN, Kagan R, Joseph L, et al. The psychological burden of peanut allergy as perceived by adults with peanut allergy and the parents of peanut-allergic children. Clin Exp Allergy 2000;30:1135–43.
7. DunnGalvin A, de BlokFlokstra BM, Burks AW, et al. Food allergy QoL questionnaire for children aged 0-12 years: content, construct, and cross-cultural validity. Clin Exp Allergy 2008;38:977–86.
8. Flokstra-de Blok BM, DunnGalvin A, Vlieg-Boerstra BJ, et al. Development and validation of the self-administered food allergy quality of life questionnaire for adolescents. J Allergy Clin Immunol 2008;122:139–44, 144.e1–2.
9. King RM, Knibb RC, Hourihane JO. Impact of peanut allergy on quality of life, stress and anxiety in the family. Allergy 2009;64:461–8.
10. Cummings AJ, Knibb RC, King RM, et al. The psychosocial impact of food allergy and food hypersensitivity in children, adolescents and their families: a review. Allergy 2010;65:933–45.
11. Flokstra-de Blok BM, van der Velde JL, Vlieg-Boerstra BJ, et al. Health-related quality of life of food allergic patients measured with generic and disease-specific questionnaires. Allergy 2010;65:1031–8.
12. van der Velde JL, Flokstra-de Blok BM, Vlieg-Boerstra BJ, et al. Development, validity and reliability of the food allergy independent measure (FAIM). Allergy 2010;65:630–5.
13. Knibb RC, Ibrahim NF, Stiefel G, et al. The psychological impact of diagnostic food challenges to confirm the resolution of peanut or tree nut allergy. Clin Exp Allergy 2012;42:451–9.
14. van der Velde JL, Dubois AE, Flokstra-de Blok BM. Food allergy and quality of life: what have we learned? Curr Allergy Asthma Rep 2013;13:651–61.
15. Franxman T, Howe L, Teich E, et al. Oral food challenge and food allergy quality of life in caregivers of food allergic children. J Allergy Clin Immunol Pract 2015;3:50–6.
16. Howe L, Franxman T, Teich E, et al. What affects quality of life among caregivers of food allergic children? Ann Allergy Asthma Immunol 2014;113:69–74.

17. Muraro A, Dubois AE, Dunngalvin A, et al. EAACI food allergy and anaphylaxis guidelines. Food allergy health-related quality of life measures. Allergy 2014; 69(7):845–53.
18. Salvilla SA, Dubois AE, Flokstra-de Blok BM, et al. Disease-specific health-related quality of life instruments for IgE-mediated food allergy. Allergy 2014;69:834–44.
19. Sampson HA, Aceves S, Bock SA, et al. Food allergy: a practice parameter update-2014. J Allergy Clin Immunol 2014;134:1016–25.e43.
20. Burks AW, Laubach S, Jones SM. Oral tolerance, food allergy, and immunotherapy: implications for future treatment. J Allergy Clin Immunol 2008;121: 1344–50.
21. Mondoulet L, Dioszeghy V, Ligouis M, et al. Epicutaneous immunotherapy on intact skin using a new delivery system in a murine model of allergy. Clin Exp Allergy 2010;40:659–67.
22. Senti G, von Moos S, Tay F, et al. Determinants of efficacy and safety in epicutaneous allergen immunotherapy: summary of three clinical trials. Allergy 2015;70: 707–10.
23. Mondoulet L, Dioszeghy V, Puteaux E, et al. Specific epicutaneous immunotherapy prevents sensitization to new allergens in a murine model. J Allergy Clin Immunol 2015;135:1546–57.e4.
24. Jones SM, Burks AW, Dupont C. State of the art on food allergen immunotherapy: oral, sublingual, and epicutaneous. J Allergy Clin Immunol 2014;133:318–23.
25. Nurmatov U, Venderbosch I, Devereux G, et al. Allergen-specific oral immunotherapy for peanut allergy. Cochrane Database Syst Rev 2012;(9):CD009014.
26. Sampson HA. Peanut oral immunotherapy: is it ready for clinical practice? J Allergy Clin Immunol Pract 2013;1:15–21.
27. Greenhawt MJ, Vickery BP. Allergist-reported trends in the practice of food allergen oral immunotherapy. J Allergy Clin Immunol Pract 2015;3:33–8.
28. Greenhawt MJ. STOPping peanut allergy: the saga of food oral immunotherapy. Lancet 2014;383:1272–4.
29. Greenhawt MJ. Oral and sublingual peanut immunotherapy is not ready for general use. Allergy Asthma Proc 2013;34:197–204.
30. Muraro A, Halken S, Arshad SH, et al. EAACI food allergy and anaphylaxis guidelines. Primary prevention of food allergy. Allergy 2014;69:590–601.
31. de Silva D, Geromi M, Halken S, et al. Primary prevention of food allergy in children and adults: systematic review. Allergy 2014;69:581–9.
32. Fleischer DM, Spergel JM, Assa'ad AH, et al. Primary prevention of allergic diseases through nutritional interventions. J Allergy Clin Immunol Pract 2013;1: 29–36.
33. Chan ES, Cummings C, Canadian Paediatric Society, Community Paediatrics Committee and Allergy Section. Dietary exposures and allergy prevention in high-risk infants: a joint statement with the Canadian Society of Allergy and Clinical Immunology. Paediatr Child Health 2013;18:545–54.
34. Du Toit G, Katz Y, Sasieni P, et al. Early consumption of peanuts in infancy is associated with a low prevalence of peanut allergy. J Allergy Clin Immunol 2008; 122(5):984–91.
35. Koplin JJ, Osborne NJ, Wake M, et al. Can early introduction of egg prevent egg allergy in infants? A population-based study. J Allergy Clin Immunol 2010;126: 807–13.
36. Katz Y, Rajuan N, Goldberg MR, et al. Early exposure to cow's milk protein is protective against IgE-mediated cow's milk protein allergy. J Allergy Clin Immunol 2010;126:77–82.e1.

37. Palmer DJ, Metcalfe J, Makrides M, et al. Early regular egg exposure in infants with eczema: a randomized controlled trial. J Allergy Clin Immunol 2013;132: 387–92.e1.
38. DuToit G, Roberts G, Sayre PH, et al. Randomized trial of peanut consumption in infants at risk for peanut allergy. N Engl J Med 2015;372:803–13.
39. Nwaru BI, Hickstein L, Panesar SS, et al. The epidemiology of food allergy in Europe: a systematic review and meta-analysis. Allergy 2014;69:62–75.
40. Osborne NJ, Koplin JJ, Martin PE, et al. Prevalence of challenge-proven IgE-mediated food allergy using population-based sampling and predetermined challenge criteria in infants. J Allergy Clin Immunol 2011;127:668–76.
41. Venter C, Hasan Arshad S, Grundy J, et al. Time trends in the prevalence of peanut allergy: three cohorts of children from the same geographical location in the UK. Allergy 2010;65:103–8.
42. Sicherer SH, Muñoz-Furlong A, Godbold JH, et al. US prevalence of self-reported peanut, tree nut, and sesame allergy: 11-year follow-up. J Allergy Clin Immunol 2010;125:1322–6.
43. Soller L, Ben-Shoshan M, Harrington DW, et al. Overall prevalence of self-reported food allergy in Canada. J Allergy Clin Immunol 2012;130:986–8.
44. Amoah AS, Obeng BB, Larbi IA, et al. Peanut-specific IgE antibodies in asymptomatic Ghanaian children possibly caused by carbohydrate determinant cross-reactivity. J Allergy Clin Immunol 2013;132:639–47.
45. Brough HA, Simpson A, Makinson K, et al. Peanut allergy: effect of environmental peanut exposure in children with filaggrin loss-of-function mutations. J Allergy Clin Immunol 2014;134:867–75.e1.
46. American Academy of Pediatrics, Committee on Nutrition. Hypoallergenic infant formulas. Pediatrics 2000;106:346–9.
47. Host A, Koletzko B, Dreborg S, et al. Dietary products used in infants for treatment and prevention of food allergy. Joint Statement of the European Society for Pediatric Allergology and Clinical Immunology (ESPACI) Committee on Hypoallergenic Formulas and the European Society for Pediatric Gastroenterology, Hepatology and Nutrition (ESPGHAN) Committee on Nutrition. Arch Dis Child 1999;81:80–4.
48. Zeiger RA. Food allergen avoidance in the prevention of food allergy in infants and children. Pediatrics 2003;111:1662–71.
49. Committee on Toxicity of Chemicals in Food, Consumer Products and the Environment. Peanut allergy. London: Department of Health; 1998. Available at: http://webarchive.nationalarchives.gov.uk/20120209132957/http://cot.food.gov. uk/pdfs/cotpeanutall.pdf.
50. Greer FR, Sicherer SH, Burks AW. Effects of early nutritional interventions on the development of atopic disease in infants and children: the role of maternal dietary restriction, breastfeeding, timing of introduction of complementary foods, and hydrolyzed formulas. Pediatrics 2008;121:183–91.
51. Agostoni C, Decsi T, Fewtrell M, et al. Complementary feeding: a commentary by the ESPGHAN committee on nutrition. J Pediatr Gastroenterol Nutr 2008;46:99–110.
52. Australasian Society of Clinical Immunology and Allergy (ASCIA). ASCIA infant feeding advice. Available at: http://www.allergy.org.au/images/stories/aer/ infobulletins/2010pdf/ASCIA_Infant_Feeding_Advice_2010.pdf. Accessed April 2, 2015.
53. Du Toit G, Roberts G, Sayre PH, et al. Identifying infants at high risk of peanut allergy: the Learning Early About Peanut Allergy (LEAP) screening study. J Allergy Clin Immunol 2013;131:135–43.

54. Joseph CL, Ownby DR, Havstad SL, et al. Early complementary feeding and risk of food sensitization in a birth cohort. J Allergy Clin Immunol 2011;127:1203–10.
55. Gruchalla RS, Sampson HA. Preventing peanut allergy through early consumption—ready for prime time? N Engl J Med 2015;372:875–7.
56. Greenhawt M, Chan ES, Fleischer DM. Looking before you LEAP [letter to the editor]. N Engl J Med 2015;372:2163–6.
57. Pongracic JA, Bock SA, Sicherer SH. Oral food challenge practices among allergists in the United States. J Allergy Clin Immunol 2012;129:564–6.
58. Tey D, Allen KJ, Peters RL, et al. Population response to change in infant feeding guidelines for allergy prevention. J Allergy Clin Immunol 2014;133:476–84.
59. Clayton HB, Li R, Perrine CG, et al. Prevalence and reasons for introducing infants early to solid foods: variations by milk feeding type. Pediatrics 2013;131:e1108–14.
60. Fleischer DM, Sicherer SH, Greenhawt MJ, et al. Consensus communication on early peanut introduction and the prevention of peanut allergy in high-risk infants. J Allergy Clin Immunol 2015;136:258–61.

Mechanisms of Oral Tolerance

Scott P. Commins, MD, PhD

KEYWORDS

- Mucosal • Food allergy • Tolerance • Autoimmunity • Oral antigen

KEY POINTS

- The gut has adapted a unique set of immune cells and sites to respond to antigens appropriately.
- Numerous characteristics of antigens are important for the induction of oral tolerance.
- Use of the oral route to establish tolerance holds promise for food-based antigens as well as other disease states.

INTRODUCTION

Oral tolerance is the active process by which the immune system does not respond to an orally administered antigen. The number of studies addressing oral tolerance in humans is surprisingly limited despite the extensive literature from murine models. In fact, animal models have largely been used to study both the mechanism of sensitization to food as well as the resulting allergic response from consuming a food allergen. Most available animal models of food allergy require an artificial sensitization method and may provide only limited insight into the sensitization phase of human food allergic disease. Thus, food allergy researchers have sought to develop an animal model that more closely mimics the sensitization of humans to food antigens. Until such a model, there may not be specific answers to the precise mechanisms that result in establishing oral tolerance or that lead to a break in tolerance. This review provides an overview of some available animal models, comments on other disease states and relevant models, and comments on possible future directions.

Disclosure: National Institutes of Health grant recipient (K08 AI085190); UpToDate author.
Department of Medicine, University of North Carolina School of Medicine, Division of Rheumatology, Allergy and Immunology, 3300 Thurston Building, CB 7280, Chapel Hill, NC 27599-7280, USA
E-mail address: scottcommins@virginia.edu

Pediatr Clin N Am 62 (2015) 1523–1529
http://dx.doi.org/10.1016/j.pcl.2015.07.013
0031-3955/15/$

ROLE OF THE GUT IMMUNE SYSTEM

The gut-associated lymphoid tissue (GALT) is the largest immune system in the body.[1] Approximately 30 kg of food proteins reach the human intestine during a year, and 130 to 190 g of these proteins are absorbed daily in the gut.[2] The microbiota in the intestine is an additional major source of natural antigenic stimulation with a perhaps underappreciated number of bacteria colonizing the human intestinal mucosa ($\sim 10^{12}$ microorganisms per gram of stool).[3] The physiologic role of the GALT is the ingestion of dietary antigens in a manner that does not result in untoward immune reactions and protection of the organism from pathogens. This represents a careful balancing act, as the mucosal barriers are thin and vulnerable to pathogenic infection. It should be noted that tolerance to food protein affects local and systemic immune responses, whereas tolerance to gut bacteria in the colon does not attenuate systemic responses. Despite these distinct and active processes, the GALT is primarily a tolerogenic environment.

The features of the gut immune system that are important participants in creating the tolerogenic environment have been studied and discussed.[4] Briefly, the inductive sites for immune responses in the gut are Peyer patches and mesenteric lymph nodes (MLNs). MLNs develop distinct from Peyer patches and peripheral lymph nodes and serve as a crossroads between the peripheral and mucosal recirculation pathways. To induce a mucosal immune response, an antigen must gain access to antigen-presenting cells by penetrating the mucus layer and then the intestinal epithelial cell barrier. Dendritic cells (DCs) themselves sample luminal contents by extending their processes through the epithelium without disruption of tight junctions.[5,6] Another important component of the GALT is the intraepithelial lymphocytes (IELs), which serve to regulate intestinal homeostasis, maintain epithelial barrier function, respond to infection, and regulate adaptive and innate immune responses.[7] Most IELs are CD8+ T cells, which express $\alpha\beta$ or $\gamma\delta$ T-cell receptors (TCRs). Of note, it has been reported that depletion of $\gamma\delta$ T cells impairs induction of oral tolerance.[8] Thus, the combination of commensals, T cells, and DCs set up a tolerogenic environment in the gut.[6,9,10] Major factors that condition the gut to be a tolerogenic environment are interleukin-10, retinoic acid, and transforming growth factor-β (TGF-β), which serves as a switch factor for immunoglobulin (Ig)A, the predominant immunoglobulin of the gut.[11]

REGULATORY T CELLS

It is now recognized that there are multiple mechanisms of oral tolerance, and one of the prime determinants is the dose of antigen fed.[4,12–19] Low doses favor the induction of regulatory T cell (Tregs), whereas higher doses favor the induction of anergy or deletion.[20] These mechanisms are not exclusive, especially at higher doses. One of the major mechanisms of oral tolerance is the induction of Treg cells, a process that is related to the gut DCs and linked to both TGF-β and retinoic acid.[10,17,21] Specifically, it has been shown that mucosal DCs induce forkhead box P3 (Foxp3) Tregs via the production of TGF-β, but that concomitant retinoic acid signaling boosted this process.[22] In fact, all major classes of Tregs can be induced or activated by oral (mucosal) antigen.[23–27] Even CD8+ Tregs have been shown to play a role in oral tolerance.[28,29] Interestingly, CD8+ T cells have been shown to recall a tolerant or hyporesponsive phenotype following immune stimulation, suggesting that epigenetic mechanisms are in place to maintain tolerance.[30] As future work progresses, it remains to be elucidated whether similar mechanisms may account for failure of programmed reactive cells to maintain hyporesponsiveness following oral immunotherapy.

ANERGY

T-cell unresponsiveness or anergy is one of the primary mechanisms by which tolerance is maintained in self-reactive lymphocytes and anergy is induced in high-dose oral tolerance. The upregulation of anergy-associated genes is largely dependent on nuclear factor of activated T cells.[31] Orally tolerized T cells can form conjugates with antigen-presenting cells, but they are defective in immunologic synapse formation.[32] Similarly, T cells made anergic in vivo following oral antigen can inhibit the migration of responsive T cells in an antigen-independent fashion, indicating that hyporesponsive T cells have broad tolerogenic signals.[33] Using a murine model to examine the role of the thymus in high-dose oral tolerance, researchers found that thymectomized animals were not protected from autoimmune disease.[34] The thymus was actually found to be an important site for the development of CD4+CD25+ Tregs after oral antigen.[34] In fact, clonal deletion was found in the periphery but not the thymus, suggesting that high-dose oral tolerance not only induces deletion but may lead to CD4+CD25+ Tregs that resemble natural Foxp3+ Tregs.[34] These observations are in keeping with results from high-dose oral immunotherapy studies that have reported increased CD4+CD25+ Foxp3+ Tregs in subjects with clinical hyporesponsiveness.[35]

LESSONS LEARNED FROM ORAL ANTI-CD3

The investigation of oral tolerance has classically involved the administration of oral antigen followed by challenge with same/similar antigen (albeit usually in an adjuvant) to demonstrate antigen-specific tolerance. One interesting experimental system that has been used to study T-cell function in oral tolerance is the use of TCR transgenic mice, in which all T cells have a common TCR. Using such mice, Dr Weiner and colleagues[36] investigated how oral administration of an antigen affected specific T-cell subsets. These investigators showed a dose-dependent induction of Tregs to the fed antigen. In similar mice that have ovalbumin-specific TCR, high-dose oral administration of ovalbumin led to deletion of Treg subsets.[37]

To translate these findings to humans, it first had to be known whether it was possible to trigger the TCR in wild-type mice in the gut and induce Tregs without using cognate antigen. Previous work had established that anti-CD3 binds to the ε chain of the TCR and, given intravenously, deletes T cells and has been shown to be an effective treatment for type 1 diabetes in the nonobese diabetic mouse.[38] It was hypothesized that oral administration of anti-CD3 monoclonal antibody would replace the use of a cognate antigen to trigger the TCR and lead to induction of Tregs when given orally. Using an autoimmune encephalitis murine model, Ochi and colleagues[39] found that oral anti-CD3 suppressed both clinical and pathologic features of the disease. Notably, there was a dose effect observed with disease suppression by oral anti-CD3 at lower, but not higher doses.[39] The scientists suggested these findings were consistent with the classic paradigm of oral tolerance: induction of Tregs is seen at lower but not higher doses.[19,20,37] Potentially important for all researchers interested in oral tolerance, it demonstrated that induction of Tregs by oral anti-CD3 was not simply related to administering large amounts of antibody to overwhelm breakdown in the gut.[39] Also of significance was the finding that the Fc portion of anti-CD3 was not required, as anti-CD3 Fab'2 fragment was active orally and induced Tregs.[39] The effects of these and similar experiments raise the question of whether it is more advantageous to induce antigen-specific versus antigen nonspecific Tregs for the treatment of relevant diseases, which is an issue being addressed in ongoing trials in humans.[17]

Box 1
Characteristics of hepatic function and structure that may favor tolerance

Liver endothelial cells sample circulating antigen and act as antigen-presenting cells that lead to tolerance[45]

Kupffer cells and conventional dendritic cells favor tolerance during antigen presentation[45]

Plasmacytoid dendritic cells are abundant in the liver and support systemic tolerance[21]

SITE OF TOLERANCE TO ORAL ANTIGENS: GUT VERSUS SYSTEMIC

One of the characteristic features of oral tolerance to soluble antigens is that it can involve the entire animal.[16] This is difficult to explain, however, as current thought focuses on anatomic compartmentalization within the mucosal immune system. In other words, antigen uptake and recognition are believed to be restricted to the GALT, MLNs, DCs, and intestinal epithelial cells (discussed previously), therefore limiting the effects to the intestinal mucosa. A possible explanation, and one that our laboratory and others are examining, is that orally administered antigens may disseminate systemically via blood and/or lymph.[40–43] In fact, earlier studies suggest that food protein can be detected in the blood of mice and humans soon after eating.[40,43] Furthermore, serum from protein-fed mice can induce antigen-specific tolerance in naive recipients, indicating the presence of "tolerogenic material."[44] This raises the important question of how and where an absorbed antigen can contribute to establishing oral tolerance.

One potential site is the liver. Administration of antigen directly into the portal vein, which drains blood from the intestine to the liver, is well known to induce antigen-specific tolerance.[45] Conversely, directing blood flow away from the liver by portocaval shunting prevents the induction of oral tolerance.[46,47] Liver has several features that could serve to promote tolerance (**Box 1**). Antigen reaching beyond the liver into peripheral lymph nodes and spleen might be expected to induce tolerance in these sites, as it will be presented by resident DCs in the absence of costimulation, leading to the induction of anergy or Tregs.[16]

There is certainly evidence to the contrary, in that systemic dissemination of fed antigen is not important for oral tolerance. For example, transport of antigen from the lamina propria into the MLNs by CD103+ DCs was found to be crucial for inducing the systemic effects of oral tolerance.[48] Moreover, the chemokine receptor CCR7 is required for continual migration of DCs into draining lymph nodes, and genetic deficiency in CCR7 prevented the recognition of fed antigen by T cells in the MLNs and impaired the induction of oral tolerance.[49,50] Other reports also have focused on MLNs having a central role in oral tolerance induction.[50,51] At this time it is unclear why there appears to be discordant findings about the relative roles of intestinal anatomic compartmentalization (eg, GALT, MLNs) versus more widespread dissemination of antigen (eg, to the liver). Possible reasons for the discrepant results include (1) the concentration of antigen reaching the circulation, (2) nature of the antigen, (3) dose of antigen ingested, and (4) the microbiome of the animals.[19,48,50]

SUMMARY

Despite the extensive literature on the effectiveness of oral tolerance to treat diseases in animals, this approach has yet to successfully translate to clinical treatment of IgE-mediated food allergy or even food hypersensitivity. With the advent of technologies such as mass cytometry and single-cell gene expression profiling applied to food allergy, we can only expect to reach a better understanding of cellular processes regulating oral tolerance. In the coming years, it will likely be time for the next phase of human studies of mucosal tolerance. The establishment of immunologic markers will provide the basis for dosing and measuring the effect of clinical trials. Although one of the major goals of future immunotherapy might be to induce Tregs, food allergy researchers must also be cognizant of the role of IgE-producing cells and their location; yet, to date, there are no specific methods to do this in vivo. The challenge is ours, therefore, to design or use clinical syndromes that can elucidate unknown aspects of oral tolerance and, specifically, breaks in tolerance that manifest as food allergy.

REFERENCES

1. Moog F. The lining of the small intestine. Sci Am 1981;245(5):154–8, 160, 162 et passiom.
2. Brandtzaeg P. Development and basic mechanisms of human gut immunity. Nutr Rev 1998;56(1 Pt 2):S5–18.
3. Macfarlane GT, Macfarlane S. Human colonic microbiota: ecology, physiology and metabolic potential of intestinal bacteria. Scand J Gastroenterol Suppl 1997;222:3–9.
4. Mowat AM. Anatomical basis of tolerance and immunity to intestinal antigens. Nat Rev Immunol 2003;3(4):331–41.
5. Mowat AM, Donachie AM, Parker LA, et al. The role of dendritic cells in regulating mucosal immunity and tolerance. Novartis Found Symp 2003;252:291–302 [discussion: 302–5].
6. Rescigno M. Functional specialization of antigen presenting cells in the gastrointestinal tract. Curr Opin Immunol 2010;22(1):131–6.
7. Sheridan BS, Lefrançois L. Intraepithelial lymphocytes: to serve and protect. Curr Gastroenterol Rep 2010;12(6):513–21.
8. Ke Y, Pearce K, Lake JP, et al. Gamma delta T lymphocytes regulate the induction and maintenance of oral tolerance. J Immunol 1997;158(8):3610–8.
9. Strober W. The multifaceted influence of the mucosal microflora on mucosal dendritic cell responses. Immunity 2009;31(3):377–88.
10. Izcue A, Coombes JL, Powrie F. Regulatory T cells suppress systemic and mucosal immune activation to control intestinal inflammation. Immunol Rev 2006;212:256–71.
11. Li MO, Flavell RA. TGF-beta: a master of ali T cell trades. Cell 2008;134(3):392–404.
12. Mowat AM. Basic mechanisms and clinical implications of oral tolerance. Curr Opin Gastroenterol 1999;15(6):546–56.
13. Vickery BP, Burks AW. Immunotherapy in the treatment of food allergy: focus on oral tolerance. Curr Opin Allergy Clin Immunol 2009;9(4):364–70.
14. Peron JP, de Oliveira AP, Rizzo LV. It takes guts for tolerance: the phenomenon of oral tolerance and the regulation of autoimmune response. Autoimmun Rev 2009;9(1):1–4.
15. Wang J, Toes RE. Mechanisms of oral tolerance revisited. Arthritis Res Ther 2008;10(2):108.
16. Pabst O, Mowat AM. Oral tolerance to food protein. Mucosal Immunol 2012;5(3):232–9.
17. Weiner HL, da Cunha AP, Quintana F, et al. Oral tolerance. Immunol Rev 2011;241(1):241–59.

18. Burks AW, Laubach S, Jones SM. Oral tolerance, food allergy, and immunotherapy: implications for future treatment. J Allergy Clin Immunol 2008;121(6): 1344–50.
19. Chen YH, Weiner HL. Dose-dependent activation and deletion of antigen-specific T cells following oral tolerance. Ann N Y Acad Sci 1996;778:111–21.
20. Friedman A, Weiner HL. Induction of anergy or active suppression following oral tolerance is determined by antigen dosage. Proc Natl Acad Sci U S A 1994; 91(14):6688–92.
21. Dubois B, Joubert G, Gomez de Agüero M, et al. Sequential role of plasmacytoid dendritic cells and regulatory T cells in oral tolerance. Gastroenterology 2009; 137(3):1019–28.
22. Mucida D, Park Y, Kim G, et al. Reciprocal TH17 and regulatory T cell differentiation mediated by retinoic acid. Science 2007;317(5835):256–60.
23. Chen Y, Kuchroo VK, Inobe J, et al. Regulatory T cell clones induced by oral tolerance: suppression of autoimmune encephalomyelitis. Science 1994;265(5176): 1237–40.
24. Zhang ZJ, Davidson L, Eisenbarth G, et al. Suppression of diabetes in nonobese diabetic mice by oral administration of porcine insulin. Proc Natl Acad Sci U S A 1991;88(22):10252–6.
25. Miller A, Lider O, Roberts AB, et al. Suppressor T cells generated by oral tolerization to myelin basic protein suppress both in vitro and in vivo immune responses by the release of transforming growth factor beta after antigen-specific triggering. Proc Natl Acad Sci U S A 1992;89(1):421–5.
26. Thorstenson KM, Khoruts A. Generation of anergic and potentially immunoregulatory CD25+CD4 T cells in vivo after induction of peripheral tolerance with intravenous or oral antigen. J Immunol 2001;167(1):188–95.
27. Tsuji NM, Mizumachi K, Kurisaki J. Interleukin-10-secreting Peyer's patch cells are responsible for active suppression in low-dose oral tolerance. Immunology 2001;103(4):458–64.
28. Chen Y, Inobe J, Weiner HL. Induction of oral tolerance to myelin basic protein in CD8-depleted mice: both CD4+ and CD8+ cells mediate active suppression. J Immunol 1995;155(2):910–6.
29. Lider O, Santos LM, Lee CS, et al. Suppression of experimental autoimmune encephalomyelitis by oral administration of myelin basic protein. II. Suppression of disease and in vitro immune responses is mediated by antigen-specific CD8+ T lymphocytes. J Immunol 1989;142(3):748–52.
30. Schietinger A, Delrow JJ, Basom RS, et al. Rescued tolerant CD8 T cells are preprogrammed to reestablish the tolerant state. Science 2012;335(6069): 723–7.
31. Macián F, García-Cózar F, Im SH, et al. Transcriptional mechanisms underlying lymphocyte tolerance. Cell 2002;109(6):719–31.
32. Ise W, Nakamura K, Shimizu N, et al. Orally tolerized T cells can form conjugates with APCs but are defective in immunological synapse formation. J Immunol 2005;175(2):829–38.
33. Mirenda V, Millington O, Lechler RI, et al. Tolerant T cells display impaired trafficking ability. Eur J Immunol 2005;35(7):2146–56.
34. Song F, Guan Z, Gienapp IE, et al. The thymus plays a role in oral tolerance in experimental autoimmune encephalomyelitis. J Immunol 2006;177(3):1500–9.
35. Vickery BP, Scurlock AM, Kulis M, et al. Sustained unresponsiveness to peanut in subjects who have completed peanut oral immunotherapy. J Allergy Clin Immunol 2014;133(2):468–75.

36. Chen Y, Inobe J, Kuchroo VK, et al. Oral tolerance in myelin basic protein T-cell receptor transgenic mice: suppression of autoimmune encephalomyelitis and dose-dependent induction of regulatory cells. Proc Natl Acad Sci U S A 1996; 93(1):388–91.
37. Chen Y, Inobe J, Marks R, et al. Peripheral deletion of antigen-reactive T cells in oral tolerance. Nature 1995;376(6536):177–80.
38. Chatenoud L, Bluestone JA. CD3-specific antibodies: a portal to the treatment of autoimmunity. Nat Rev Immunol 2007;7(8):622–32.
39. Ochi H, Abraham M, Ishikawa H, et al. Oral CD3-specific antibody suppresses autoimmune encephalomyelitis by inducing CD4+ CD25- LAP+ T cells. Nat Med 2006;12(6):627–35.
40. Husby S, Jensenius JC, Svehag SE. Passage of undegraded dietary antigen into the blood of healthy adults. Quantification, estimation of size distribution, and relation of uptake to levels of specific antibodies. Scand J Immunol 1985;22(1): 83–92.
41. Commins SP, James HR, Stevens W, et al. Delayed clinical and ex vivo response to mammalian meat in patients with IgE to galactose-alpha-1,3-galactose. J Allergy Clin Immunol 2014;134(1):108–15.
42. Warshaw AL, Walker WA. Intestinal absorption of intake antigenic protein. Surgery 1974;76(3):495–9.
43. Walker WA, Isselbacher KJ. Uptake and transport of macromolecules by the intestine. Possible role in clinical disorders. Gastroenterology 1974;67(3):531–50.
44. Peng HJ, Turner MW, Strobel S. The generation of a 'tolerogen' after the ingestion of ovalbumin is time-dependent and unrelated to serum levels of immunoreactive antigen. Clin Exp Immunol 1990;81(3):510–5.
45. Thomson AW, Knolle PA. Antigen-presenting cell function in the tolerogenic liver environment. Nat Rev Immunol 2010;10(11):753–66.
46. Callery MP, Kamei T, Flye MW. The effect of portacaval shunt on delayed-hypersensitivity responses following antigen feeding. J Surg Res 1989;46(4): 391–4.
47. Yang R, Liu Q, Grosfeld JL, et al. Intestinal venous drainage through the liver is a prerequisite for oral tolerance induction. J Pediatr Surg 1994;29(8):1145–8.
48. Pabst O, Bernhardt G, Förster R. The impact of cell-bound antigen transport on mucosal tolerance induction. J Leukoc Biol 2007;82(4):795–800.
49. Förster R, Davalos-Misslitz AC, Rot A. CCR7 and its ligands: balancing immunity and tolerance. Nat Rev Immunol 2008;8(5):362–71.
50. Worbs T, Bode U, Yan S, et al. Oral tolerance originates in the intestinal immune system and relies on antigen carriage by dendritic cells. J Exp Med 2006;203(3): 519–27.
51. Spahn TW, Weiner HL, Rennert PD, et al. Mesenteric lymph nodes are critical for the induction of high-dose oral tolerance in the absence of Peyer's patches. Eur J Immunol 2002;32(4):1109–13.

Current Options for the Treatment of Food Allergy

Bruce J. Lanser, MD[a,b],*, Benjamin L. Wright, MD[c,d], Kelly A. Orgel, MS[c],
Brian P. Vickery, MD[c], David M. Fleischer, MD[a,e]

KEYWORDS

- Food allergy/hypersensitivity • Anaphylaxis • Food allergy treatment
- Immunotherapy • Desensitization • Tolerance • Probiotics • Omalizumab

KEY POINTS

- The standard of care for the management of food allergies is education, avoidance of trigger foods, and treatment of allergic reactions due to accidental ingestion.
- Oral, sublingual, and epicutaneous immunotherapy are all investigational treatment modalities primarily performed in research settings.
- Evidence from clinical trials suggests that oral immunotherapy and possibly sublingual immunotherapy can effectively desensitize many subjects to trigger foods. A subset of desensitized subjects may achieve sustained unresponsiveness after withdrawal of therapy.
- Nonspecific immunotherapy and other emerging therapies using modified food antigens may also be options for treatment, but they are currently limited to early clinical or preclinical trials.

INTRODUCTION

The increase in food allergy in the United States and throughout the world is a growing public health concern. From 1997 to 2007, the prevalence of food allergy in children increased by 18%.[1] An estimated 15 million Americans have a food allergy,

Disclosure Statement: B.J. Lanser, K.A. Orgel, and B.P. Vickery have nothing to disclose. B.L. Wright's fellowship is supported by an NIH training grant (T32AI007062). D.M. Fleischer is on the Research Advisory Board of Food Allergy Research and Education and the Medical Advisory Board of Food Allergy and Anaphylaxis Connection Team; has received research support from Monsanto Company and Receptos; is employed by University Physicians, Inc, University of Colorado Denver School of Medicine; has consultant arrangements with LabCorp; has received payment for lectures from Nestle Nutrition Institute; and has received royalties from UpToDate.
[a] Department of Pediatric, University of Colorado Denver School of Medicine, Aurora, CO, USA;
[b] National Jewish Health, 1400 Jackson Street, J322, Denver, CO 80206, USA; [c] Department of Pediatric, University of North Carolina at Chapel Hill School of Medicine, Campus Box #7231, Chapel Hill, NC 27599, USA; [d] Allergy, Asthma & Clinical Immunology, Mayo Clinic, 13400 East Shea Boulevard, Scottsdale, AZ 85259, USA; [e] Children's Hospital Colorado, 13123 E. 16th Ave, B518, Aurora, CO 80045, USA
* Corresponding author. 1400 Jackson Street, J322, Denver, CO 80206.
E-mail address: lanserb@njhealth.org

Pediatr Clin N Am 62 (2015) 1531–1549
http://dx.doi.org/10.1016/j.pcl.2015.07.015
0031-3955/15/$ – see front matter © 2015 Elsevier Inc. All rights reserved.

pediatric.theclinics.com

accounting for approximately 8% of children and 5% of adults.[2] Although most reactions from accidental ingestions are typically mild and self-limited, severe cases of anaphylaxis are associated with peanut, tree nuts, and shellfish and have resulted in fatalities.[3] Appropriately, there has been an increase in research for food allergy treatments. Current guidelines for food allergy management include education, strict avoidance, nutritional monitoring, appropriate treatment of anaphylaxis with injectable epinephrine, and regular follow-up with an allergy specialist.[4] In this review, the authors seek to update the previous article on food allergy therapy from this series, highlighting key clinical trials and emerging approaches for the treatment of food allergies.[5]

STANDARD OF CARE

At present, there is no cure for food allergy. Diagnosis and management are focused on identification of triggers and targeted dietary elimination.[4] Patients are encouraged to read ingredient labels, avoid cross-contamination, and consult with a nutritionist to ensure adequate growth. They are taught to recognize anaphylaxis and administer injectable epinephrine. In principle, strict dietary elimination should protect an individual from immunoglobulin (Ig) E–mediated reactions; however, in practice, patients with food allergies experience multiple exposures following diagnosis from both accidental and nonaccidental ingestions.[6,7] Constant vigilance and perpetual risk produce significant anxiety. Quality-of-life surveys among children with food allergies and their parents suggest this anxiety leads to restriction of daily activities.[8,9] Avoidance measures can also result in nutritional deficits and growth impairment.[10]

IMMUNOTHERAPY BACKGROUND

Oral immunotherapy (OIT) is not conceptually new, as instructions for treatment of egg sensitivity with egg white are recorded in the Babylonian Talmud.[11] There are reports of physicians attempting food desensitization published as early as 1905 with varied success (**Table 1**). Investigators demonstrated that patients were able to tolerate foods after a period of gradual incremental exposure, usually occurring over a period of months to years.[12] Clinical texts through the mid-twentieth century reference hyposensitization to foods as a treatment for food allergy, although its effectiveness remained in question. In the 1980s, European investigators renewed interest in OIT after publishing positive results from small case series.[13,14] These early reports and studies paved the way for more systematic investigation of immunotherapy as an active treatment for food allergy. An understanding of the pathogenesis of IgE-mediated disease and mechanisms of desensitization has elucidated pathways for targeted approach. Interestingly, many questions raised by early investigators continue to elude researchers today (**Box 1**).

   In an effort to answer these questions, researchers are now performing clinical trials in humans, predominantly with OIT, sublingual immunotherapy (SLIT), and epicutaneous immunotherapy (EPIT). It is important to note that these 3 most commonly considered methods of immunotherapy are allergen-specific, meaning that the therapy is only effective for the particular food given. Nonspecific therapies such as monoclonal antibodies to IgE have also been used to alter host immune responses. Second-generation OIT trials are beginning to use specific and nonspecific approaches in tandem to increase safety and efficacy.

IMMUNOTHERAPY MECHANISMS

Immunotherapy is based on the principle that incremental exposure to a given antigen can render an individual temporarily less reactive to that antigen (eg, desensitization)

Table 1
Early history of allergen immunotherapy for food allergy

Year	Summary of Key Findings
1905	Finkelstein conceptualizes OIT. He successfully desensitizes nurslings with "milk idiosyncrasy" by gradually administering increasing drops of milk.[15]
1908	Schofield treats a 13-year-old patient with egg allergy over an 8-mo period by incrementally increasing small amounts of raw egg disguised in pill form.[13]
1912	Schloss describes a patient with allergies to egg, oat, and almond, which he orally desensitizes to egg. Sensitivity to almond and oat also decreases during this treatment. He uses skin testing to guide up-dosing during therapy.[16]
1920	Schloss reports 5 patients with egg allergy treated with subcutaneous injection of ovomucoid. He also describes 12 children with food allergies successfully desensitized using OIT.[17]
1920	Park describes oral desensitization of a child with hypersensitiveness to cow's milk. Pallor and drowsiness were noted during build-up phase.[18]
1926	Stuart and Farnham advise treatment of food allergies by the oral method at an early age. In cases of milk or egg sensitization, their recommendation is enthusiastic because treatments are "simple and regularly successful."[19]
1930	Freeman performs rush inoculation over 8 d with cod fish juices in a 7-y-old boy with fish sensitivity. The patient is subsequently started on a fish diet and prescribed an ounce of cod-liver oil daily. A concurrent egg allergy resolves with this therapy.[20]
1935	Keston, Waters, and Hopkins report effectively desensitizing 50 cases of food allergy to milk, wheat, egg, orange, tomato, or cocoa and publish oral desensitization protocols to each of these foods.[21]
1940	Edwards describes successful oral desensitization of 11 of 12 patients with milk allergy using protocols published by Keston et al.[22]

and eventually result in longer-lasting changes. Although the exact mechanisms are unknown, some of the immunologic changes that occur have been elucidated **(Fig. 1)**.[23] Early on, repeated administration of increasing immunotherapy doses suppressed basophil and mast cell reactivity. Interleukin-10 is produced, presumably by lymphocytes, which is thought to suppress allergic responses and drive production of IgG4 antibody. Initially, immunotherapy increased the production of antigen-specific IgA, IgG1, IgG4, and IgE, although IgE tends eventually to decline to below baseline values in response to therapy (around 12–18 months). Ultimately, these changes result

Box 1
Key questions

- Can true immune tolerance be achieved through food desensitization?
- What is the preferred route for antigen administration?
- Do clinical outcomes improve if immunotherapy is started earlier in life?
- How long must therapy continue in order to achieve a permanent effect?
- What differences exist between children who naturally outgrow food sensitivity and those who are desensitized?
- Does immunotherapy hasten the development of immunologic tolerance in children who will ultimately outgrow a food allergy?

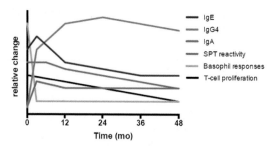

Fig. 1. Approximate changes seen in immunologic parameters for food allergy while undergoing immunotherapy. Notably, basophil reactivity declines relatively quickly. IgG4 and IgE increase, although ultimately IgE will decrease. SPT, skin prick test.

in a decrease in tissue mast cells and eosinophils, accounting for clinical hyporesponsiveness to antigen exposure and diminished skin prick test reactivity.

DESENSITIZATION VERSUS TOLERANCE

Interpretation of food allergy literature requires understanding of an important distinction between the concepts of clinical desensitization and tolerance. Desensitization refers to a reversible state induced by short-term exposure to an allergen. Once administration of the allergen is discontinued, the previous level of clinical reactivity returns. An analogy would be the brief desensitization protocols widely used to manage patients with certain drug allergies. On the other hand, therapeutic tolerance would suggest that the immunotherapy treatment has induced disease-modifying changes that will persist even after the treatment is discontinued. Importantly, some individuals, regardless of treatment, will spontaneously develop immune tolerance and naturally outgrow their food sensitivity. Although eventual tolerance to milk and egg are relatively common, peanut, tree nut, and seafood allergies tend to persist over time.[2]

Incomplete understanding of the immunologic changes induced by immunotherapy, and whether these changes truly reflect immune tolerance, has led to the emergence of the term sustained unresponsiveness (SU). SU refers to the ability to successfully consume the treated allergen during an oral food challenge (OFC) performed typically 1 to 4 weeks after stopping active treatment. Importantly, many of the studies addressed in this review have only measured desensitization as a primary outcome. Only a few trials have addressed whether OIT results in SU, and none have done so in a rigorous, placebo-controlled fashion.[23]

ORAL IMMUNOTHERAPY

Milk, egg, and peanut are the most studied foods in OIT trials. Most modern studies have been single-food OIT trials; as a result, these 3 major foods will be discussed separately. Overall, OIT trials have a dropout rate of 15% to 20%.[24] Moreover, several studies have observed spontaneous resolution of food allergy among subjects receiving placebo. This finding is consistent with observational studies of the natural history of peanut allergy, for example, which have found spontaneous resolution in about 20% of individuals.[25]

General conclusions regarding efficacy are difficult to draw from the current literature because success rates for OIT have been defined differently. Ideally, subjects completing a course of immunotherapy should be able to incorporate culprit foods into their diets, consuming them ad libitum without symptoms. However, most studies only approximate the inclusion of the culprit food ad libitum in subjects' diets. Studies often define success in terms of reaching a target maintenance dose or passing an endpoint challenge; therefore, it is important to interpret results in the context of the selected outcome measures. Overall safety of immunotherapy is also somewhat variable among studies, with adverse events not always being categorized in the same way (eg, many exclude oral itching). The lack of natural history or control groups as comparisons in many studies has also limited the determination of safety. Safety and efficacy are discussed further with regards to specific studies.

In addition to significant heterogeneity and varied primary endpoints, published trials have other scientific shortcomings. Most clinical protocols incorporate a crossover design that allows subjects in the placebo group to be reassigned to the treatment arm after a desensitization challenge. Although this may facilitate subject recruitment and retention and satisfy ethical concerns associated with repeatedly challenging subjects treated with placebo, it does not allow for comparisons between subjects who successfully complete immunotherapy and those who might have developed natural tolerance. **Table 2** provides a general overview of study design for OIT.

Despite the paucity of data supporting tolerance induction, some argue that OIT protects against accidental ingestions and improves quality of life, thus justifying its incorporation into clinical practice.[26,27] It is clear from multiple studies that OIT increases reaction thresholds, but there are no good data to prove this protects from reactions due to accidental ingestions. OIT has also not been thoroughly studied in subjects who are the most sensitive. A history of severe anaphylaxis is often a criterion for exclusion, while these patients might benefit the most from food immunotherapy.

Milk

Cow's milk (CM) is the most common food allergy in early childhood. It is also one of the most important foods to reintroduce into the diets of children with food allergies, because children who must avoid milk are at an increased risk for significantly decreased weight, height, and body mass index–for-age percentiles.[28,29] A recent systematic review and meta-analysis examined 6 randomized, controlled trials conducted between 2007 and 2012. Pooled data demonstrated a 10-fold increased likelihood of achieving desensitization to CM in children undergoing CM OIT than in non-OIT-treated patients. Subjects with CM allergy who underwent milk OIT tended to tolerate more milk protein, although these data did not reach statistical significance. A wide range of children received treatment with epinephrine during OIT trials (6.7%–30.8% of children); however, most reactions were mild.[30]

Maintenance of desensitization after CM OIT has been evaluated in 2 recent studies. A study published in 2013 evaluated 2 different CM maintenance regimens. Thirty-two children with milk allergy were randomized after successfully completing

Table 2
Overview of oral immunotherapy

Phase	Length	Description
Modified rush	1 d	Minute quantities given and dose is escalated over a period of several hours (6–8 doses)
Build-up period	6–9 mo	Daily doses taken at home with gradual increases performed under clinical observation every 1–2 wk
Maintenance	Months to years	Target dose of allergen consumed daily at home

CM OIT and achieving desensitization, defined as consumption of 200 mL of CM. For 1 year, 16 patients continued daily maintenance ingestion of 150 to 200 mL of CM (group A), while the other 16 ingested the same amount twice weekly (group B). Both groups were also allowed to consume CM ad libitum. The primary outcome was maintenance of desensitization without symptoms on CM ingestion. Three subjects were lost to follow-up (1 in group A and 2 in group B). Adverse events were similar between groups, and none discontinued therapy due to adverse events or noncompliance. The authors concluded that twice-weekly ingestion of a maintenance dose seems to be equally effective at safely maintaining desensitization as the daily regimen, with 9 of 15 subjects in group A and 9 of 15 subjects in group B consuming CM without symptoms. It is important to note the absence of a placebo group or a group exclusively consuming CM ad libitum. Moreover, differences in the quantity of CM consumed ad libitum between groups were not assessed.[31]

In contrast, a retrospective study examined 32 patients who had successfully completed CM OIT under 2 different protocols (16 from each), with follow-up ranging from 1.3 to 5.3 years. Twenty-two percent of subjects limited their consumption of CM due to symptoms, and only 31% of subjects tolerated full servings of CM with minimal or no symptoms. One subject required multiple doses of epinephrine for ongoing symptoms. Both studies provide important data that must be considered before starting OIT. Strict adherence to daily maintenance dosing may be difficult for children and families for a variety of reasons (eg, illness, travel, strenuous exercise, menses, food aversion). The same may be true for regular incorporation of trigger foods after OIT. It is also clear from these data that satisfactory long-term outcomes after CM immunotherapy appear to be dependent on ongoing exposure, which is difficult for some individuals. Importantly, some subjects who had been classified as protocol-defined successes in the trial seemed to have relapsed completely.[32]

Egg

In 2012, a multicenter study by the Consortium for Food Allergy Research (CoFAR) randomized 55 subjects with egg allergy (placebo 15, treatment 40). After 22 months of OIT using a daily maintenance dose of 2 g of egg white powder, 30 subjects (75%) passed a desensitization challenge (10 g of egg powder). After 6 to 8 weeks off treatment, just 11 of 29 subjects tolerated this same amount of egg. Using intention-to-treat analysis, 28% had developed SU. This study revealed differences in rates of desensitization after OIT for 10 months (55% passed a 5-g challenge) and 22 months (75% passed a 10-g challenge), suggesting that continued allergen administration over a prolonged period might improve efficacy. None of the subjects in the placebo arm passed the challenge at 10 months.[33] In a more recent, smaller open trial of egg OIT, Meglio and colleagues[34] achieved desensitization rates of 80% (8/10, active treatment) versus 20% (2/10, placebo) after 6 to 9 months of OIT.

A 2014 *Cochrane Review* analyzed 4 randomized, controlled trials of egg OIT. Only the CoFAR trial mentioned earlier included a placebo arm, whereas the other 3 compared subjects on OIT versus standard avoidance diet. Of the 100 patients receiving OIT in the 4 studies, 69% experienced adverse events, with 5% requiring epinephrine. Overall, 44% could tolerate a partial serving of egg, while 39% could tolerate a whole egg. However, because of the small sample size, low quality of evidence, and methodological differences, the only conclusion that could be drawn was that desensitization seems to be possible in a large number of egg-allergic patients, but adverse events remain a significant concern.[35]

Peanut

Although less common than milk and egg allergy, peanut allergy is less likely to resolve spontaneously; as a result, it may be easier to study the effects of treatment in peanut-allergic subjects. The only double-blind, placebo-controlled (DBPC) trial of OIT for peanut allergy was conducted in 2011 and assessed desensitization. Twenty-eight subjects (ages 1–16) were randomized to receive peanut OIT (n = 19) or placebo (n = 9). Three subjects (16%) in the OIT group discontinued treatment because of side effects, but all remaining participants tolerated a maintenance dose of 4000 mg of peanut protein and completed 12 months of therapy. Each of the treatment subjects passed an OFC with 5000 mg of peanut protein after 1 year of therapy, compared with 280 mg in the placebo group (range, 0–1900 mg; P<.001).[36]

The first study to investigate SU to peanut was published in 2014. In this open, non-placebo-controlled trial of peanut OIT, 24 of 39 (61.5%) subjects completed therapy for up to 5 years. Of these 24, 12 (50% per protocol, and 31% by intention to treat) were able to consume 5000 mg of peanut protein and 8000 to 10,000 mg of peanut butter after stopping OIT for 4 weeks. Thus, 12 patients were considered to achieve SU. These patients were subsequently instructed to incorporate peanut into their diet ad libitum at least several days per week. Questionnaire follow-up completed by 87.5% of the SU patients revealed that none experienced any allergic reactions due to peanut exposure, with a median follow-up time of 40 months.[37]

Another study in 2014 evaluated immunologic parameters and the possibility of SU to peanut after OIT or SLIT. Gorelik and colleagues[38] found a greater effect for OIT than SLIT, but both demonstrated suppression of basophil activity and decreased Th2 responses to peanut. However, these changes were not preserved in some patients while on maintenance and waned in others after stopping immunotherapy. Despite the lack of a placebo group and its crossover design, the data strongly suggest that immunologic changes associated with SU may not be truly sustained in most patients.

The recent STOP II trial conducted in the United Kingdom was a 2-phase, randomized, controlled crossover trial of 99 children with peanut allergy (ages 7–16). During phase I, subjects were allocated to active treatment (n = 49) or elimination (n = 50). After an OFC at 6 months, placebo subjects were reallocated to the treatment arm for phase II. The primary outcome measure of the study was the proportion of subjects able to tolerate 1400 mg of peanut protein following 6 months of OIT with 800 mg of peanut protein daily. Despite the lower maximum daily dose than that used in other OIT trials, 62% (24/39) of the treatment group was able to tolerate 1400 mg of peanut protein (approximately 10 peanuts) and were considered to be desensitized, while none of the placebo group passed the OFC. By the end of phase II, however, 84% of the active group and 91% of the control group were able to tolerate the daily maintenance doses. The study did not have participants stop OIT and thus did not assess for SU. Adverse reactions were higher in the treatment group as expected, although they were mild, primarily consisting of oral pruritus and abdominal pain.[39]

The findings described have led some clinicians to incorporate OIT into routine clinical practice.[40] A retrospective chart review of peanut OIT used in clinical practice, not as research, following different protocols in multiple clinical sites was recently published. Results for 352 patients showed that 85% reached maintenance dosing, but actual dose and length of maintenance therapy differed by site. The authors argue that OIT is safe for use in clinical practice given the low rate of epinephrine administration (0.7 per 1000 escalation doses, 0.2 per 1000 maintenance doses). However, other adverse reactions were not reported, and there is no evidence that accidental exposures were reduced or any other benefits were achieved.[41] In addition, other studies have reported significantly higher rates of allergic reactions among OIT participants compared with those avoiding the food.[42] Quality-of-life changes with OIT have also not been significantly observed, despite the assumption of improved quality of life with OIT. The Food Allergy Quality of Life Questionnaire was used before and after egg OIT in 22 children and their parents. They found only minimal improvement in health-related quality of life as rated by the parents, whereas children reported a benefit in terms of dietary restriction, but a negative impact by allergic reactions due to OIT.[43] More data conclusively demonstrating safety and efficacy are needed in order to justify routine clinical use of OIT outside of a research setting.[44]

EXTENSIVELY HEATED MILK AND EGG AS ORAL IMMUNOTHERAPY

Baking egg or milk proteins decreases their allergenicity, likely due to alteration of conformational epitopes. However, heating alone does not reduce the allergenicity of all proteins; in fact, with limited heat application, some foods can form neoepitopes, increasing their allergenicity.[45] Baking food proteins with wheat may also confer a matrix effect in which the wheat-protein complex alters sequential IgE-binding epitopes that are unaffected by heat alone. This decreased allergenicity is sufficient for many patients to tolerate the trigger food on a regular basis.[46] There is evidence to suggest that regular consumption of baked egg- and milk-containing products may help patients outgrow these allergies more quickly, although this evidence is weakened by the lack of an appropriate control group. Several studies have demonstrated that regular ingestion of baked egg or milk may hasten and increase rates of SU to nonbaked egg or milk when compared with strict avoidance. These studies have also shown that consumption of baked egg or milk decreases skin prick test size and increases IgG4. As seen in OIT, specific IgE increases initially and ultimately decreases with time. Although tolerance to baked goods may be associated with a milder clinical phenotype, these data suggest that introduction of baked allergens may actually alter the natural history of egg and milk allergies.[47]

Introduction of baked egg or milk into the diets of allergic children should be performed cautiously. Although some studies suggest that some patients can perform these OFCs at home, passage rates range from 60%[48] to 85%, and up to 20% of failures to baked egg require epinephrine.[49] Ideally, patients should be evaluated by an allergist and undergo a medically supervised OFC before introducing baked allergens.

MULTIPLE FOOD ORAL IMMUNOTHERAPY

Although OIT for single allergens shows promise, up to 30% of children with food allergy are sensitive to more than one allergen,[50] and in highly atopic populations, this proportion may be greater than 50%.[51] Results from a phase I trial of multifood OIT were recently published. Forty participants (ages 4–46) were recruited, and a DBPC OFC to peanut was performed at enrollment. Additional reported food allergies were documented with subsequent DBPC OFCs. Twenty-five subjects were started on multifood OIT after demonstrating 1 or more food allergies in addition to peanut allergy. The remaining 15 subjects were diagnosed with peanut allergy alone and allocated to single allergen OIT. Doses of each allergen were escalated until a maintenance dose of 4000 mg was reached. Adverse reaction rates did not differ significantly between groups, and the dropout rates were similar. Two subjects from each group required treatment with epinephrine for OIT dose-related reactions.[52] This study suggests the safety of multifood OIT is comparable to peanut OIT, but further randomized trials are needed to demonstrate efficacy.

SUBLINGUAL IMMUNOTHERAPY

The first study evaluating food SLIT was performed in Europe for hazelnut allergy. SLIT for pollen allergy had been widely used in Europe before this study, and the US Food and Drug Administration (FDA) recently approved its use with tablets for grass and ragweed allergies (dust mite remains in development). Like OIT, SLIT takes advantage of allergen exposure through the oral mucosa, which is thought to be tolerogenic. Liquid doses are delivered to the surface under the tongue, where antigen-presenting cells (ie, Langerhans cells) take up the antigen.[53] Extract concentrations and the volume of liquid that can be held under a patient's tongue have limited the utility of SLIT. Unlike OIT doses that range from milligrams to grams, SLIT doses typically range from micrograms to milligrams at maintenance. Although the quantity of antigen delivered is smaller with SLIT, the oral mucosa is exposed to undigested antigen, in contrast to OIT, which exposes the antigen to gastric digestion.[54] Clinical trials investigating the safety and efficacy of SLIT in the treatment of food allergies have been limited to studies on hazelnut[55] and peach allergy,[56] which is not reviewed here, as well as milk and peanut, that are discussed later.

Results of DBPC, randomized trials examining the use of SLIT in peanut allergy have been published. In 2011, Kim and colleagues[57] published a study in which 18 children (ages 1–11) completed 12 months of dosing followed by a DBPC OFC. Eleven subjects were randomized to active treatment with peanut with a goal dose of 2500 μg daily, while 7 subjects were randomized to placebo. Compliance was similar between the groups, with only 0.26% of peanut doses requiring treatment with antihistamines and 0.02% of home doses requiring albuterol for minor wheeze. The median cumulative tolerated dose after 1 year of SLIT therapy in the peanut group was 1710 mg of peanut protein, compared with 85 mg for the placebo group.

The largest published SLIT study was performed in 40 peanut-allergic subjects (ages 12–37 years) by the CoFAR group in 2013. The first phase was a randomized, DBPC study for the first 44 weeks using a daily dose of 1386 μg. After 44 weeks of therapy, subjects completed a 5 g DBPC OFC to peanut. No subjects were able to consume the full 5 g of peanut powder (~50% peanut protein), but 14 (70%) peanut SLIT subjects were able to consume at least 10-fold more peanut powder than at baseline (responders), compared with 3 (15%) placebo SLIT subjects. In the second phase, the placebo group crossed over to active treatment to a higher daily dose of peanut SLIT of 3696 μg. This group completed a subsequent crossover 5 g DBPC OFC after 44 weeks. At this challenge, 7 of the 16 (44%) subjects who crossed over to active treatment were considered responders. After 68 weeks of treatment in the original active peanut SLIT group, the median successfully consumed dose increased from 496 mg at 44 weeks to 996 mg ($P = .05$); 5 subjects were able to consume the full 5 g, with one subject consuming 10 g, suggesting that longer-term therapy may confer increased dose threshold. There was a high dropout rate among the 40 children, but this was largely due to personal reasons rather than side effects. In the first phase, 40.1% of peanut SLIT doses resulted in mild symptoms, but this decreased to 3.3% when oropharyngeal reactions were excluded. One subject on peanut SLIT in phase 1 did require epinephrine during up-dosing and was withdrawn from active therapy. Side effects were similar after crossover: 35.8% of doses after week 44 elicited symptoms, but only 1.1% of doses elicited symptoms when oropharyngeal symptoms were excluded, and no reactions required epinephrine. Children with a history of life-threatening reactions were excluded for safety.[25] This group may be the most likely to undertake SLIT and achieve clinically significant results.

SLIT may ultimately represent a safer method of immunotherapy for patients with a history of severe allergy who cannot tolerate OIT, or as a bridge to OIT to decrease side effects and improve safety, but it may never be the most effective method to induce clinically significant desensitization or SU given the lower daily maintenance doses used. Further investigation into this possibility is needed as well as the duration of therapy required and any potential lasting effects of SLIT. Unfortunately, recently published follow-up data from the previously cited CoFAR SLIT study demonstrate substantial rates of nonadherence and lower rates of SU (10.8%) than seen in OIT.[58] Given that indefinite exposure is likely necessary to maintain whatever treatment benefits are achieved, this is a concerning finding. Studies directly comparing SLIT and OIT are discussed in the next section.

SUBLINGUAL IMMUNOTHERAPY VERSUS ORAL IMMUNOTHERAPY

In a DBPC pilot study comparing SLIT and OIT, 21 children with peanut allergy were randomized to receive active SLIT/placebo OIT or active OIT/placebo SLIT. Although adverse reactions and withdrawal were less common among the active SLIT group, reaction thresholds were significantly higher in the OIT group (141- versus 22-fold, $P = .01$), and SLIT overall was not significantly superior to placebo.[59] A retrospective comparison was carried out among peanut-allergic subjects who had completed 2 years of therapy, with 23 subjects in the OIT group and 27 subjects in the SLIT group. Safety was not directly compared, but the amount of peanut protein tolerated was higher in the OIT group and showed less variability, while changes in immunologic parameters (eg, IgE, IgG4, basophil reactivity) were greater in the OIT group.[60]

Another comparison of SLIT and OIT was performed for CM allergy as an open-label, randomized study. Thirty children were randomized to SLIT or SLIT converting to OIT at a lower and a higher dose, with a period off-therapy after about 15 months of maintenance in all groups. Adverse events led 2 children from the OIT group to withdraw. All children who reached maintenance were able to tolerate a higher amount of CM protein, and the amount increased with time. After 60 weeks, 60% of the SLIT group tolerated at least 10 times baseline CM protein, whereas 90% of the OIT group did the same, but this was not statistically significant ($P = .053$). After 6 weeks off therapy, only 1 in 10 children in the SLIT group maintained SU, whereas 8 of 20 in the OIT group had SU to CM, but again this was not significant ($P = .09$). Notably, 2 children reacted after only 1 week off therapy. Limitations to this study include small sample size and lack of power as well as lack of a placebo group.[61] These early results suggest that despite a poorer safety profile, OIT is more effective than SLIT in inducing desensitization.

EPICUTANEOUS IMMUNOTHERAPY

EPIT is an alternative approach to oral methods that is performed by repeated application of an allergen to intact skin. This approach is accomplished through a novel and proprietary epicutaneous delivery system (EDS) successfully developed in animal models.[62] The EDS uses a circular disc spray-dried with allergen. Perspiration solubilizes the allergen, which is then disseminated into the stratum corneum. Food EPIT is ongoing in phase 1 and 2 trials, and it is important to note that there are few peer-reviewed results published in the literature to date. Pilot studies have found that it is relatively well-tolerated with very few systemic reactions and no reports of anaphylaxis. Reactions are primarily mild, cutaneous symptoms, including erythema, pruritus, and flares of atopic dermatitis.[63,64]

However, these studies have failed to show a statistically significant increase in the amount of food tolerated by milk- and peanut-allergic subjects treated with EPIT. The phase 1 CM EPIT pilot study was only performed for 3 months, which may not be long enough to show a significant effect. Nineteen subjects were randomized to milk EPIT (n = 10) or placebo (n = 9), with OFC before and after the use of EPIT. The mean cumulative tolerated dose was 12-fold higher in the active group versus 8% in the placebo, which was not statistically different (P = .13). Subjects in the active treatment group had a higher risk of local eczema at the site of antigen delivery. Interestingly, in one child, they observed a decrease in the minimum amount of CM protein that was tolerated after undergoing EPIT, compared with pre-EPIT CM OFC.[64] The potential for increased sensitization with cutaneous exposure is a concern with EPIT in light of the dual exposure hypothesis proposed by Lack.[65] The hypothesis proposes that low-dose cutaneous exposure to a food can increase allergic sensitization, while oral/gastrointestinal exposure leads to tolerance.

The peanut EPIT pilot study followed children for 18 months of therapy and found a progressively increasing amount of peanut protein that was tolerated in the active group, but again it was not statistically significant.[64] There are currently 3 clinical trials underway that will investigate various doses, safety, and efficacy, with 1 in Europe and 2 in the United States. If successful, these studies, and others performed for inhalant allergy, could suggest that EPIT may be a viable and safe treatment option for food allergy.

NONSPECIFIC IMMUNOTHERAPY
Anti-Immunoglobulin E Therapy

Use of anti-IgE as monotherapy for food allergy was first investigated in a DBPC trial of the humanized, monoclonal, anti-IgE antibody TNX-901. Anti-IgE significantly increased reaction thresholds to peanut flour by 76% in the active group, although the trial was terminated early before completing subject recruitment.[66] More recent phase I trials have used omalizumab as an adjunct to OIT, and these studies are discussed next. Subjects are generally pretreated with omalizumab for 2 to 5 months during a washout period and then continued on therapy until a maintenance dose of OIT is reached.

A pilot study in 13 children with peanut allergy demonstrated that omalizumab in conjunction with peanut OIT was effective at decreasing initial reactions and allowed for a more rapid build-up phase, with 92% of children achieving maintenance. Reactions were rare and mild during the study; however, after omalizumab was stopped, half of the children experienced reactions, and 17% required epinephrine. Notably, this small sample of patients had an overall higher total and peanut-specific IgE level than many other OIT studies.[67]

CM OIT was studied with omalizumab in 11 patients. After a 9-week lead-in on omalizumab, they underwent rush CM desensitization. Reactions were again rare and relatively mild, with only 4 reactions requiring epinephrine, which is similar to other studies. Unlike in the peanut study, increased reactions were not experienced after stopping omalizumab. The study is limited by a small sample size and lack of placebo group, and baseline OFCs were not performed, so the significance in the amount of CM protein tolerated after OIT cannot be established.[68]

A larger, phase I study examined the use of omalizumab as an adjunct to multiple food OIT. Twenty-five subjects were desensitized to up to 5 different foods. Doses of each allergen were escalated until a maintenance dose of 4000 mg was reached. Reactions were experienced by 5.3% of subjects, and this rate decreased over time. No subjects had serious adverse events while on omalizumab, although one patient did have a serious reaction requiring epinephrine off omalizumab in the maintenance phase.[69]

These studies suggest that omalizumab may be useful as an adjunct to other forms of immunotherapy. Aside from being relatively safe and well tolerated, it confers several benefits over immunotherapy alone, including decreased initial reactions, shorter escalation phases, and more patients reaching higher cumulative doses during rush desensitization. However, further investigation is needed to identify the appropriate dose, duration of pretreatment, and optimal length of use during therapy. Omalizumab is currently only FDA-approved in patients aged 12 years and older with severe atopic asthma or chronic idiopathic urticaria. The lack of a clinical indication for use in food allergy and cost has restricted its use to a research setting thus far.

Chinese Herbal Formula

Interest in complementary and alternative therapies and encouraging data from mouse models have led to clinical trials investigating the use of Chinese herbal therapy as a treatment of food allergy. Food allergy herbal formula-2 (FAHF-2), a compound containing 9 different traditional Chinese herbs, has been shown to be safe in preclinical and pilot studies. Some efficacy was seen in food-allergic mice treated with FAHF-2.[70] Preliminary results of phase 2 trials in humans reveal that the treatment is safe. However, at the dose used in this study, there was no statistically significant benefit observed in the treatment group. Notably, there was poor adherence among the treatment group given the large number of capsules required.[71] The major advantage of this therapy is that it is nonspecific, and could, therefore, be used to treat individuals with multiple food allergies if efficacy can be demonstrated with other herbal formulations and dosing regiments that are in preclinical studies.[70]

Table 3 provides an overview of the major forms of immunotherapy discussed earlier, with a summary of the advantages and disadvantages of each.

Probiotics

Probiotic supplementation has been examined in several allergic diseases, including asthma and atopic dermatitis, with mixed results. A recent meta-analysis including 21 studies found a significant decrease in the risk of atopic sensitization (positive skin prick test or elevated specific IgE) to common allergens, but not specifically to food. They found that prenatal and postnatal administration caused a significant reduction in sensitization. However, probiotics did not protect subjects from developing asthma or wheeze.[72] Despite mixed results, probiotics remain an area of interest as a nonspecific form of immunotherapy.

One of the largest and most rigorous studies on probiotics was published in 2009, evaluating 119 infants with CM allergy. This randomized, DBPC study demonstrated no increase in tolerance to CM after 6 months of probiotic supplementation.[73] More recently, a study of 55 infants with CM allergy was randomized to receive extensively hydrolyzed casein formula, with or without probiotic supplementation, for 6 months. They found statistically significantly higher rates of tolerance to CM at 6 and 12 months of therapy in the probiotic groups; however, greater differences were seen for those infants who had non-IgE-mediated allergy to CM.[74]

Probiotics have also been used as an adjunct to peanut OIT. A DBPC trial randomized 62 subjects with peanut allergy to receive probiotics plus peanut OIT (PPOIT) or placebo over an 18-month period. Maintenance therapy was then stopped for 2 to 5 weeks, and subjects underwent an OFC. Possible SU was achieved in 82.1% receiving PPOIT and 3.6% receiving placebo (P<.001). Nine children would need to be treated for 7 to achieve

Table 3
Immunotherapy summary: pro/con

Method	Advantages	Disadvantages
OIT	• Can give larger maintenance doses (g) than SLIT/EPIT (mg) • More effective than SLIT	• Greatest side effects • Not tolerated in 15%–20% of subjects • Potential for iatrogenic EoE • Requires long-term adherence
SLIT	• Fewer side effects than OIT • Not tolerated in 5% of subjects	• Only able to reach small maintenance doses (mg) • Not as effective as OIT • Requires long-term adherence
EPIT	• May have fewer side effects than SLIT and OIT • May be safer in broader clinical settings	• Only able to reach small maintenance doses (mg) • May only be as effective as SLIT, likely less than OIT • May not be safe in patients with atopic dermatitis
Allergen-nonspecific therapies (eg, omalizumab, Chinese herbal formula)	• Potentially desensitize to all food allergens • May have the fewest side effects	• May have the poorest efficacy, potentially limiting use to adjunct therapy • Omalizumab is not currently approved by the US FDA for food allergy and is cost-prohibitive

SU (1.27; 95% confidence interval, 1.06–1.59). Unfortunately, the PPOIT group was not compared with OIT alone, so it is impossible to determine the independent effect of probiotics.[75] Carefully designed trials with appropriate controls are necessary for defining the effect of probiotic supplementation on food allergy.

EOSINOPHILIC ESOPHAGITIS AND FOOD IMMUNOTHERAPY

Although OIT has not been studied as a treatment of eosinophilic esophagitis (EoE) (rather, food avoidance is one treatment option), it deserves special consideration in the realm of OIT. The development of EoE has been observed in a small number of patients undergoing OIT for food allergy. Most of the current literature regarding this phenomenon consists of case reports and small case series. A recent systematic review with meta-analysis found one randomized clinical trial with 40 patients in which one child developed EoE. Three other full-length articles also met inclusion criteria, for a total of 6 of 179 patients developing EoE attributed to food OIT. According to their analysis, the incidence of EoE on OIT was 2.7%; however, they note considerable limitations. A significant drawback to these reports is that subjects are rarely screened for EoE before beginning clinical OIT trials due to the costs and risks associated with endoscopy. Given the frequency of comorbid IgE-mediated food allergy in patients with EoE, is it unclear whether the EoE was induced by OIT or existed as subclinical disease before treatment. Given available evidence, the risk of developing EoE while on OIT should not preclude further investigation, but it should be recognized as a potential adverse outcome and monitored in clinical research trials.[76]

Despite this risk of EoE while undergoing food OIT, baked milk may be safe to include in the diets of children with concomitant CM allergy and EoE. A small retrospective

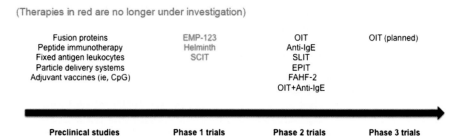

(Therapies in red are no longer under investigation)

Fusion proteins	EMP-123	OIT	OIT (planned)
Peptide immunotherapy	Helminth	Anti-IgE	
Fixed antigen leukocytes	SCIT	SLIT	
Particle delivery systems		EPIT	
Adjuvant vaccines (ie, CpG)		FAHF-2	
		OIT+Anti-IgE	

| Preclinical studies | Phase 1 trials | Phase 2 trials | Phase 3 trials |

Fig. 2. Many preclinical studies are in process as well as phase 2 trials as discussed. OIT will move into phase 3 trials. Other studies have not progressed beyond phase 1 studies due to safety or efficacy concerns. EMP-123, E-coli encapsulated, recombinant Modified Peanut proteins Ara h 1, Ara h 2, Ara h 3.

study in children with EoE, without IgE-mediated food allergy, found that 73% of patients maintained histologic remission of EoE while eating 2 to 3 servings per week of baked milk for 6 weeks.[77] It remains to be seen if the same is true for baked egg.

FAILED METHODS OF IMMUNOTHERAPY

Several additional methods have been attempted as food allergy therapy, with significant safety concerns or lack of efficacy. Given the effectiveness of subcutaneous immunotherapy (SCIT) in treating venom and environmental allergies, researchers hypothesized that subcutaneous injection of food antigens would yield similar results. In a study published in 1997, peanut SCIT was performed in 12 patients. Although some efficacy was established, a high rate of systemic reactions prevented patients from reaching or continuing maintenance dosing. Following an anaphylaxis-related death of a patient who was mistakenly given a higher dose of peanut, it was concluded that peanut SCIT carried an unacceptable risk of severe reactions, preventing its continued clinical use.[78]

Escherichia coli (E-coli) encapsulated, recombinant Modified Peanut proteins Ara h 1, Ara h 2, Ara h 3 (EMP-123). EMP-123 is a novel form of immunotherapy that has not progressed beyond phase 1 trials due to safety concerns. EMP-123 is a rectally administered peanut vaccine comprising 3 recombinant modified peanut antigens (Ara h 1, 2, and 3) encapsulated within heat/phenol-inactivated *Escherichia coli*. Although the vaccine was safe in healthy control subjects, peanut-allergic subjects experienced significant adverse events; half of the 10 subjects terminated dosing early, and 2 suffered anaphylaxis requiring epinephrine.[79] Both of these studies are important for historical consideration as well as potential future use if adjunctive therapies prove to minimize adverse reactions.

PRECLINICAL STUDIES

In addition to the ongoing studies mentioned previously, a variety of potential methods of immunotherapy are in development and preclinical trials. A summary is included in **Fig. 2**. Some of these methods may represent promising future directions in food allergy, requiring continued rigorous investigation.

SUMMARY

Immunotherapy for food allergy remains a promising area for future clinical application. Many of the questions posed by early investigators remain unanswered. Clinical trials have provided some insight as to viable treatment options for food allergy immunotherapy. At this point, the following conclusions can be made based on current evidence:

- Desensitization can be achieved in most subjects receiving OIT and SLIT. Among desensitized individuals, a small subset may achieve SU.
- Because of the absence of large controlled studies that include a natural history group, it cannot be definitively concluded that the number of subjects who achieve SU on OIT is greater than the number of individuals who would naturally outgrow their food allergy.
- When compared with OIT, SLIT offers an enhanced safety profile at the expense of decreased efficacy.
- Attempts at desensitization may be more effective and rapid if omalizumab is used as an adjunct.
- Adverse effect profiles for all forms of food allergy immunotherapy are still being characterized, because the population that may benefit most from these therapies (those with a history of severe anaphylaxis) has been excluded from nearly all studies. Potential links between OIT and the development of EoE also require further investigation.

Continued investigation may reveal that among the variety of methods, certain forms may be best suited for certain foods or subsets of patients with or without adjunctive therapy. Given outstanding questions regarding safety and efficacy, food allergy immunotherapy requires further investigation before incorporation into routine clinical practice.

REFERENCES

1. Branum AM, Lukacs SL. Food allergy among children in the United States. Pediatrics 2009;125:1549–55.
2. Sicherer SH, Sampson HA. Food allergy: epidemiology, pathogenesis, diagnosis and treatment. J Allergy Clin Immunol 2014;133(2):291–307.
3. Bock SA, Munoz-Furlong A, Sampson HA. Further fatalities caused by anaphylactic reactions to food, 2001–2006. J Allergy Clin Immunol 2007; 119:1016–8.
4. Sampson HA, Aceves S, Bock SA, et al. Food allergy: a practice parameter update-2014. J Allergy Clin Immunol 2014;134(5):1016–25.e43.
5. Nowak-Wegrzyn A, Muraro A. Food allergy therapy: is a cure within reach? Pediatr Clin North Am 2011;58:511–30.
6. Fleischer DM, Perry TT, Atkins D, et al. Allergic reactions to foods in preschool-aged children in a prospective observational food allergy study. Pediatrics 2012; 130:e25–32.
7. Sampson MA, Munoz-Furlong A, Sicherer SH. Risk-taking and coping strategies of adolescents and young adults with food allergy. J Allergy Clin Immunol 2006; 117:1440–5.
8. Primeau MN, Kagan R, Joseph L, et al. The psychological burden of peanut allergy as perceived by adults with peanut allergy and the parents of peanut-allergic children. Clin Exp Allergy 2000;30:1135–43.
9. Sicherer SH, Noone SA, Munoz-Furlong A. The impact of childhood food allergy on quality of life. Ann Allergy Asthma Immunol 2001;87:461–4.
10. Christie L, Hine RJ, Parker JG, et al. Food allergies in children affect nutrient intake and growth. J Am Diet Assoc 2002;102:1648–51.

11. Goldstein GB, Heiner DC. Clinical and immunological perspectives in food sensitivity. A review. J Allergy 1970;46:270–91.
12. Schofield AT. A case of egg poisoning. Lancet 1908;1:715.
13. Patriarca C, Romano A, Venuti A, et al. Oral specific hyposensitization in the management of patients allergic to food. Allergol Immunopathol (Madr) 1984;12: 275–81.
14. Patriarca G, Schiavino D, Nucera E, et al. Food allergy in children: results of a standardized protocol for oral desensitization. Hepatogastroenterology 1998; 45:52–8.
15. Freier S, Kletter B. Milk allergy in infants and young children. Current knowledge. Clin Pediatr 1970;9:449–54.
16. Schloss OM. A case of allergy to common foods. Am J Dis Child 1912;3:341.
17. Schloss OM. Allergy in infants and children. Am J Dis Child 1920;19:433–55.
18. Park EA. A case of hypersensitiveness to cow's milk. Am J Dis Child 1920;3:341.
19. Stuart HC, Farnham M. Acquisition and loss of hypersensitiveness. Am J Dis Child 1926;32:341–9.
20. Freeman J. "Rush" inoculation, with special reference to hay-fever treatment. Lancet 1930;215:744–7.
21. Keston BM, Waters I, Hopkins JG. Oral desensitization to common foods. J Allergy 1935;6:431–6.
22. Edwards HE. Oral desensitization in food allergy. Can Med Assoc J 1940;43: 234–6.
23. Rachid R, Umetsu DT. Immunological mechanisms for desensitization and tolerance in food allergy. Semin Immunopathol 2012;34(5):689–702.
24. Khoriaty E, Umetsu DT. Oral immunotherapy for food allergy: towards a new horizon. Allergy Asthma Immunol Res 2013;5(1):3–15.
25. Fleischer DM, Burks AW, Vickery BP, et al. Sublingual immunotherapy for peanut allergy: a randomized, double-blind, placebo-controlled multicenter trial. J Allergy Clin Immunol 2013;131:119–27.
26. Mansfield LE. Oral immunotherapy for peanut allergy in clinical practice is ready. Allergy Asthma Proc 2013;34:205–9.
27. Factor JM, Mendelson L, Lee J, et al. Effect of oral immunotherapy to peanut on food-specific quality of life. Ann Allergy Asthma Immunol 2012;109:348–52.e2.
28. Robbins KA, Wood RA, Keet CA. Milk allergy is associated with decreased growth in US children. J Allergy Clin Immunol 2014;134:1466–8.
29. Hobbs CB, Skinner AC, Burks AW, et al. Food allergies affect growth in children. J Allergy Clin Immunol Pract 2015;3:133–4.e1.
30. Calatayud CM, Garcia AM, Aragones AM, et al. Safety and efficacy profile and immunological changes associated with oral immunotherapy for IgE-mediated cow's milk allergy in children: systematic review and meta-analysis. J Investig Allergol Clin Immunol 2014;24:298–307.
31. Pajno GB, Caminiti L, Salzano G, et al. Comparison between two maintenance feeding regimens after successful cow's milk oral desensitization. Pediatr Allergy Immunol 2013;24:376–81.
32. Keet CA, Seopaul A, Knorr S, et al. Long-term follow-up of oral immunotherapy for cow's milk allergy. J Allergy Clin Immunol 2013;132:737–9.
33. Burks AW, Jones SM, Wood RA, et al. Oral immunotherapy for treatment of egg allergy in children. N Engl J Med 2012;367:233–43.
34. Meglio P, Giampietro PG, Carello R, et al. Oral food desensitization in children with IgE-mediated hen's egg allergy: a new protocol with raw hen's egg. Pediatr Allergy Immunol 2013;24:75–83.

35. Ramantsik O, Bruschettini M, Tosca MA, et al. Oral and sublingual immunotherapy for egg allergy [review]. Cochrane Database Syst Rev 2014;(11):CD010638.

36. Varshney P, Jones SM, Scurlock AM, et al. A randomized controlled study of peanut oral immunotherapy: clinical desensitization and modulation of the allergic response. J Allergy Clin Immunol 2011;127:654–60.

37. Vickery BP, Scurlock AM, Kulis M, et al. Sustained unresponsiveness to peanut in subjects who have completed peanut oral immunotherapy. J Allergy Clin Immunol 2014;133:468–75.

38. Gorelik M, Narisety SD, Guerrerio AL, et al. Suppression of the immunologic response to peanut during immunotherapy is often transient. J Allergy Clin Immunol 2015;135(5):1283–92.

39. Anagnostou K, Islam S, King Y, et al. Assessing the efficacy of oral immunotherapy for the desensitisation of peanut allergy in children (STOP II): a phase 2 randomised control trial. Lancet 2014;383:1297–304.

40. Greenhawt MJ, Vickery BP. Allergist-reported in the practice of food allergen oral immunotherapy. J Allergy Clin Immunol Pract 2015;3:33–8.

41. Wasserman RL, Factor JM, Baker JW, et al. Oral immunotherapy for peanut allergy: multipractice experience with epinephrine-treated reactions. J Allergy Clin Immunol Pract 2014;2:91–6.

42. Keet CA, Wood RA. Emerging therapies for food allergy. J Clin Invest 2014;124:1880–6.

43. Vazquez-Ortiz M, Alvaro M, Piquer M, et al. Impact of oral immunotherapy on quality of life in egg allergic children. Pediatr Allergy Immunol 2015;26(3):291–4.

44. Wood RA, Sampson HA. Oral immunotherapy for the treatment of peanut allergy: is it ready for prime time? J Allergy Clin Immunol Pract 2014;2:97–8.

45. Shin M, Lee J, Ahn K, et al. The influence of the presence of wheat flour on the antigenic activities of egg white proteins. Allergy Asthma Immunol Res 2013;5:42–7.

46. Nowak-Wegrzyn A, Fiocchi A. Rare, medium, or well done? The effect of heating and food matrix on food protein allergenicity. Curr Opin Allergy Clin Immunol 2009;9:234–7.

47. Huang F, Nowak-Wegrzyn A. Extensively heated milk and egg as oral immunotherapy. Curr Opin Allergy Clin Immunol 2012;12:283–92.

48. Tan JW, Campbell DE, Turner PJ, et al. Baked egg food challenges – clinical utility of skin test to baked egg and ovomucoid in children with egg allergy. Clin Exp Allergy 2013;43:1189–95.

49. Bartnikas LM, Sheehan WJ, Larabee KS, et al. Ovomucoid is not superior to egg white testing in predicting tolerance to baked egg. J Allergy Clin Immunol Pract 2013;1:354–60.

50. Gupta RS, Springston EE, Warrier MR, et al. The prevalence, severity, and distribution of childhood food allergy in the United States. Pediatrics 2011;128:e9–17.

51. Sampson HA, Ho DG. Relationship between food-specific IgE concentrations and the risk of positive food challenges in children and adolescents. J Allergy Clin Immunol 1997;100:444–51.

52. Begin P, Winterroth LC, Dominguez T, et al. Safety and feasibility of oral immunotherapy to multiple allergens for food allergy. Allergy Asthma Clin Immunol 2014;10:1.

53. Akdis CA, Barlan IB, Bahceciler N, et al. Immunological mechanisms of sublingual immunotherapy. Allergy 2006;61(Suppl 81):11–4.

54. Untersmayr E, Jensen-Jarolim E. The role of protein digestibility and antacids on food allergy outcomes. J Allergy Clin Immunol 2008;121:1301–8.

55. Enrique E, Pineda F, Malek T, et al. Sublingual immunotherapy for hazelnut food allergy: a randomized, double-blind, placebo-controlled study with a standardized hazelnut extract. J Allergy Clin Immunol 2005;116:1073–9.

56. Garrido-Fernandez S, Garcia BE, Sanz ML, et al. Are basophil activation and sulphidoleukotriene determination useful tests for monitoring patients with peach allergy receiving sublingual immunotherapy with a Pru p 3-enriched peach extract? J Investig Allergol Clin Immunol 2014;24:106–13.

57. Kim EH, Bird JA, Kulis M, et al. Sublingual immunotherapy for peanut allergy: clinical and immunologic evidence of desensitization. J Allergy Clin Immunol 2011; 127:640–6.e1.

58. Burks AW, Wood RA, Jones SM, et al. Sublingual immunotherapy for peanut allergy: long-term follow-up of a randomized multicenter trial. J Allergy Clin Immunol 2015;135(5):1240–8.e1–3.

59. Narisety SD, Frischmeyer-Guerrerio PA, Keet CA, et al. A randomized, double-blind, placebo-controlled pilot study of sublingual versus oral immunotherapy for the treatment of peanut allergy. J Allergy Clin Immunol 2015;135(5):1275–82.e1–6.

60. Chin SJ, Vickery BP, Kulis MD, et al. Sublingual versus oral immunotherapy for peanut-allergic children: a retrospective comparison. J Allergy Clin Immunol 2013;132:476–8.e2.

61. Keet CA, Frischmeyer-Guerrerio PA, Thyagarajan A, et al. The safety and efficacy of sublingual and oral immunotherapy for milk allergy. J Allergy Clin Immunol 2012;129:448–55.

62. Mondoulet L, Dioszeghy V, Ligouis M, et al. Epicutaneous immunotherapy on intact skin using a new delivery system in a murine model of allergy. Clin Exp Allergy 2010;40:659–67.

63. Dupont C, Kalach N, Soulaines P, et al. Cow's milk epicutaneous immunotherapy in children: a pilot trial of safety, acceptability, and impact on allergic reactivity. J Allergy Clin Immunol 2010;125:1165–7.

64. Dupont C, Bourrier T, de Blay F, et al. Peanut epicutaneous immunotherapy (EPIT) in peanut allergic children: 18 months treatment in the Arachild Study. J Allergy Clin Immunol 2014;133:AB102.

65. Lack G. Update on risk factors for food allergy. J Allergy Clin Immunol 2012;129: 1187–97.

66. Leung DY, Sampson HA, Yunginger JW, et al. Effect of anti-IgE therapy in patients with peanut allergy. N Engl J Med 2003;348:986–93.

67. Schneider LC, Rachid R, LeBovidge J, et al. A pilot study of omalizumab to facilitate rapid oral desensitization in high-risk peanut allergic patients. J Allergy Clin Immunol 2013;132:1368–74.

68. Nadeau KC, Schneider LC, Hoyte L, et al. Rapid oral desensitization in combination with omalizumab therapy in patients with cow's milk allergy. J Allergy Clin Immunol 2011;127:1622–4.

69. Begin P, Dominguez T, Wilson SP, et al. Phase 1 results of safety and tolerability in a rush oral immunotherapy protocol to multiple foods using omalizumab. Allergy Asthma Clin Immunol 2014;10:7.

70. Wang J, Xiu-Min LI. Chinese herbal therapy for the treatment of food allergy. Curr Allergy Asthma Rep 2012;12:332–8.

71. Wang J, Jones SM, Pongracic JA, et al. Safety, clinical and immunologic efficacy of a Chinese herbal medicine (Food Allergy Herbal Formula-2) for food allergy. J Allergy Clin Immunol 2015;135:AB234.

72. Elazab N, Mendy A, Gasana J, et al. Probiotic administration in early life, atopy and asthma: a meta-analysis of clinical trials. Pediatrics 2013;132: e666–76.

73. Se Soh, Aw M, Chong YS, et al. Probiotic supplementation in the first 6 months of life in at risk Asian infants – effects on eczema and atopic sensitization at the age of 1 year. Clin Exp Allergy 2009;39:571–8.

74. Canani RB, Nocerino R, Terrin G. Effect of Lactobacillus GG on tolerance acquisition in infants with cow's milk allergy: a randomized trial. J Allergy Clin Immunol 2012;129:580–2.e5.

75. Tang MLK, Ponsonby A-L, Orsini F, et al. Administration of a probiotic with peanut oral immunotherapy: a randomized trial. J Allergy Clin Immunol 2015;135(3): 737–44.e8.

76. Lucendo AJ, Arias A, Tenias JM. Relation between eosinophilic esophagitis and oral immunotherapy for food allergy: a systematic review with meta-analysis. Ann Allergy Asthma Immunol 2014;113:624–9.

77. Leung J, Hundal NV, Katz AJ, et al. Tolerance of baked milk in patients with cow's milk-mediated eosinophilic esophagitis. J Allergy Clin Immunol 2013;132:1215–6.

78. Nelson HS, Lahr J, Rule R, et al. Treatment of anaphylactic sensitivity to peanuts by immunotherapy with injections of aqueous peanut extract. J Allergy Clin Immunol 1997;99:744–51.

79. Wood RA, Sicherer SH, Burks AW, et al. A phase 1 study of heat/phenol-killed, E. coli-encapsulated, recombinant modified peanut proteins Ara h 1, Ara h 2, and Ara h 3 (EMP-123) for the treatment of peanut allergy. Allergy 2013;68:803–8.

Index

Note: Page numbers of article titles are in **boldface.**

A

Abdominal pain
  in anaphylaxis, 1381, 1388
  in FPIES, 1465–1466
Absolute neutrophil count, for FPIES, 1471
Actinobacteria, allergic disease prevalence and, 1480–1485
Adaptive immune development, microbiome and, 1480–1481
Adjuvants, in oral tolerance, 1365–1368
Adverse food reactions
  definition of, 1378–1379
  differential diagnosis of, 1410
Advocacy, for allergy management, 1436
Albuterol, 1416
Allergens, exposure to, in oral tolerance, 1367
Allergist
  referral to, 1419
  role in school environment, 1430–1433
Allergy clinic, testing in, 1413–1415
Allergy-directed elimination diets, 1400–1401
Alpha-lactalbumin, in oral tolerance, 1368
Alternative and complementary medicine, 1542
American Academy of Allergy, Asthma, and Immunology, 1417
  breastfeeding guidelines of, 1502–1503
  food introduction guidelines of, 1512
  school emergency care plans of, 1429
American Academy of Pediatrics
  food introduction recommendations of, 1511
  school emergency care plans of, 1429, 1431
American Medical Association, school care plans of, 1431
Americans with Disabilities Act, food allergy rules of, 1429, 1433, 1437
Anaphylaxis, **1377–1392,** 1411
  diagnosis of, 1385–1386
  emergency care plans for, 1429–1434
  epinephrine for, 1415–1417, 1429–1437
  in school environment, **1425–1439**
  pathophysiology of, 1369–1370
  preparedness for, 1429–1434
  prevention of, 1426–1437
  quality of life issues in, 1457–1459
  signs and symptoms of, 1369, 1380, 1382–1386
Anergy, in oral tolerance, 1527
Angioedema, 1379–1380, 1411

Pediatr Clin N Am 62 (2015) 1551–1562
http://dx.doi.org/10.1016/S0031-3955(15)00165-0
0031-3955/15/$ – see front matter © 2015 Elsevier Inc. All rights reserved.

pediatric.theclinics.com

Moving?

Make sure your subscription moves with you!

To notify us of your new address, find your **Clinics Account Number** (located on your mailing label above your name), and contact customer service at:

Email: journalscustomerservice-usa@elsevier.com

800-654-2452 (subscribers in the U.S. & Canada)
314-447-8871 (subscribers outside of the U.S. & Canada)

Fax number: 314-447-8029

Elsevier Health Sciences Division
Subscription Customer Service
3251 Riverport Lane
Maryland Heights, MO 63043